AF564592

Atlas of Pediatric and Adolescent Gynecology

Atlas of Pediatric and Adolescent Gynecology

Second Edition

Editors

Corazon Yabes-Almirante MD MSc PhD FPOGS FPCS FIFEPAG
Center Chief, Perinatal-Neonatology-Pediatric Gynecology Center
Philippine Children's Medical Center
Founding Head, Pediatric and Adolescent Gynecology Unit
Philippine Children's Medical Center, Department of Health, Republic of the Philippines
Founding President, Pediatric and Adolescent Gynecology Society of the Philippines (PAGSPHIL)
Founding President, Philippine Society of Ultrasound in
Clinical Medicine (PSUCMI) under AFSUMB and WFUMB, Philippines

Franklin P Atencio MD FPOGS FPCS
Founding President, Philippine Society of Pelvic Surgeons
Founding Vice-President, Pediatric and Adolescent
Gynecology Society of the Philippines (PAGSPHIL)
Fellow, International Gynecologic Cancer Society
Project Director, Advanced Pelvic Surgery, East Avenue Medical Center, Philippines

Blanca C de Guia MD MSc FPOGS FPSREI FPSGE FPSUOG FIFEPAG
Professor, Section of Reproductive Endocrinology and Infertility
Department of Obstetrics and Gynecology
University of the Philippines College of Medicine and the Philippine General Hospital
Head, Pediatric and Adolescent Gynecology Unit, Philippine Children's Medical Center, Philippines

Foreword

Emil Javier

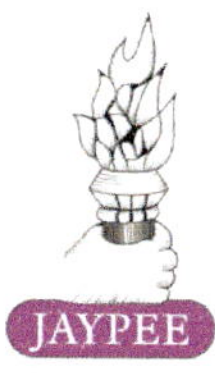

JAYPEE BROTHERS MEDICAL PUBLISHERS
The Health Sciences Publisher
New Delhi | London

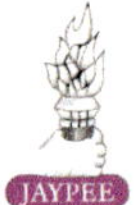

Jaypee Brothers Medical Publishers (P) Ltd

Headquarters
EMCA House, 23/23-B
Ansari Road, Daryaganj
New Delhi 110 002, India
Landline: +91-11-23272143,
+91-11-23272703+91-11-23282021,
+91-11-23245672
e-mail: jaypee@jaypeebrothers.com

Corporate Office
4838/24, Ansari Road, Daryaganj
New Delhi 110 002, India
Phone: +91-11-43574357
Fax: +91-11-43574314
e-mail: jaypee@jaypeebrothers.com

Overseas Office
JP Medical Ltd.
83, Victoria Street, London
SW1H 0HW (UK)
Phone: +44-20 3170 8910
e-mail: info@jpmedpub.com

EU GPSR Authorised Representative
Logos Europe, 9 rue Nicolas Poussin
17000, La Rochelle, France
Phone: +33 (0) 6 67 93 73 78
e-mail: contact@logoseurope.eu

Website: www.jaypeebrothers.com
Website: www.jaypeedigital.com

Inquiries for bulk sales may be solicited at: jaypee@jaypeebrothers.com

Atlas of Pediatric and Adolescent Gynecology

First Edition: 2009

Second Edition: 2012, Reprint: **2026**

ISBN 978-93-5025-641-1

Printed in India

Contributors

Alicia Berbano-Tamesis
MD FPPS
Director, Dr Fe Del Mundo
Children's Hospital
Head, Adolescent Center
Philippine Children's Medical Center
Philippines

Angela Sison Aguilar
MD FPOGS FPSREI FIFEPAG FPSGE
Associate Professor
Section of Reproductive
Endocrinology and Infertility
Department of Obstetrics and Gynecology
UP College of Medicine and the
Philippine General Hospital
Philippines

Annebelle Dimatulac-Aherrera
MD FPOGS FIFEPAG
Vice-Chair, Department of
Obstetrics and Gynecology
Makati Medical Center, Philippines

Bernadette J Madrid
MD FPPS
Director, UP Manila Child Protection Unit
Clinical Associate Professor
Department of Pediatrics
Philippine General Hospital, Philippines

Blanca C de Guia
MD MSc FPOGS FPSREI FPSGE FPSUOG
FIFEPAG
Professor, Section of Reproductive
Endocrinology and Infertility
Department of Obstetrics and Gynecology
University of the Philippines College of
Medicine and the Philippine
General Hospital
Head, Pediatric and Adolescent
Gynecology Unit
Philippine Children's Medical Center
Philippines

Corazon Yabes-Almirante
MD MSc PhD FPOGS FPCS FIFEPAG
Center Chief, Perinatal-Neonatology-
Pediatric Gynecology Center
Philippine Children's Medical Center
Founding Head, Pediatric and
Adolescent Gynecology Unit
Philippine Children's Medical Center
Department of Health
Republic of the Philippines
Founding President, Pediatric and
Adolescent Gynecology Society of the
Philippines (PAGSPHIL)
Founding President, Philippine
Society of Ultrasound in
Clinical Medicine (PSUCMI) under AF-
SUMB and WFUMB
Philippines

David T Bolong
MD
Head, Section of Pediatric Urology
Philippine Children's Medical Center
Department of Health
Republic of the Philippines

Dianalyn G Sazon-Carlos
MD FPOGS FPSREI FPSUOG FPSGE FIFEPAG
Head, Department of
Obstetrics and Gynecology
Angles University Foundation
Medical Center
Consultant, Pediatric and Adolescent
Gynecology Unit
Philippine Children's Medical Center
Philippines

Eva Maria Cutiongco-Dela Paz
MD FPPS
Assistant Director
Institute of Human Genetics
National Institutes of Health
University of the Philippines-Manila

Franklin P Atencio
MD FPOGS FPCS
Founding President, Philippine
Society of Pelvic Surgeons
Founding Vice-President
Pediatric and Adolescent Gynecology
Society of the Philippines (PAGSPHIL)
Fellow, International Gynecologic
Cancer Society
Project Director
Advanced Pelvic Surgery
East Avenue Medical Center
Philippines

Julie Christine F Dimaano-De Torres
MD
Medical Officer
Pediatric and Adolescent Gynecology Unit
Philippine Children's Medical Center
Philippines

Lorna F Ramos-Abad
MD FPPS
Professor, Department of Pediatrics
UP College of Medicine and the
Philippine General Hospital
Head, Section of Pediatric Endocrinology
UP-PGH and Philippine Children's
Medical Center, Philippines

Maria Therese Beriña-Mallen
MD
Medical Officer
Pediatric and Adolescent Gynecology Unit
Philippine Children's Medical Center
Philippines

Marietta S Sapaula
MD FPOGS FIFEPAG
Associate Professor
St Luke's Medical Center
William H Quasha College of Medicine
Active Consultant, Department of
Obstetrics and Gynecology
St Luke's Medical Center, Philippines

Marites Miguel-Butaran
MD DPOGS
Head, Women and Child Protection Unit
Cagayan Valley Medical Center
Philippines

Merle P Tan
MD FPPS
Training Director
Child Protection Unit Network, Philippines

Ma Socorro C Bernardino
MD FPOGS FIFEPAG
Consultant, Pediatric and Adolescent Gynecology Unit
Philippine Children's Medical Center
Head, Section of Pediatric Gynecology
Department of Obstetrics and Gynecology
St Luke's Medical Center
Philippines

Rosa Maria Hipolito-Nancho
MD FPPS FIFEPAg
Professor, Department of Pediatrics
UP College of Medicine and the Philippine General Hospital
Training Officer
Division of Adolescent Medicine
Philippine Children's Medical Center
Philippines

Foreword

First edition of the book *Atlas of Pediatric and Adolescent Gynecology* was published in October 2009 and was awarded the Outstanding Book of the Year Award, 2010 by the National Academy of Science and Technology (NAST) based on the criteria of quality, originality of content, contribution to science and technology and the thoroughness of documentation.

As President of the National Academy of Science and Technology, I am happy to note that on the third year after publication, this Atlas will now be published with a world-wide readership as target because of a need for easily understandable reading in pediatric and adolescent gynecology by healthcare providers. The presentation of actual cases supplemented with ample elucidating pictures done in most chapters makes the readers learn more about the diseases being discussed. Local statistics are retrieved to show the myriad and wealth of cases seen in the Philippines.

The nineteen (19) chapters were written by 16 authors who are guardians of the pioneering specialty of Pediatric and Adolescent Gynecology, the first and only one established in 2002 at the Philippine Children's Medical Center. The specialists include: pediatric gynecologists, pediatric oncologists, urologists, endocrinologists, geneticists and adolescent specialists who are recognized leaders in their fields.

The content, the style and elegance of the book bespeaks of a genuine and enviable collaboration of the contributors. The ATLAS treats the child and the adolescent as distinct individuals with personal needs and rights that merits care and respect.

I therefore enjoin you all to read, understand and enjoy the ATLAS.

Emil Javier
President
National Academy of Science and Technology
Philippines

Preface to the Second Edition

The creation of the *Atlas of Pediatric and Adolescent Gynecology*, the first such publication in the Philippines, was received well not only by colleagues in the practice of Pediatric Gynecology and Pediatrics, but also those in the Allied Specialties, Academe, and those in the peripheral sectors dealing with social problems of children.

The Atlas received the Outstanding Book Award for 2010 from the National Academy of Science and Technology Philippines on July 15, 2010, 9 months after its launching in October 20, 2009.

This second edition will be published and distributed worldwide by Jaypee Brothers Medical Publishers (P) Ltd. Some changes are made to make the images clearer (black and white photos are replaced with colored ones); ultrasound pictures enhanced and some chapters improved.

Out of the 350 pictures in this Atlas, 70% are now printed in color. In contrast to the 1st edition where only 50% of the pictures were printed in color to save the cost of printing.

Corazon Yabes-Almirante
Franklin P Atencio
Blanca C de Guia

Preface to the First Edition

A malfunctioning computer, the threat of losing valuable pictures and data of patients, led to the development of this ATLAS. The pictures and data were quickly retrieved and transferred to CDs for review. The idea of preserving them for teaching purposes evolved. Ultrasound pictures were retrieved together with the histopathological slides of diagnosed tumors, vaginoscopy and laparoscopy videos, videos and still pictures of surgeries (laparotomies and vaginal repairs of malformations of the genital tract). These were all collated and the authors selected those that had teaching values; those that were relatively rare and those that had good follow-up.

Other specialists from other institutions such the National Institute of Health, University of the Philippines, UP Child Protection Unit, Makati Medical Center and St. Luke's Medical Center were tapped to contribute to the Atlas. Other colleagues that form part of the multidisciplinary team of Pediatric and Adolescent Gynecology Unit of the Philippine Children's Medical Center, such as the Pediatric Urologist and Adolescent Medicine specialists, were invited to write a chapter. A graphic artist, with the guidance of the authors, was hired to sketch the majority of the 27 illustrations found listed before the index.

The 19 chapters truly represent the collaborative effort of 16 specialists of varied expertise in the care of girls with gynecologic problems in the Philippines. More than 300 pictures, 50% of which are in color, and 27 illustrations are worth preserving in a book form not only for teaching purposes but for providing evidences for medical students, general medical practitioners, pediatricians, gynecologists, surgeons, parents and the girls themselves. There is hope of survival for those with cancer. Fertility can be preserved with proper diagnosis. Reconstructive and restorative surgery of the genital tract can provide sexual function. Most important of all, if you don't look for it, you won't find it—a lesson to be learned in doing a thorough examination of a girl even as a newborn and in early infancy, so that measures can be done before it is too late.

Corazon Yabes-Almirante
Franklin P Atencio
Blanca C de Guia

Acknowledgments

A pioneering work such as the *Atlas of Pediatric and Adolescent Gynecology* goes through a lot of birth pains.

We are indebted to the contributors for their dedication in finishing and polishing their chapters on time. They come from different institutions but are all Filipinos who are one in their desire to impart their expertise about this new subspecialty.

The Philippine Children's Medical Center, where the first fellowship training program for PAG in Asia and in the Philippines was born, and its Current Executive Director, Dr Julius Lecciones for the support.

To the Philippine National Academy of Science and Technology (NAST) and its president Dr Emil Javier, who believed in and gave recognition to our Atlas, highlighting its significance to Philippine medical literature.

To our patients, girls and young women, who have entrusted their bodies to our care, and from whom we derive most of our knowledge.

Contents

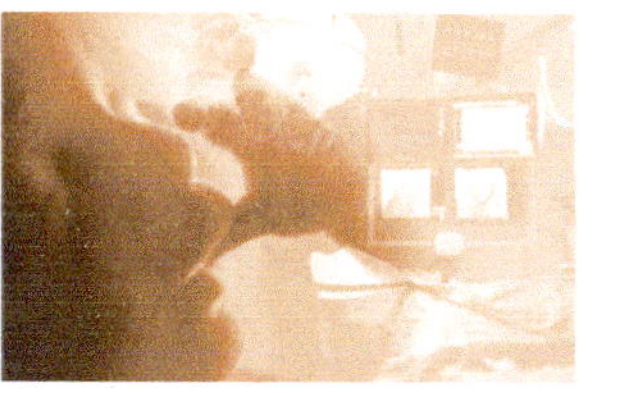

1 The Female Pediatric Patient: Normal Genitalia and Examining Techniques

Marites Miguel-Butaran

EXAMINATION OF THE PEDIATRIC PATIENT

Preparing Pediatric Patient for Examination

While performing pediatric gynecologic examination (Figs 1.1 to 1.3), it is important to gain the confidence of the child and make the process as pain-free as possible. The environment in which a child receives health care should be inviting and the medical staff child friendly in order to facilitate the examination process and make the child's first gynecologic encounter nontraumatic.

INSTRUMENTS AND SUPPLIES FOR THE PREPUBERTAL EXAMINATION

Different instruments and supplies are used for the prepubertal examination and are shown in the Figures 1.4 to 1.6.

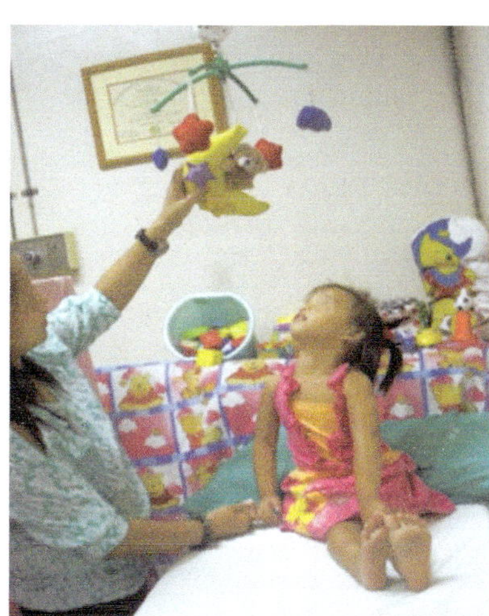

Fig. 1.2: Medical staff talking to child prior to the conduct of examination

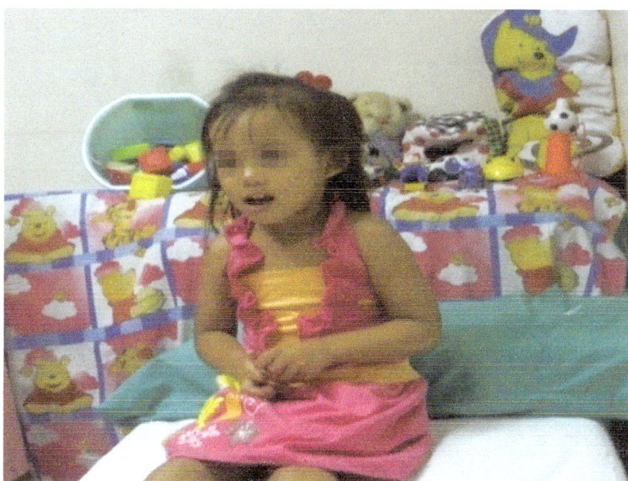

Fig. 1.1: The child in the examination area made comfortable with the toys and familiar cartoon characters

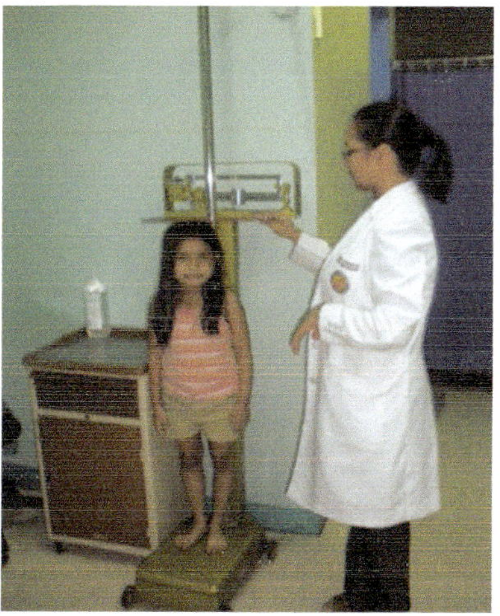

Fig. 1.3: Pediatric gynecology exam starts with general examination; starting with records of the height, weight, vital signs and physical examination with emphasis on the gynecologic examination

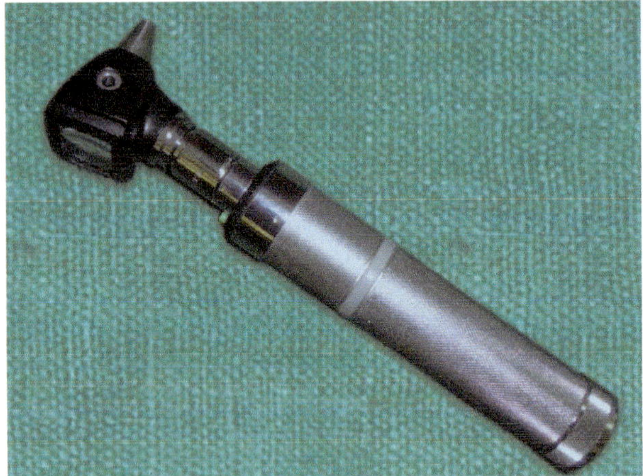

Fig. 1.4: Use of an otoscope (with removed truncated ear piece) to magnify minute tissues

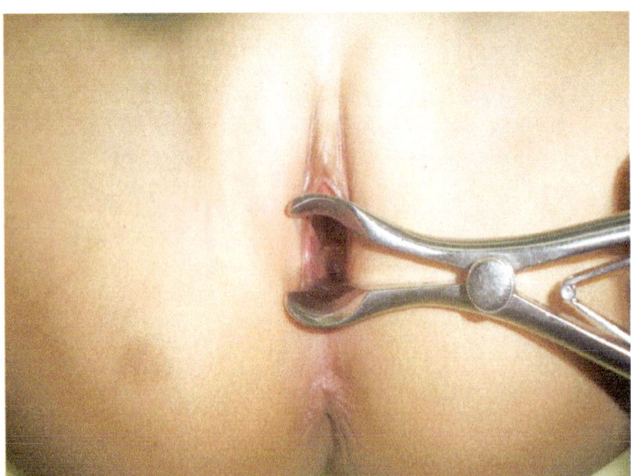

Fig. 1.5: Use of a nasal speculum to visualize the vagina of an 8-year-old child patient. It is preferable to do vaginal examination with instrumentation under anesthesia

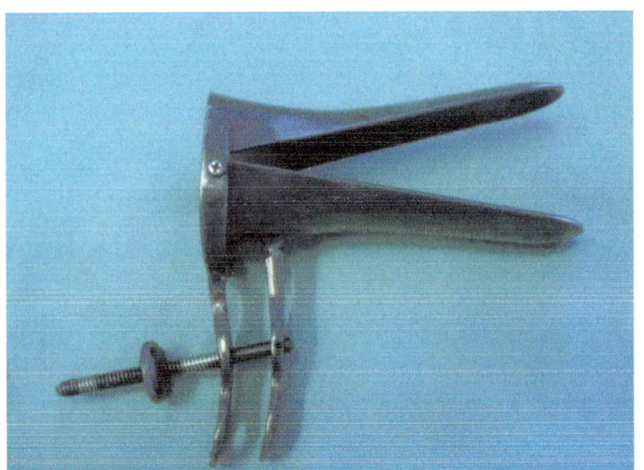

Fig. 1.6: Vaginal speculum is used to visualize the vagina and cervix in a nonvirgin adolescent. Speculum is lubricated, patient is asked to relax their pelvic diaphragm and the speculum inserted slowly with blades closed and pointed posterior toward the coccyx

DIFFERENT TECHNIQUES OF POSITIONING

There are different techniques of positioning in pediatric gynecologic examination, which are shown in the Figures 1.7 to 1.10.

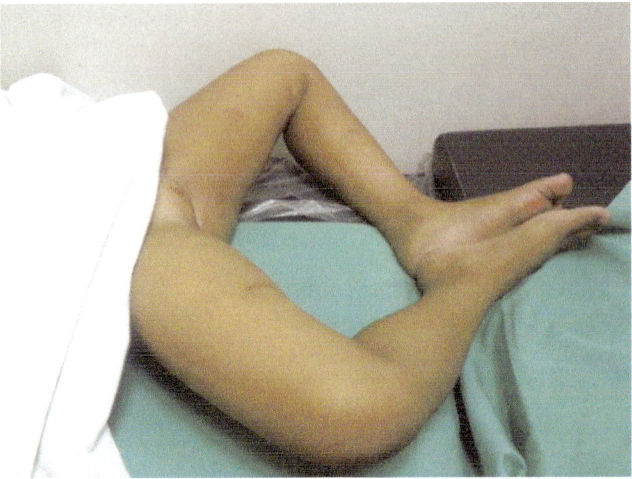

Fig. 1.7: A 3-year-old child patient in a frog leg position. Supine, with hips flexed and the soles of the feet must be meeting together. Draping the child's lower body leaves an impression that the genitalia is a special part of the body

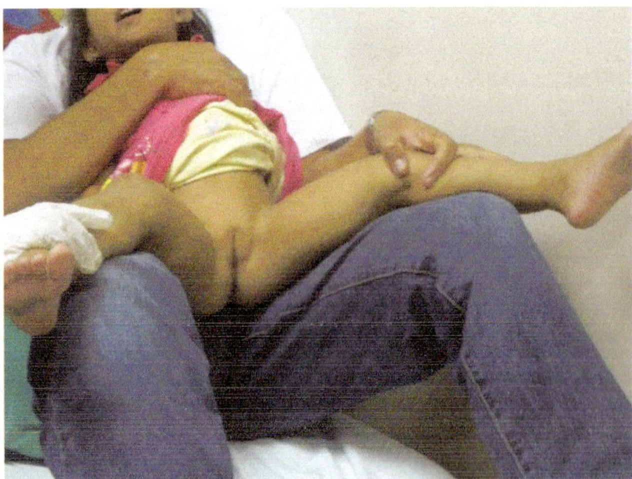

Fig. 1.8: A 3-year-old child patient is in supine position sitting on parent's lap with the legs spread out across the parent's thighs. The parent embraces and reassures the child

DIFFERENT TECHNIQUES OF VISUALIZING THE VESTIBULE

There are different methods that a doctor can use to visualize the vestibule as shown in the Figures 1.11 and 1.12.

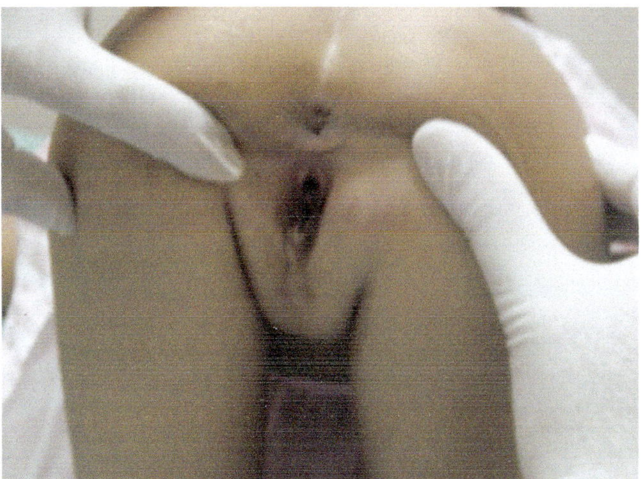

Fig. 1. 9: A 9-year-old child patient in a knee chest position. The child is in prone position with the chest resting on a pillow, back slightly swayed and the knees on the table. In this position, gravity causes the lower edge of the hymen to roll outward

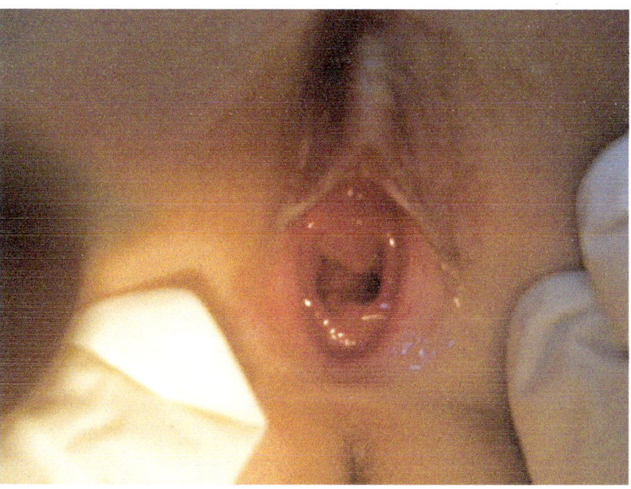

Fig. 1.11: Supine lateral spread method. The index finger of both hands is placed in the labia majora, lateral to the vestibule and slightly posterior to the vaginal orifice; the labia majora are then spread laterally and posteriorly, enough to visualize the vestibule

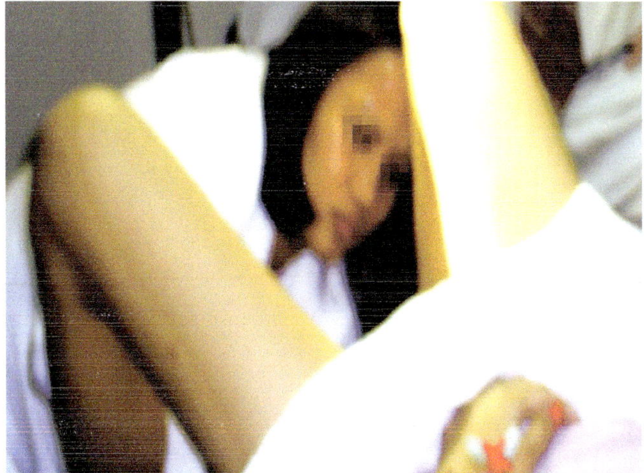

Fig. 1.10: A 15-year-old adolescent. Dorsal lithotomic position stirrups (for the older, co-operative child and the adolescent). The patient's buttocks are on the edge of the table, knee flexed and legs rest on stirrups

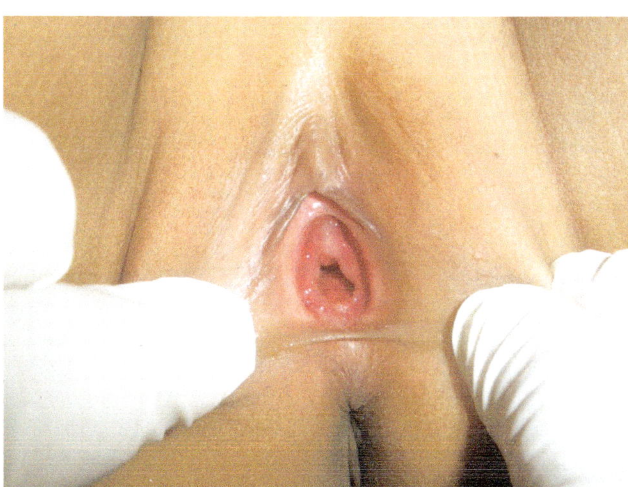

Fig. 1.12: Supine lateral traction method. The labia majora are grasped gently in the same location used for the lateral spread method, followed by gentle traction of the tissue toward the examiner and slightly posterior and lateral

OBTAINING SAMPLES

The techniques to obtain sample from the external genitalia are shown in the Figures 1.13 to 1.15.

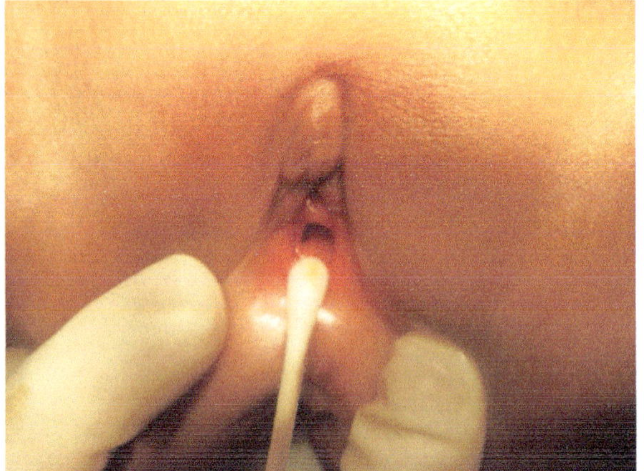

Fig. 1.13: A cotton tip applicator held near the vaginal opening while the child patient is instructed to cough out to allow vaginal fluid to egress

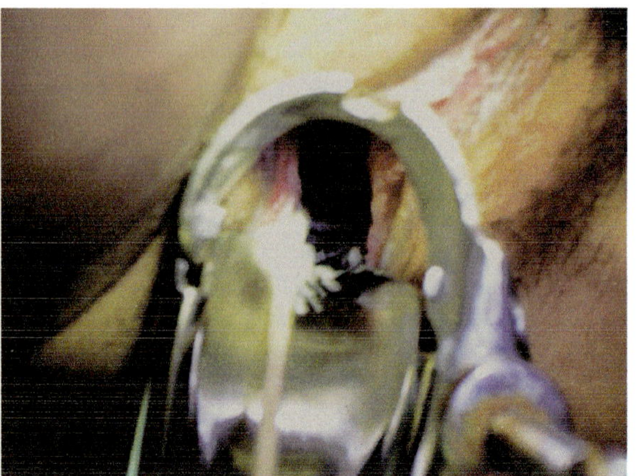

Fig. 1.14: Cervico-vaginal discharge of a 15-year-old adolescent patient is visualized by using vaginal speculum. Sample of discharge is obtained with a cotton tip swab

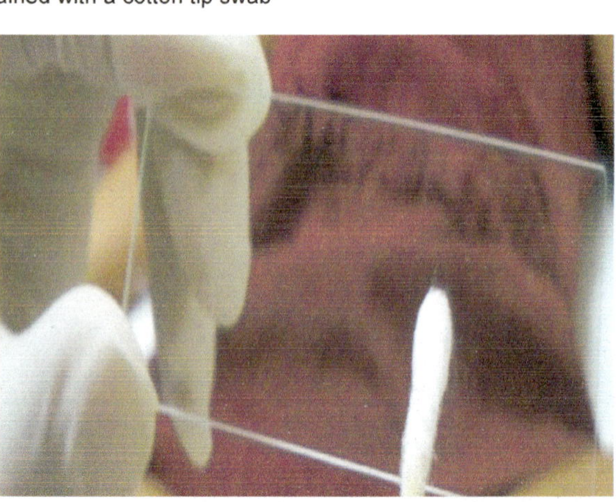

Fig. 1.15: Vaginal discharge smeared on a clear glass slide

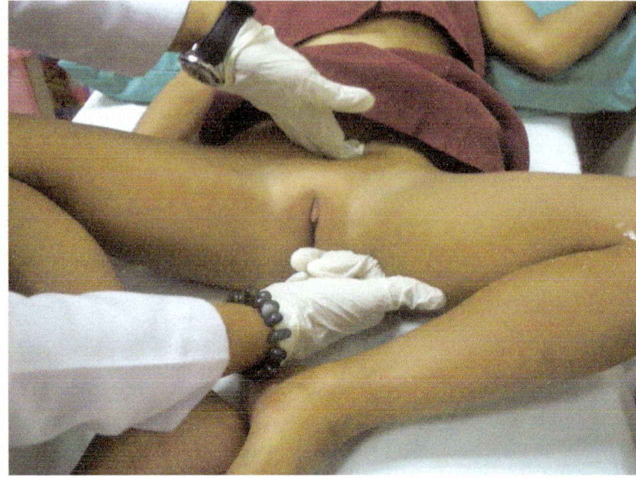

Fig. 1.16: A 6-year-old child patient undergoing recto-abdominal examination (*Photo was taken by the author from own patient, taken with permission from patient, with permission to be used for educational/ reference purposes*)

RECTO-ABDOMINAL EXAMINATION

Recto-abdominal examination of a child (Figs 1.16 and 1.17): Before performing a recto-abdominal examination to a child, the first thing to do is to ask permission and explain the examination procedure. It is important to maintain eye contact and communication while doing the examination. Wear gloves, lubricate the index finger of right hand with KY Jelly or oil then, gently insert the index finger into the rectum while the left hand is used to depress the hypogastric area. With the left hand, gently palpate for the uterus that feels like a small button.

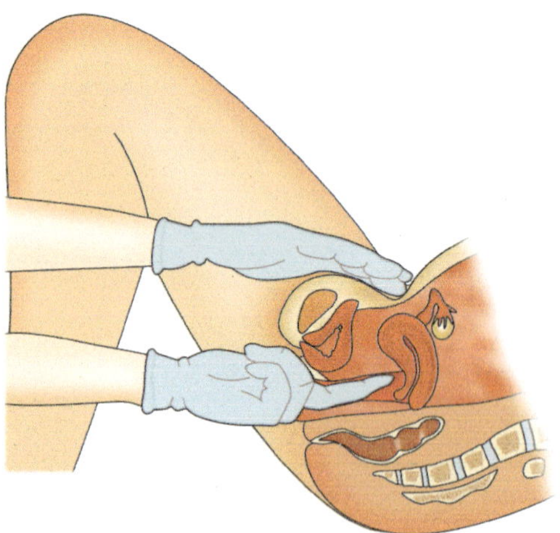

Fig. 1.17: Internal examination may be done for sexually active adolescents

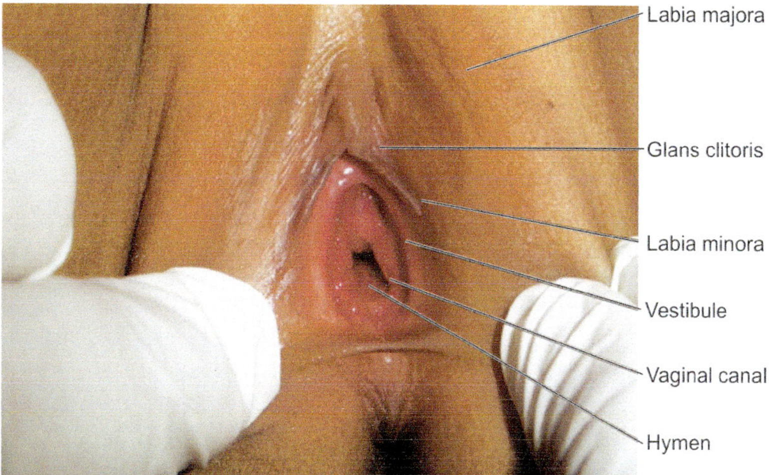

Fig. 1.18: Normal external genitalia of prepubertal child (*Photo was taken by the author from own patient, taken with permission from patient, with permission to be used for educational/reference purposes*)

NORMAL EXTERNAL GENITALIA OF A CHILD

Normal external genitalia (Figs 1.18 and 1.19): There are differences in the normal external genitalia of a prepubertal child and a neonate. In the neonate the effect of intrauterine transfer of estrogen of the mother to the fetus usually last up to two years then it gradually wanes out. As a result, estrogenized external genitalia is seen among neonates. As the child approaches the prepubertal years, estrogen effect becomes totally absent, hence the external genitalia will show an unestrogenized features such as the a thin labia majora, thin and small labia minora, a vestibule that is reddish due to the prominence of blood vessels, a hymen that is thin and inelastic, and a dry vaginal canal.

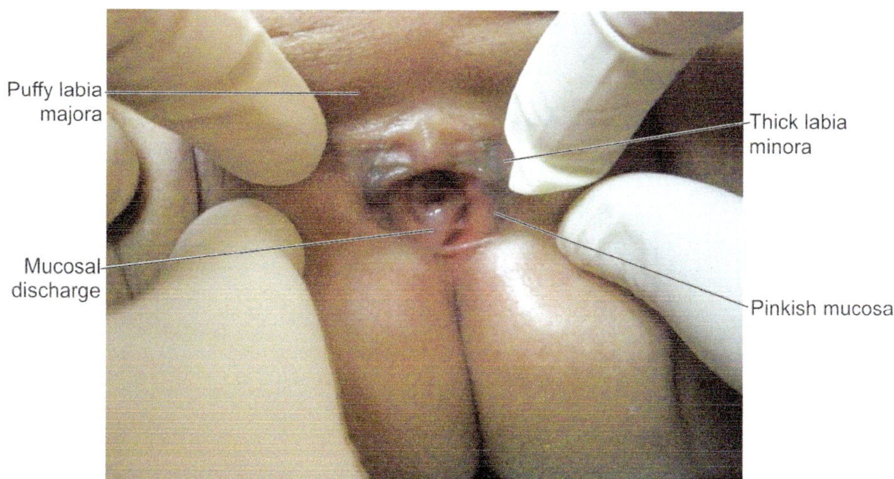

Fig. 1.19: Neonatal vulva–estrogenized, from maternal transfer in utero (*Photo was taken by the author from own patient, taken with permission from patient, with permission to be used for educational/reference purposes*)

DIFFERENT HYMENAL CONFIGURATIONS

Different hymenal configurations (Figs 1.20 to 1.23): The hymen is a thin mucosal membrane with abundant blood vessels and lines the vaginal opening. There are variation in shapes and size of the hymen, the one in this atlas are those commonly seen in our day to day practice.

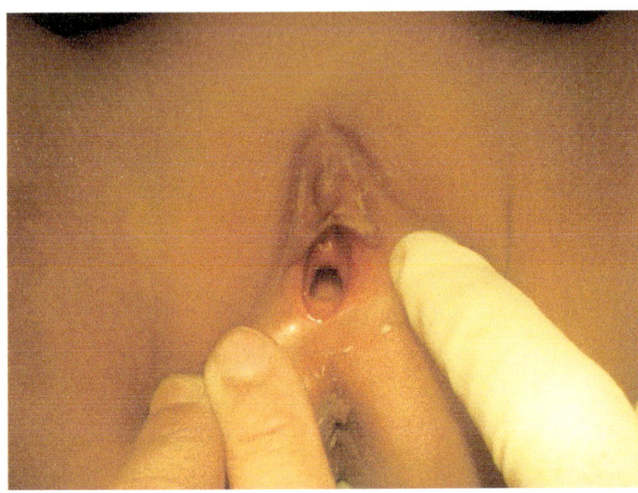

Fig. 1.20: Annular hymen—also known as circular, lunar or moon-shaped hymen (*Photo was taken by the author from own patient, taken with permission from patient, with permission to be used for educational/reference purposes*)

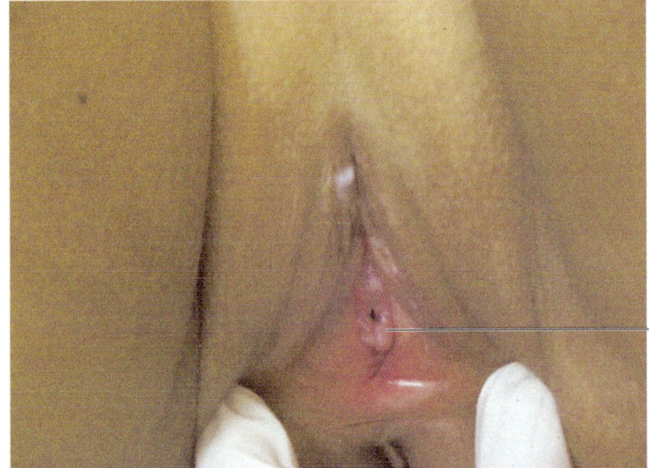

Fig. 1.21: Redundant hymen—has several folds of tissues; spread laterally to reveal the opening (*Photo was taken by the author from own patient, taken with permission from patient, with permission to be used for educational/reference purposes*)

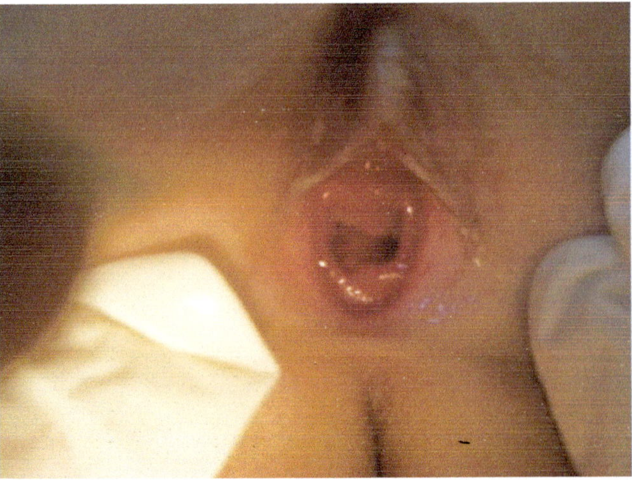

Fig. 1.22: Crescentric hymen—half moon shaped hymen (*Photo was taken by the author from own patient, taken with permission from patient, with permission to be used for educational/reference purposes*)

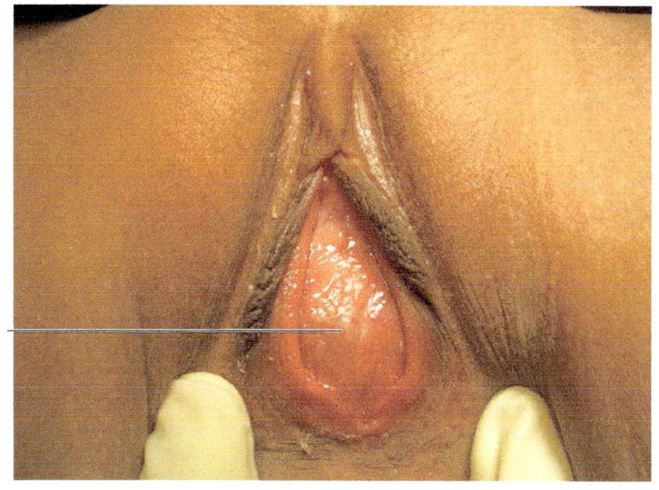

Fig. 1.23: Imperforate hymen. Vaginal opening completely closed (*Photo was taken by the author from own patient, taken with permission from patient, with permission to be used for educational/reference purposes*)

BIBLIOGRAPHY

1. Bhatnagar K. Embryology and normal anatomy. In: Sanfilippo J, et al (Eds). Pediatric and Adolescent Gynecology, 2nd edn. Philadelphia: WB Saunders Company 2001; pp. 2-17.
2. Carson S. Gynecologic examination of the adolescent. In: Carpenter S, et al (Eds). Pediatric and Adolescent Gynecology. New York; Raven Press Ltd 1992; pp. 67-76.
3. Pokorny S. Genital examination of prepubertal child and peripubertal females. In: Sanfilippo J, et al (Eds). Pediatric and Adolescent Gynecology, 2nd edn. Philadelphia: WB Saunders Company 2001; pp.182-98.
4. Wilson M. Vaginal discharge and vaginal bleeding in Childhood. In: Carpenter S, et al (Eds). Pediatric and Adolescent Gynecology. New York: Raven Press Ltd 1992;139-51.

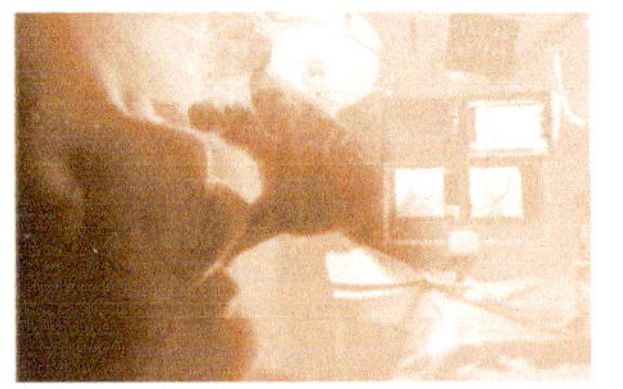

2 Sonography in Pediatric Gynecology

Corazon Yabes-Almirante

ULTRASOUND EXAMINATION OF CHILDREN WITH GYNECOLOGIC PROBLEMS

Ultrasound of children is completely different from that of adults. The ultrasound probes (Fig. 2.1) that come with the machine are often not appropriate for use in young children. The ultrasound probes available are:

1. 3–5 MHz convex probe;
2. 7.5–8.5 MHz transvaginal probe and
3. 8–10 MHz linear probe.

Hence to get the best image one has to find the right probe based on the built of the patient and the depth of the region of interest. Although pediatric gynecology ultrasound is now widely accepted as it is fast (especially in emergencies), accurate, painless, noninvasive, widely available, easy to use, less intimidating and cheaper than magnetic resonance imaging (MRI) or computed tomography (CT) scan with no ionizing radiation and no need for sedation, there are a few limitations.

Limitations of Pediatric Gynecology Ultrasound

Following are the limitations of pediatric gynecology ultrasound:

- Bladder needs to be full
- Patient's movement
- Absence of identifiable reference landmarks
- Vaginal probe cannot be used
- Abdominal ultrasound may not have the best resolution
- Dependence on operator or machine.

How to Overcome the Limitations?

The limitations can be overcome by keeping the following points in mind:

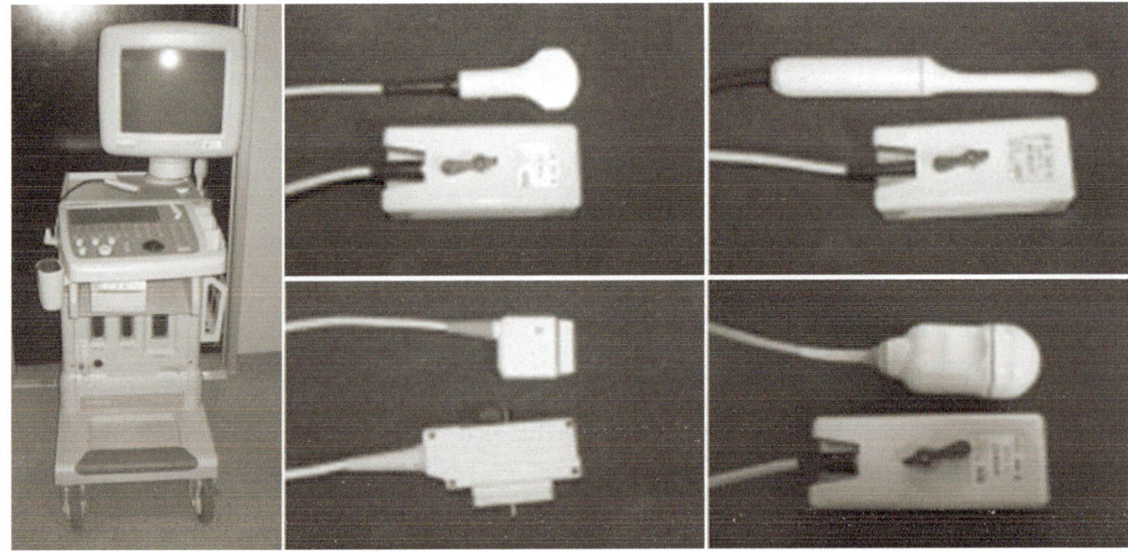

Fig. 2.1: Ultrasound machine for perinatal services and its four probes

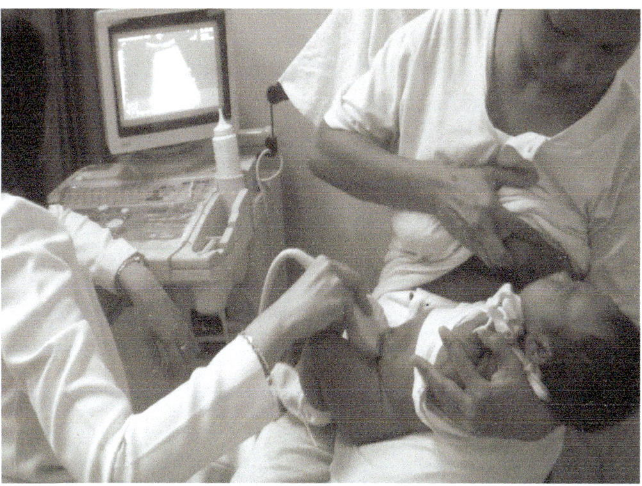

Fig. 2.2: Mother is breastfeeding the infant while ultrasound examination is going on. Mother is sitting on the table facing the sonologist. Mother cuddles the infant while breastfeeding. The sonologist places the ultrasound probe on the baby's abdomen

1. A full bladder can be replaced by water in vagina (vaginography), rectum, cloaca or utricle or urinary bladder instilled through a catheter.
2. Toys can be given to the movable child to catch his/her attention, show picture on the TV monitor so that he/she can cooperate and sedative can be given 30 minutes before examination (the best sedation for a neonate is a full stomach or breast sucking), the mother or guardian should be with the child, cuddling or, if necessary, breastfeed to the child (Fig. 2.2).
3. Use of Doppler technology to identify the blood vessel close to the organ to fast track the identification of the subject. Three-dimensional UTZ also makes the identification easier and cheaper than a CT scan or an MRI.
4. A vaginal probe can be placed transrectally to insonate the uterus and adnexa; can be placed at the perineum to insonate the lower genital tract (Figs 2.3 to 2.4A and B) (see Fig. 2.3A). This gives a more focused view in contrast to a transabdominal sonography (TAS), a panoramic view. Figure 2.4B shows the ruptured cyst at surgery. Figure 2.4A TAS image of a thin walled cyst before rupture.
5. Pediatric gynecology ultrasound needs a well trained and experienced operator as well as a high-end machine. Ultrasound examination is included in the curriculum of the fellowship training of pediatric and adolescent gynecology specialists. The high-end ultrasound machine is available at tertiary centers and a referral network should be in place.

ANATOMICAL DIFFERENCE BETWEEN ADULT AND CHILD

The sonologist must be aware of the anatomic differences between the adult and the child. Sonologist must also know the normal measurements, the growth pattern and the stages of functional development of the organs so the abnormality can be recognized. The body of the uterus, for example, varies in size in proportion to the cervix at different ages until adulthood is attained (Figs 2.5A to C). At birth the ratio of the cervix to the fundus is 1:1, premenarcheal it is 3:2, puberty it is 1:3 and in the adult it is 1:3 based on measurements of autopsy specimens (Fig. 2.6).

MEASUREMENT OF UTERUS AND OVARIES

Realtime ultrasonography made it possible to measure the uterus and the ovaries. The mean length of the uterus at

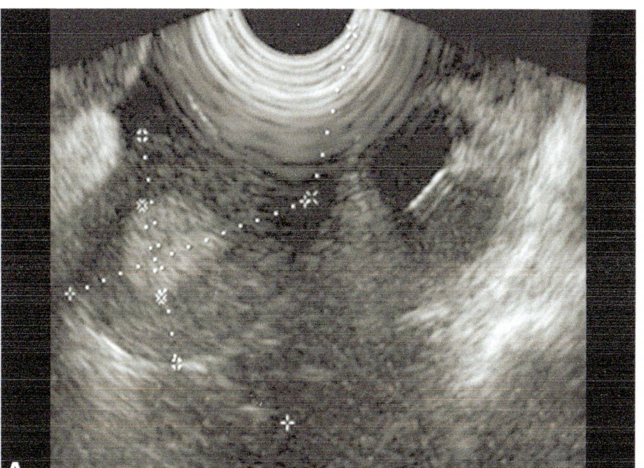

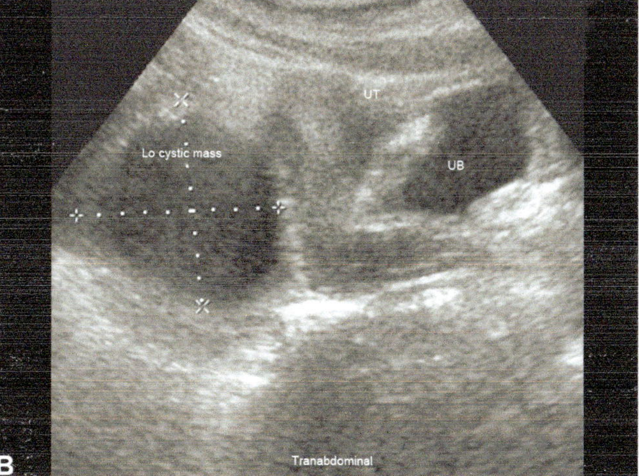

Figs 2.3A and B: Ultrasound image of transrectal insonation of genital organs compared to abdominal ultrasound: (A) Transrectal sonography (TRS) of uterus and cystic mass, focused view of thickened endometrial stripe; (B) Transabdominal sonography (TAS) image, panoramic view of cystic mass and thickened endometrium

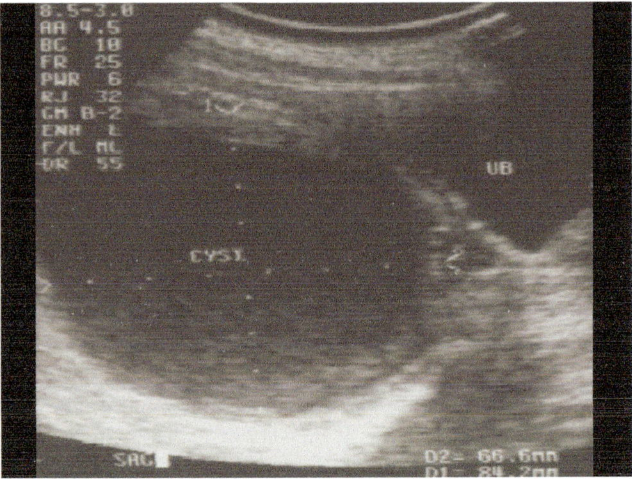

Fig. 2.4A: Transabdominal sonography (TAS) image of a thin-walled cyst before rupture

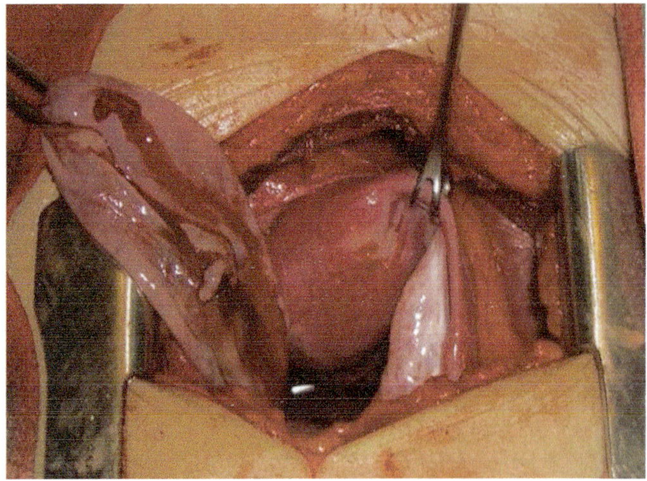

Fig. 2.4B: Emergency surgery for signs of acute abdomen; ruptured follicular cyst

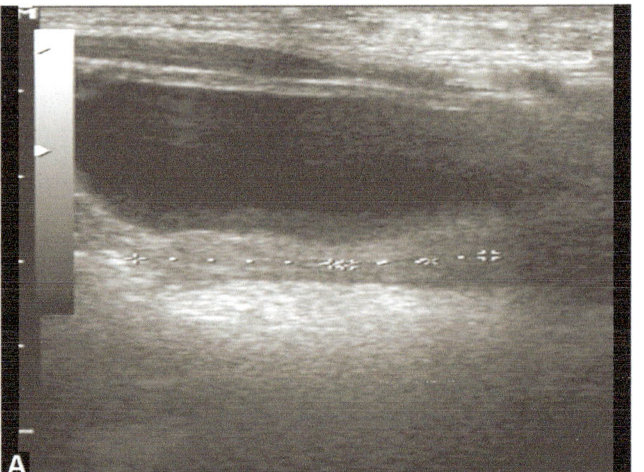

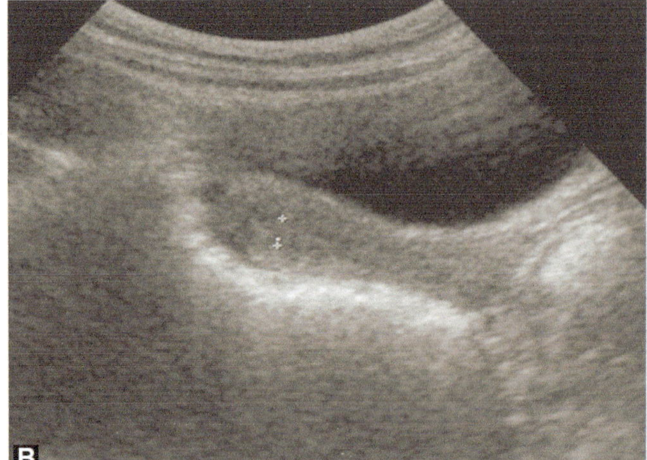

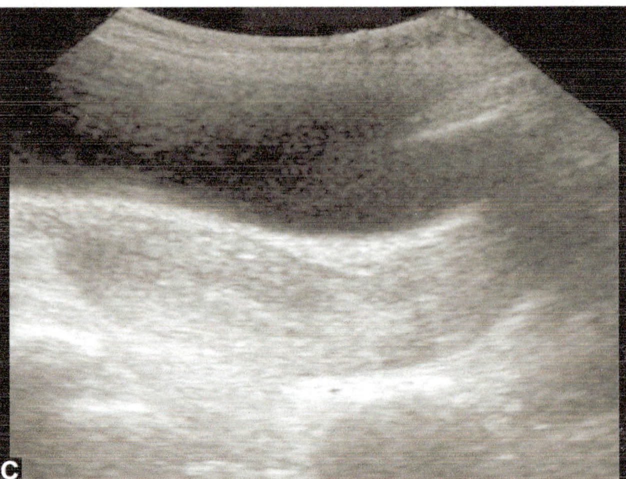

Figs 2.5A to C: Normal uterus and ovaries at different age groups: (A) Transabdominal sonography (TAS) of a newborn shows uterus to cervix ratio of 1:1; (B) TAS of a 3-year-old child, uterus to cervix ratio is 2:3; (C) TAS of a 13-year-old child, uterus to cervix ratio is 3:1;

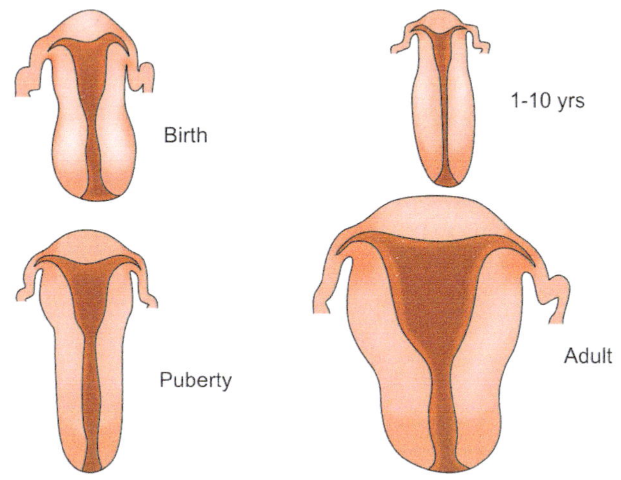

Fig. 2.6: Ratio of the cervix to the corpus uteri at birth, premenarcheal age (1–10 years), puberty and adulthood
Source: Illustration 2.6. *Courtesy*: Parsons L and Sommers S, Gynecology

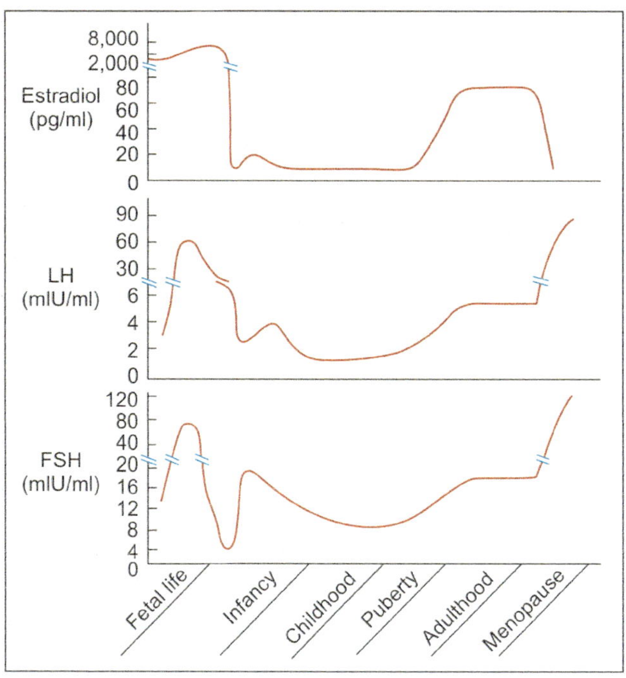

Fig. 2.7: Levels of estradiol, LH and FSH during fetal life, infancy, childhood, puberty and adulthood.
Source: Courtesy, www.medscape.com, October 2003

birth is 3.4 cm; at 1 year later is 2.8 cm and at 7 to 10 years is 3.5 cm. Ratio of fundus to the cervix grows from 0.95 to 1.25 between 1 and 4 Tanner's stage and changes from a tubular to a pear shape. Herter et al. showed better correlation of uterine length with age than uterine volume and that fundal to cervical ratio is a better marker of pubertal development up to age of 7 years (reference population study of patients with premature signs of puberty). These changes are influenced by levels of luteinizing hormone (LH), follicle stimulating hormone (FSH) and estradiol at different stages in the life of the girl child (Fig. 2.7).

CASE REVIEW

At the Pediatric and Adolescent Gynecology Unit of the Philippine Children's Medical Center, a total of 2,170 cases were seen from April 22, 2002 to December 31, 2008. Of all 32% of the cases were referred to the perinatal medical services co-operative ultrasound machine for sonography. Referrals from private physicians constitute 7% of archived digital images. A review of 701 cases below 19 years of age from digital archives of the ultrasound machine showed that there were 397 cases with measurement of the ovaries and uterus done through transabdominal sonography [TAS (238)], (Figs 2.8A and B on methods of transabdominal ensonation) transrectal sonography [TRS (79)], transperineal sonography [TPS (51)], transvaginal sonography [TVS (9)] routes with 3D (11) and Doppler

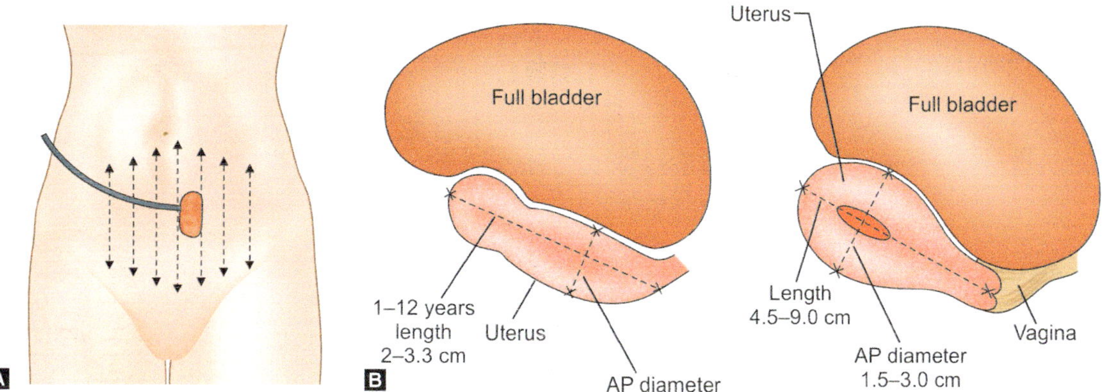

Figs 2.8A and B: Illustrations on methods of ensonations: (A) Longitudinal or Sagittal position of the probe; (B) Obtaining the uterine measurements

Table 2.1:
Ultrasound measurement of ovaries and uteri of children at different age groups and Tanner stages referred to the perinatal medical services co-operative ultrasound machine (SonoAce 8000) (April 2002–December 2008)

Tanner stages	Age (mean) (years)	Uterine length (mean) (cm)	Right ovarian volume (mean) (cm^2)	Left ovarian volume (mean) (cm^2)	Total cases (%)
Breast bud (infants)	0-1 (6.03 mos.)	2.34	1.62	1.50	29 (7.3)
I	1-7 (3.43)	2.10	1.04	1.00	74 (18.6)
II	7-13 (10)	3.19	3.58	3.03	42 (10.6)
III	9-18 (12.93)	4.30	5.67	5.40	73 (18.4)
IV	11-19 (15.8)	5.44	6.78	6.60	122 (30.7)
V	15-19 (17.19)	6.03	7.94	6.62	57 (14.4)
Total					397 (100)

Velocimetry (9). The measurements of the uterus and ovaries at different ages and Tanner stages of the children are shown in the Table 2.1.

TRANSPERINEAL SONOGRAPHY

Transperineal sonography (TPS) is done for congenital anomalies, vaginal discharge, vaginal bleeding, lower genital tract tumors, foreign body suspect and lower urinary tract anomalies.

Transperineal sonography cases were done using the perinatal medical services co-operative machine reviewed since 2002, and a total of 59 examinations were studied. These TPS were done when the patients were referred for the following complaints: absent vaginal opening, vaginal discharge, vaginal bleeding, introital mass and abdominal pain. Illustration and various TPS are shown in the Figures 2.9 to 2.12.

Technique of Transperineal Sonography

- Patient in lithotomic position
- Transducer is applied in a sagittal position between the labia majora, or directly over the labia minora
- Center of transducer is located posterior to urethra and anterior to vagina
- Mild pressure is applied with the transducer and slight alterations in transducer angle and location to visualize cervix and lower genital tract.

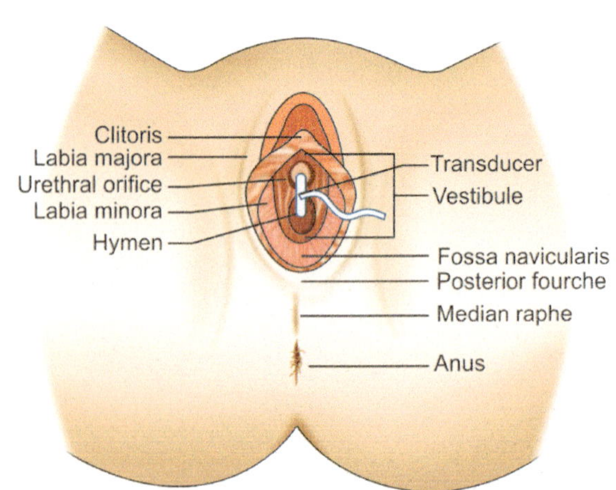

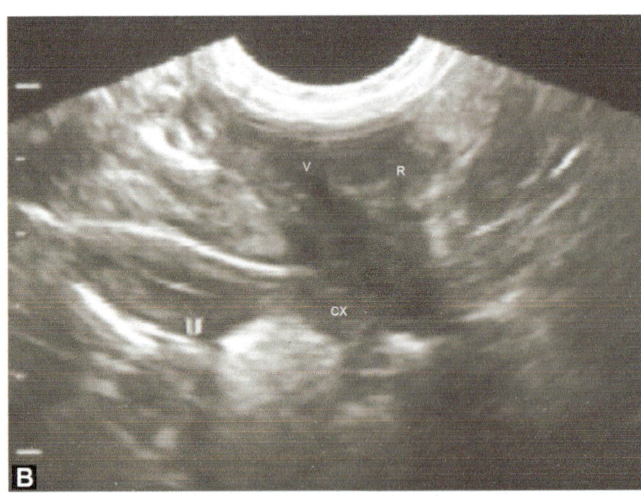

Figs 2.9A and B: Transperineal sonography (TPS): (A) Illustration on where to place the probe for TPS; Transducer 3.5, 5, 7.5 MHz depends on age and habitus of patient. Ultrasound gel is placed on the transducer, covered with rubber gloves and secured tightly. Ultrasound gel is again applied over the covering. (B) Ultrasound image of the uterus (U), vagina (V), rectum (R) and cervix (CX)

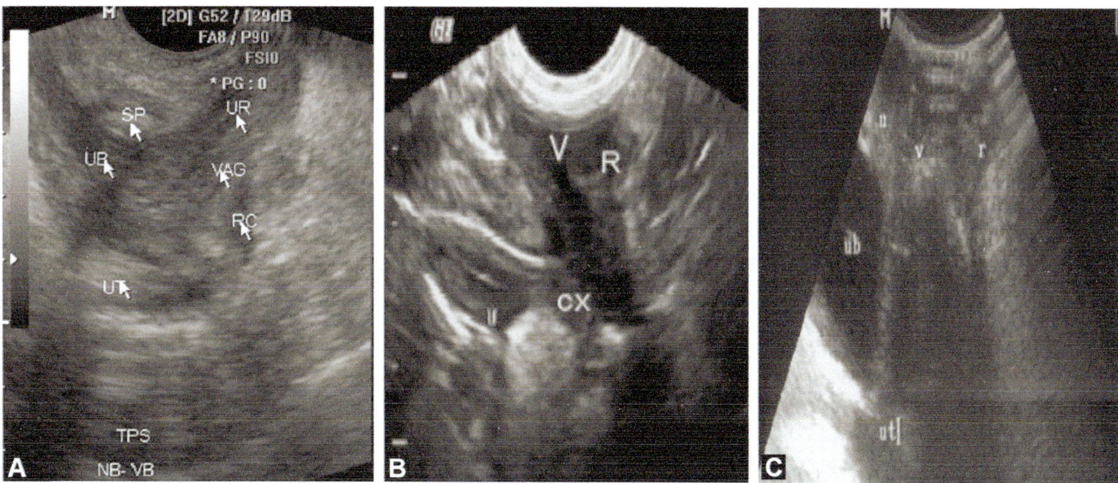

Figs 2.10A to C: Transperineal sonography (TPS): (A) Normal infant, newborn; (B) Premenarcheal, at 12 year of age; (C) Adolescent female at 19 year of age

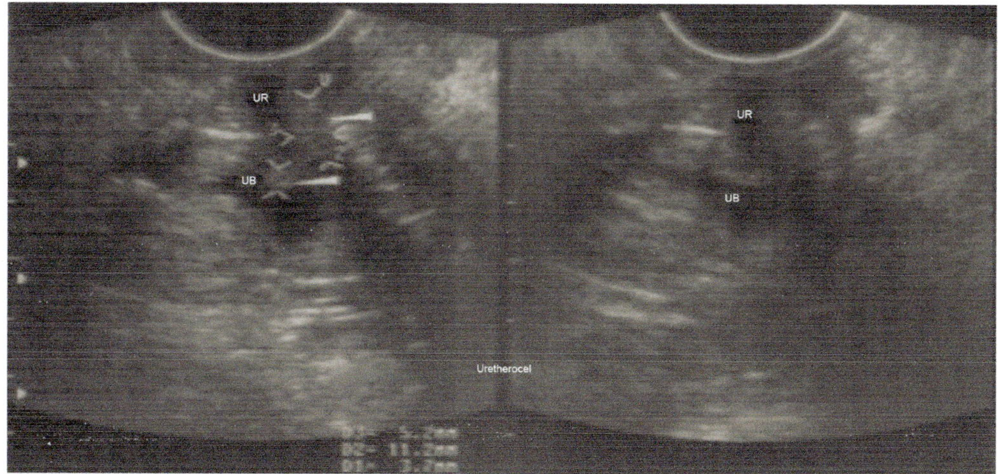

Fig. 2.11: Transperineal sonography (TPS) of an urethrocele. Arrows on the left picture point to an echogenic mass in the urethra going out of the introitus. Right picture shows a similar structure

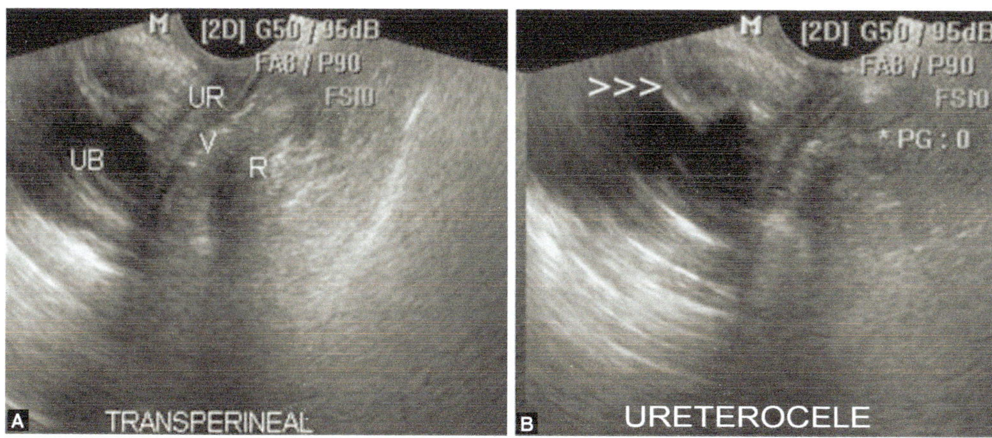

Figs 2.12A and B: (A) A transperineal sonography (TPS) of a patient with absent vaginal opening associated with cyst within the urinary bladder (arrow >); (B) Ureterocele

OVARIAN NEW GROWTH

Some cases of ovarian newgrowths are illustrated in Figures 2.13 to 2.28.

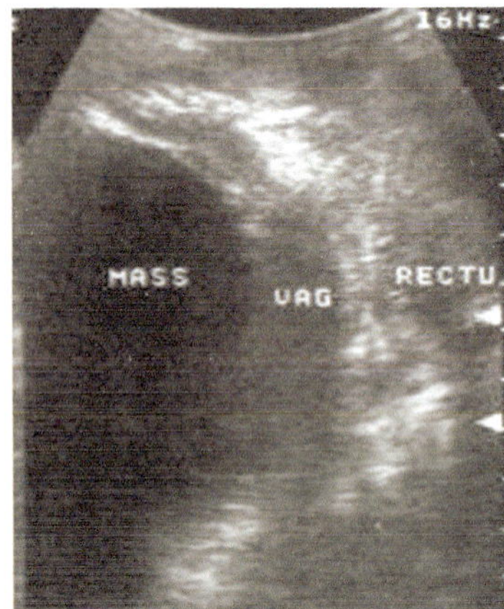

Fig. 2.13: A transperineal sonography (TPS) of an 18-year-old patient with a palpable abdominal mass. A cystic mass is confirmed

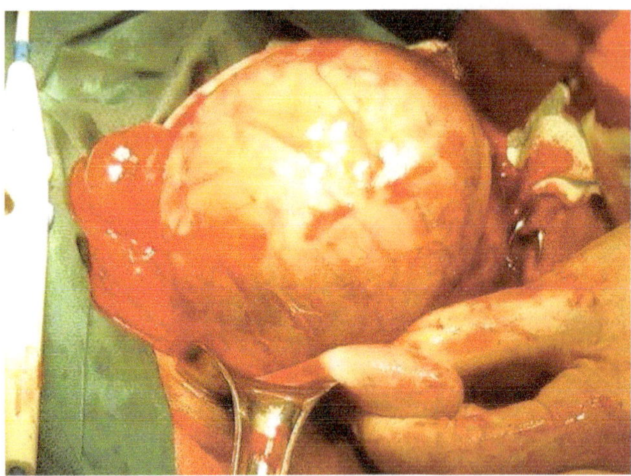

Fig. 2.14: A cystic mass is confirmed (same patient as in the Figure 2.13 at surgery)

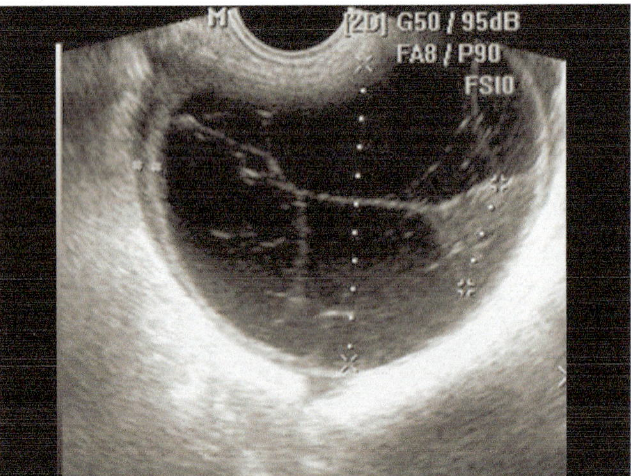

Fig. 2.15: A transabdominal sonography (TAS) of an 18-year-old patient complaining of abdominal pain and tenderness. The cyst is thin-walled with fine trabeculations

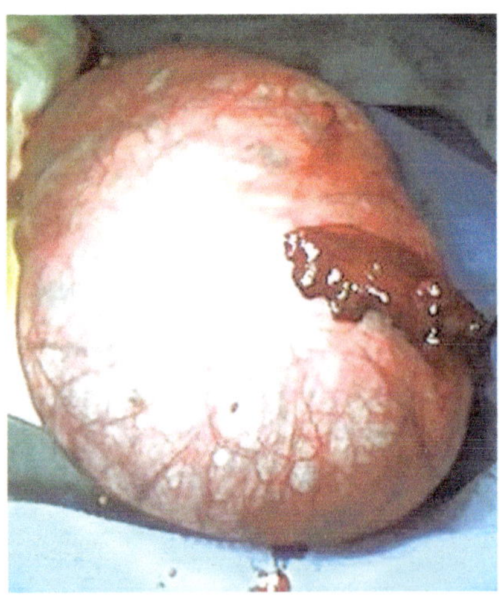

Fig. 2.16: Confirmed to be a serous cystadenoma with twisting at the time of surgery

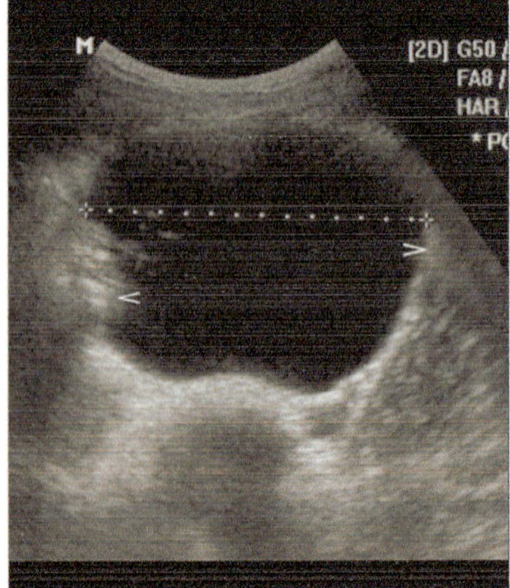

Fig. 2.17

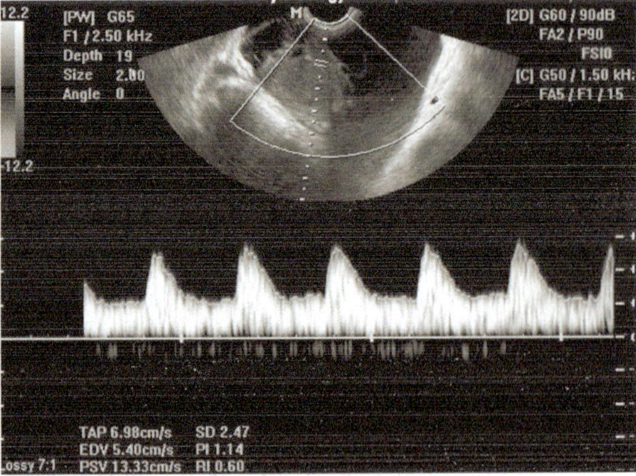

Fig. 2.18

Figs 2.17 and 2.18: A cyst in an 18-month-old infant. There is a solid component in the figure indicated by arrow < and cyst wall by >

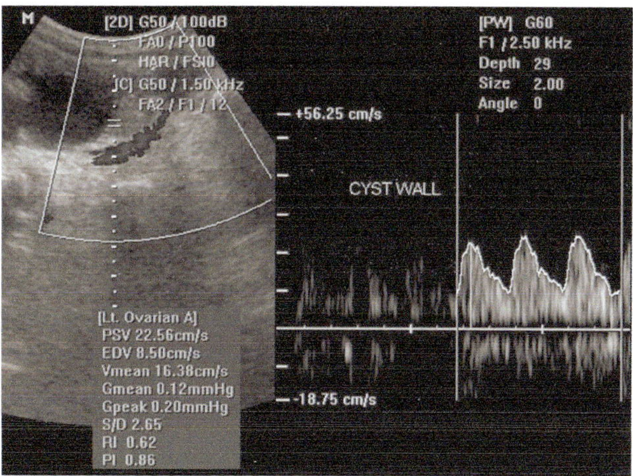

Fig. 2.19: Doppler studies do not show any abnormal flow

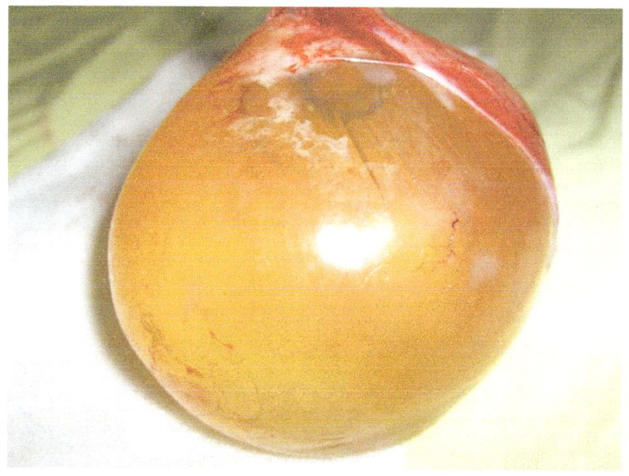

Fig. 2.20: Turns out to be a mature teratoma

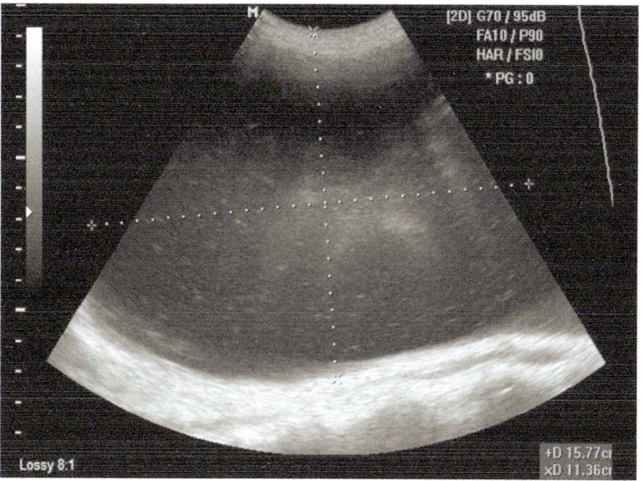

Fig. 2.21

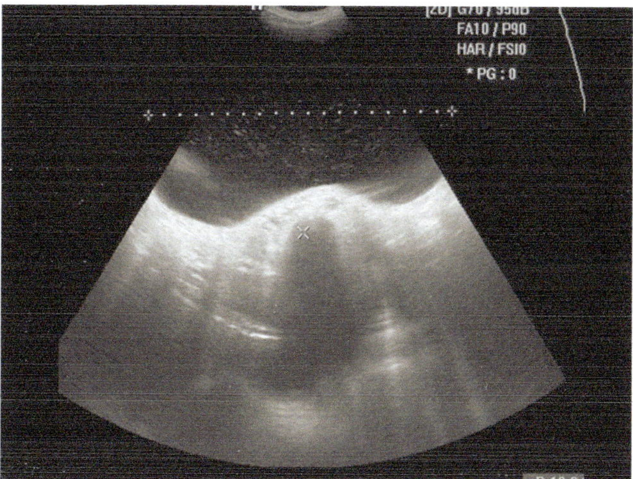

Fig. 2.22

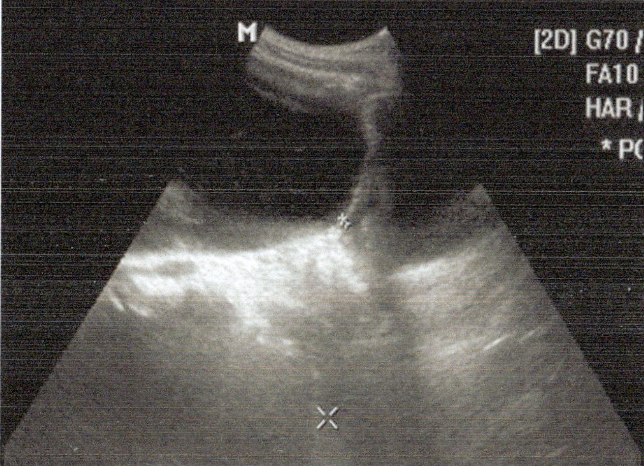

Fig. 2.23

Figs 2.21 to 2.23: Ultrasound of a 17-year-old patient with Klippel-Trenaunay-Weber syndrome shows a huge (32×19×14 cm), unilocular, thin-walled ovarian cyst, with no abnormal color flow on Doppler studies. Tumor markers (LDH, AFP, B-HCG and CA-125) are within normal limits

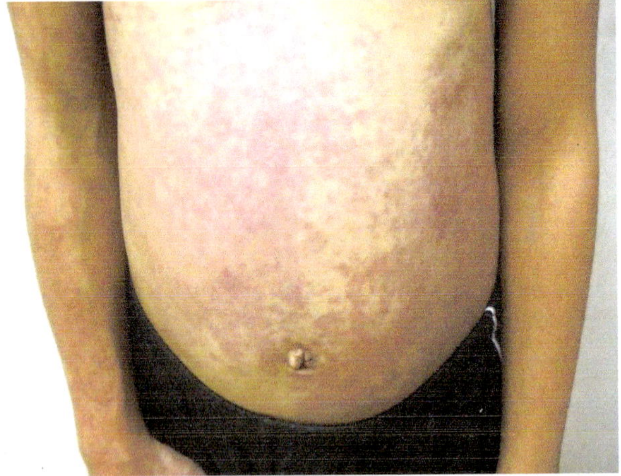

Fig. 2.24: Klippel-Trenaunay-Weber syndrome presents with port-wine stain

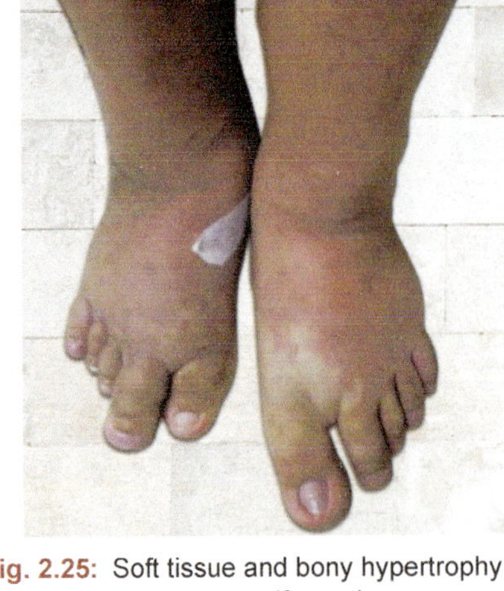

Fig. 2.25: Soft tissue and bony hypertrophy and venous malformation

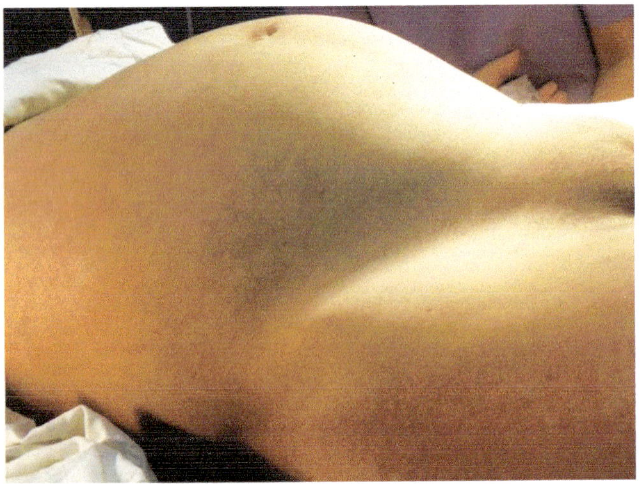

Fig. 2.26: Shows the huge abdominal mass, with the upper border extending near the subxiphoid area

In figures 2.27 and 2.28, intraoperatively, the cyst was suctioned and decompressed so as to limit the abdominal incision to the infraumbilical area. Unilateral salpingo-oophorectomy was done. Histopathological examination showed serous cystadenoma.

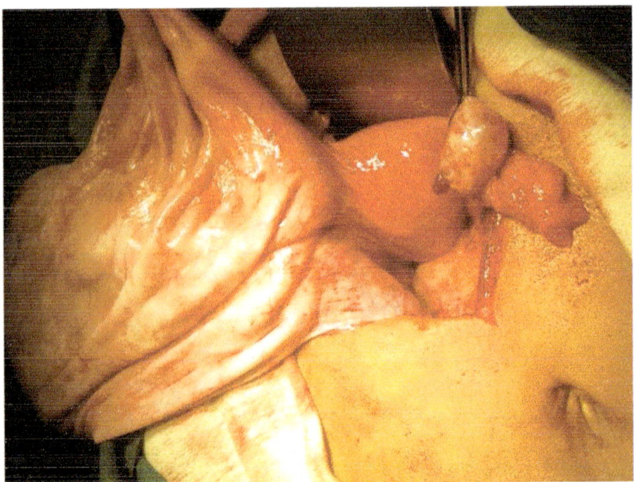

Fig. 2.27: Suction of the cyst intraoperatively

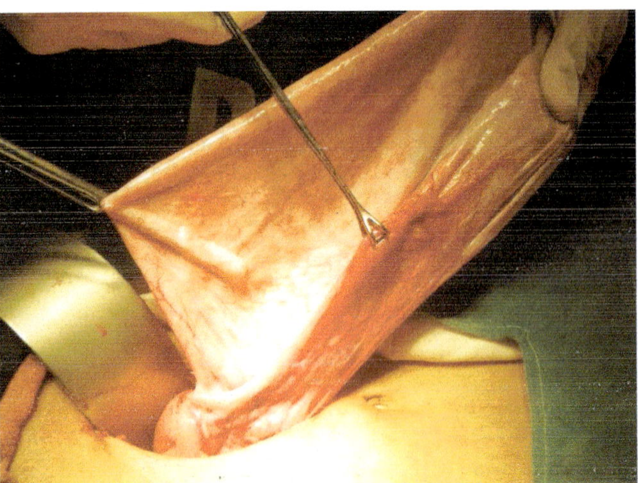

Fig. 2.28: Intraoperative decompression of the cyst

MALIGNANT TUMORS

Rhabdomyosarcoma

Rhabdomyosarcoma (Figs 2.29 to 2.31) is the third most common malignancy in children. It is derived from embryonic mesenchymal cells. Overall survival rate is 70% double that of the rates 25 years ago.

Figures 2.32 to 2.59 show ultrasound pictures and pictures of patients demonstrating various gynecological pathologies in pediatric patients.

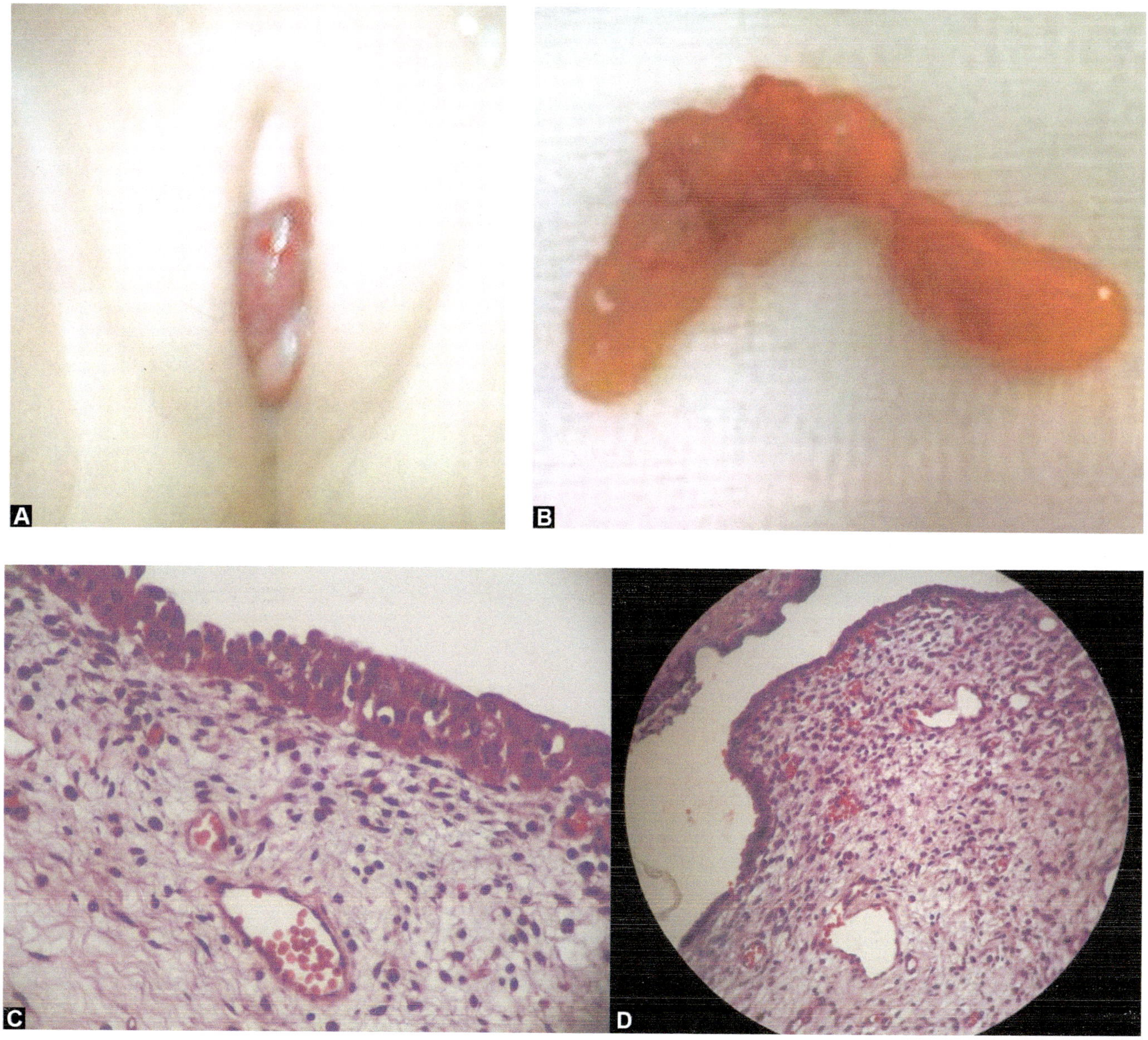

Figs 2.29A to D: Embryonal rhabdomyosarcoma: (A) Mass protruding from introitus, reddish translucent tissue in a 1-year-old; (B) Excised tissue; (C and D) Histopathology shows round and spindle cells with eosinophilic cytoplasm and hyperchromatic pleomorphic nucleus in a dense cellular area within the subepithelial area

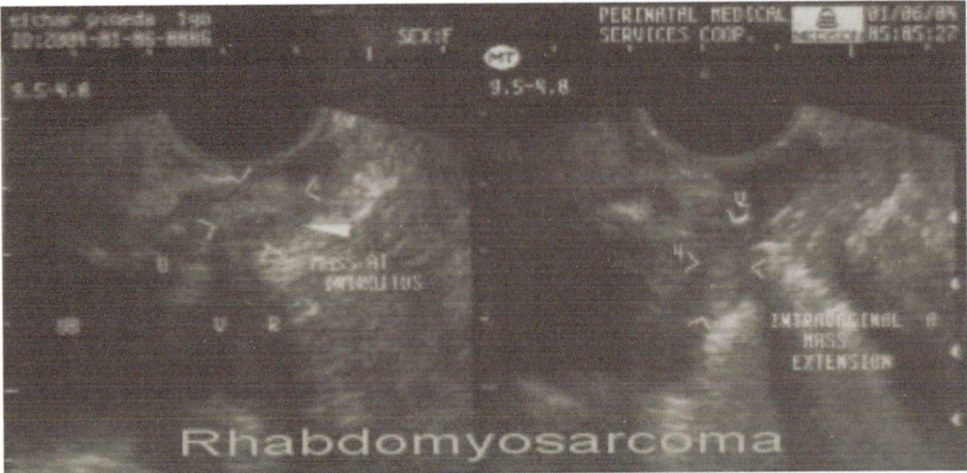

Fig. 2.30: Transperineal ultrasound shows the echogenic spindle shaped mass extending inside the vagina, defined by 4 markers. Arrow points to mass in introitus

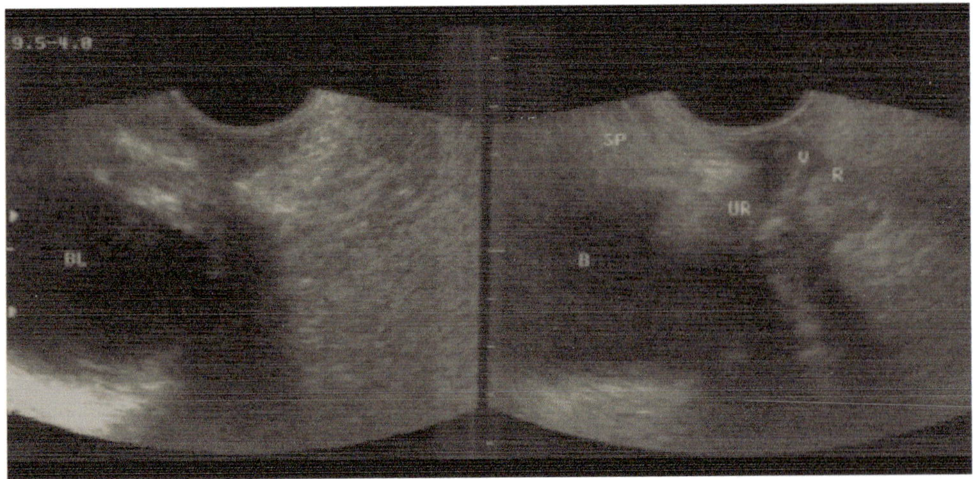

Fig. 2.31: A transperineal sonography (TPS) 1 year after excision of mass and chemotherapy shows a disease free status

Germ Cell Tumors

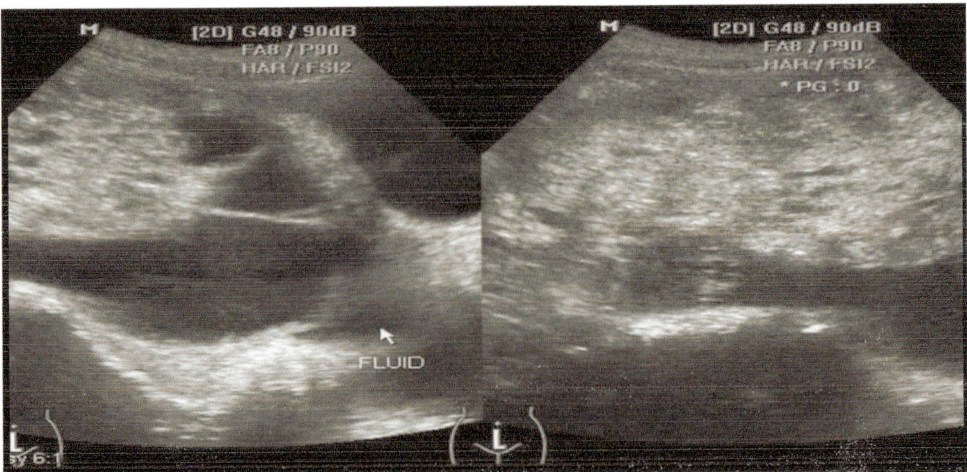

Fig. 2.32A

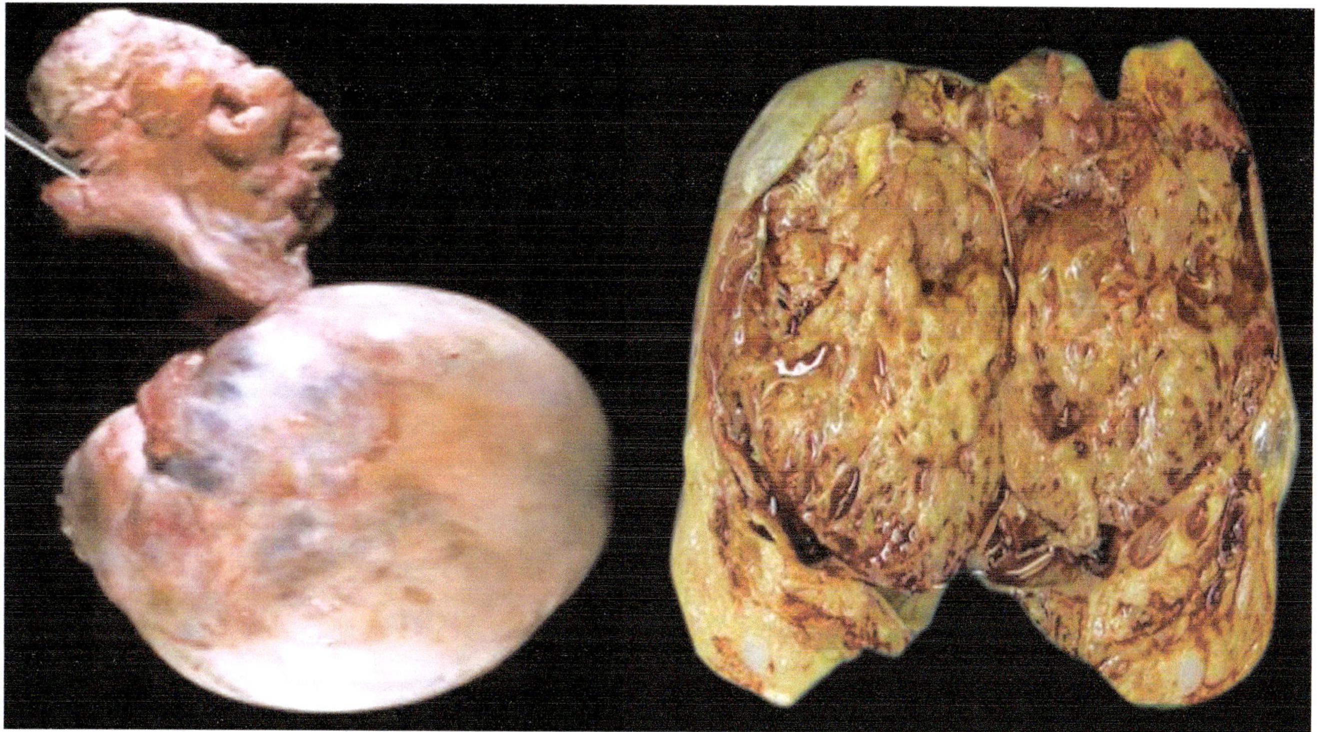

Fig. 2.32B

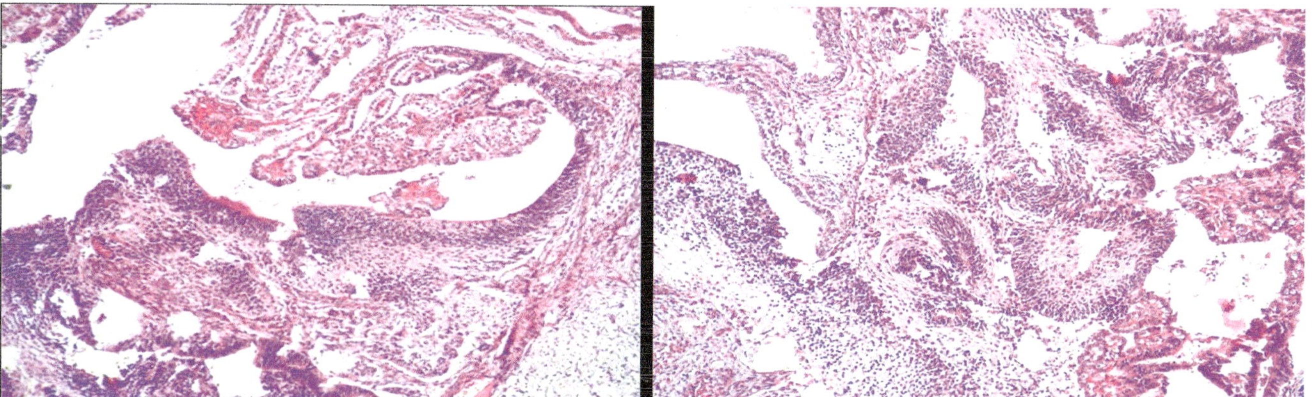

Fig. 2.32C

Figs 2.32A to C: (A) Complex abdominal mass in a 13-year-old female adolescent; (B) Cystic and solid elements of a well encapsulated mass on pelvic ultrasound and on gross examination; (C) Histopathology shows adipose and fibromuscular tissue matrix, mature and immature cartilage, hair follicle, gastrointestinal epithelium, neural elements and extensive neuroepithelial elements. Immature Teratoma

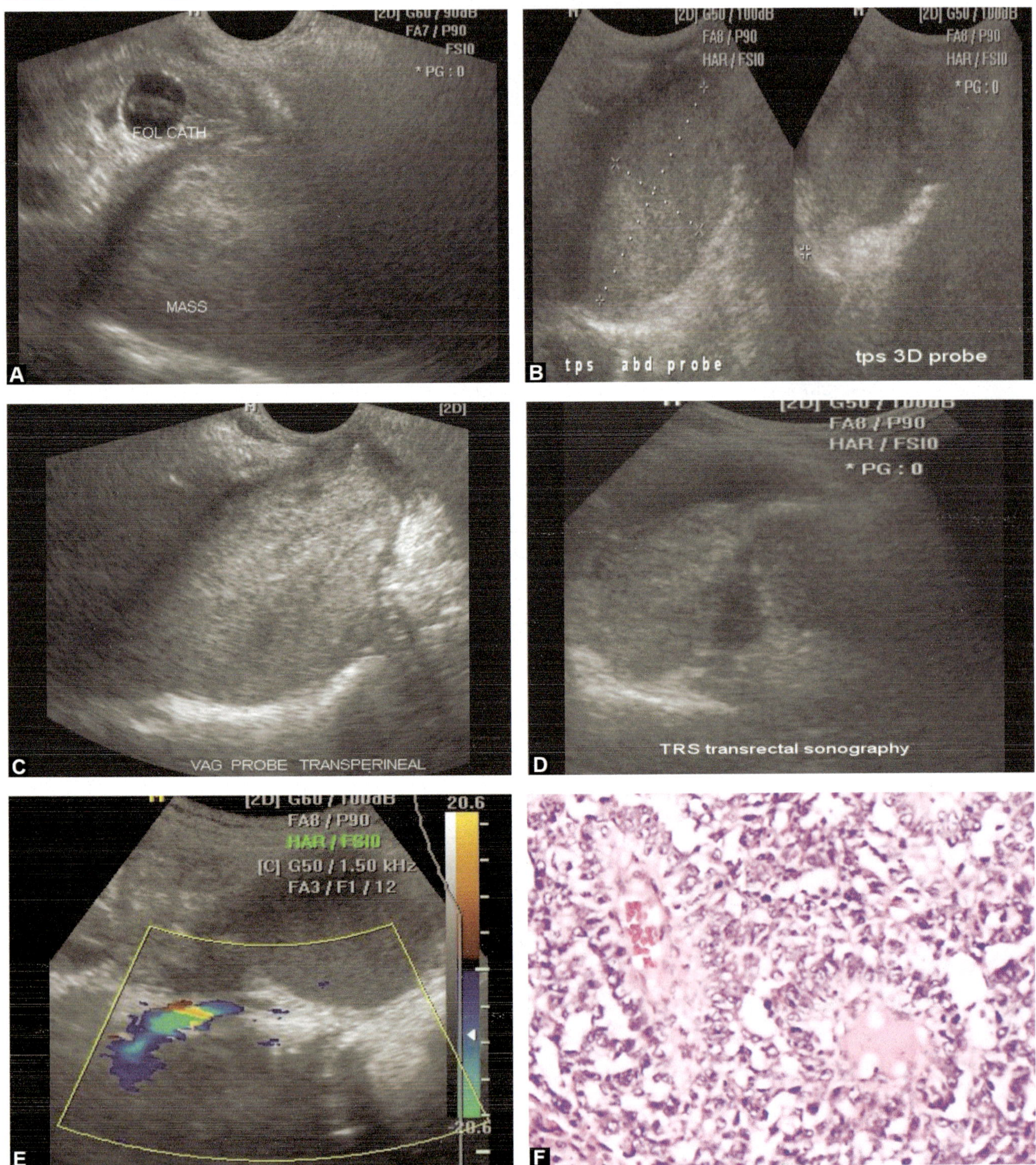

Figs 2.33A to F: Germ cell tumor (endodermal sinus tumor) in a 2-year-old child patient. Solid mass occupying vagina extending to the abdomen and to less than 1 cm from introitus: (A) Transabdominal sonography (TAS); (B) Transperineal sonography (TPS) using a convex 5 MHz probe and the other using a 3D probe; (C) TPS using vaginal probe; (D) Transrectal sonography (TRS); (E) TRS with Doppler shows a lot of blood flow and characteristic of malignancy; (F) Schiller-Duvall bodies on histopathologic examination

INFECTION AND OTHER CONDITIONS

Abdomino-pelvic Tuberculosis

Abdomino-pelvic tuberculosis is not rare in children. There are two cases confirmed by examination of ascitic fluid.

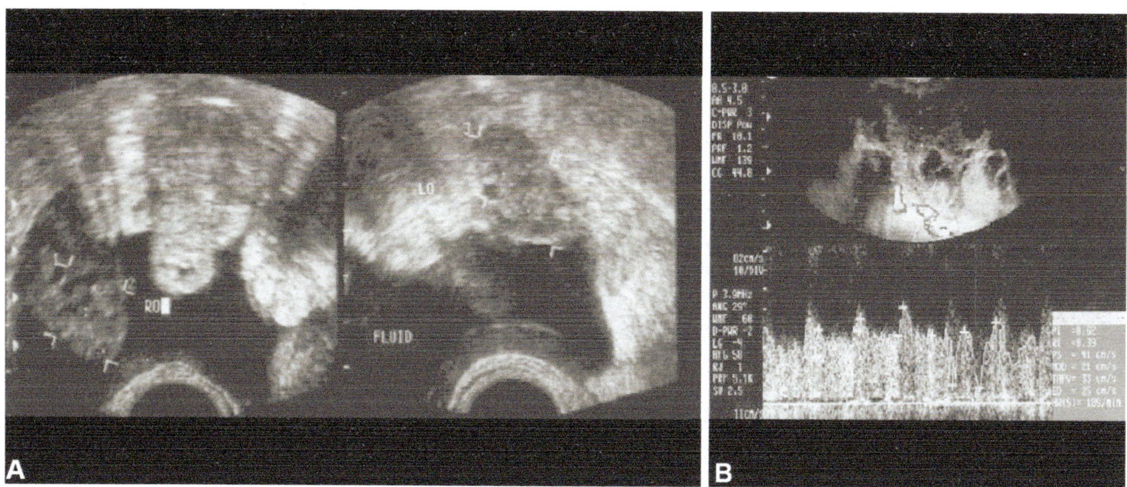

Figs 2.34A and B: (A) A 12-year-old patient with complaint of an abdominal mass and (B) A 16-year-old patient with complaint of abdominal pain. Both have ascites and have wire-looped echogenic intestines

Pelvic Abscess Due to Ruptured Appendix

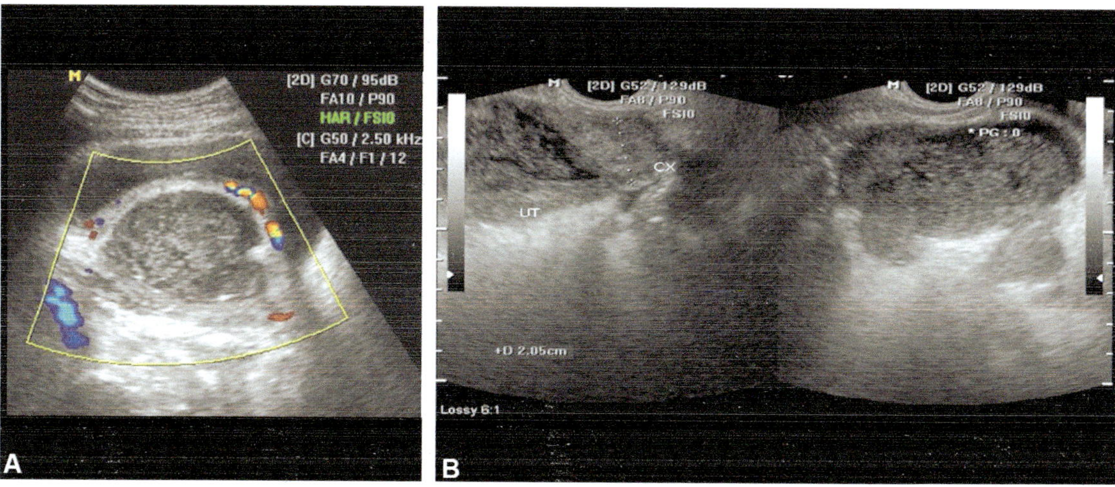

Figs 2.35A and B: A and B Blood flow in the dilated fallopian tube

CONGENITAL ANOMALIES OF THE GENITAL TRACT

Imperforate Hymen

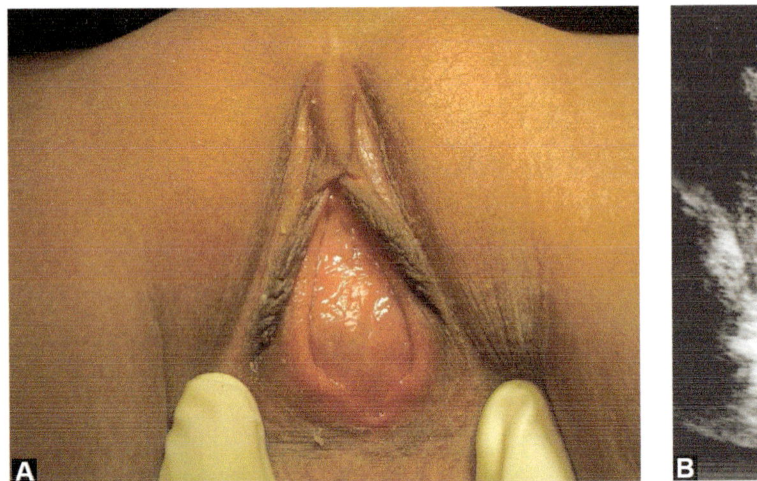

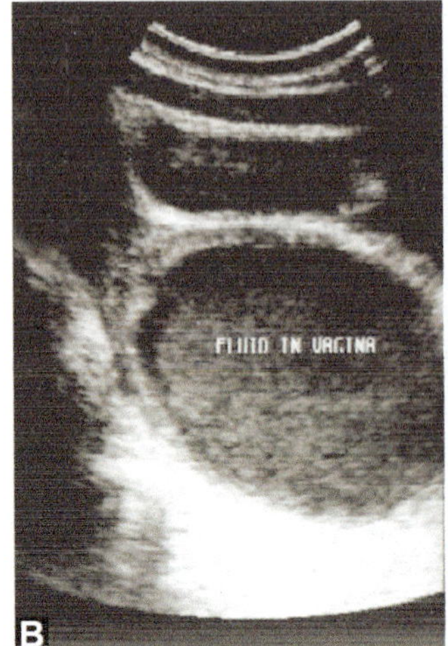

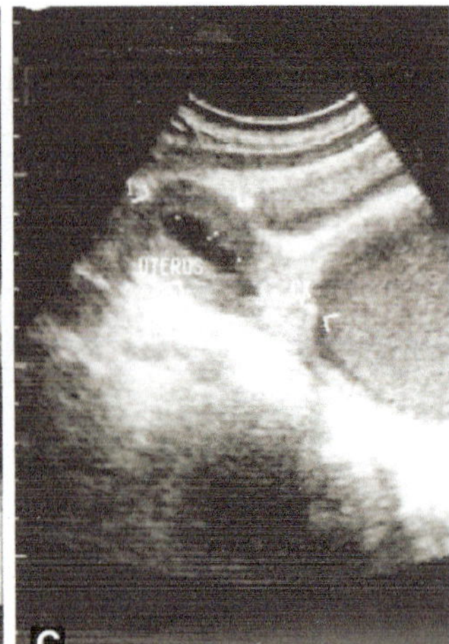

Figs 2.36A to C: Ultrasound images of an 8-year-old child: (A) Imperforate hymen; (B) Showing echogenic fluid distending both the vagina and (C) The uterine cavity

Transverse Vaginal Septum

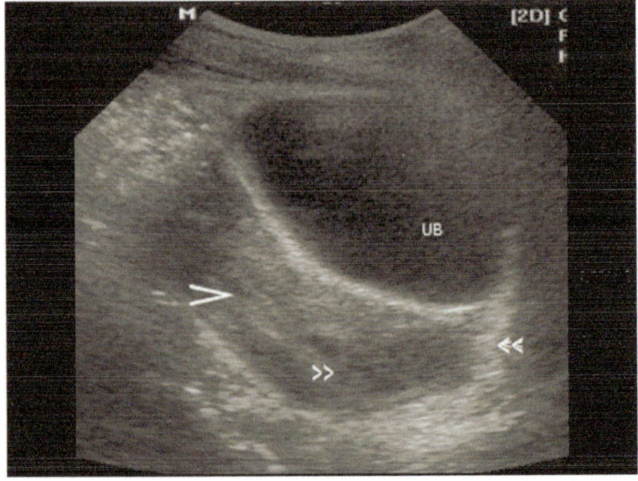

Fig. 2.37: Transverse vaginal septum with hematometra and hematocolpos in a 12-year-old girl. Transabdominal ultrasound shows the transverse septum (<<), the hematocolpos (>>), the hematometra (>) and the urinary bladder (UB)

Cloacal Malformation

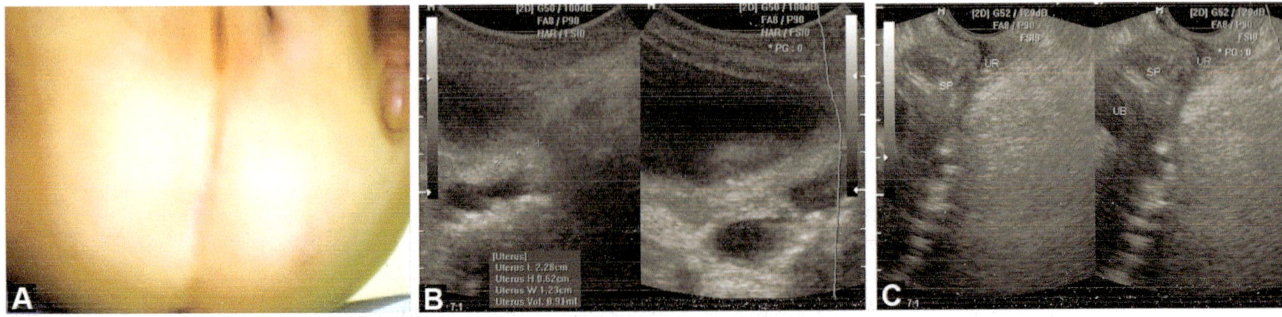

Figs 2.38A to C: Cloacal malformation in a female infant: (A) Absence of vaginal and anal opening; (B) Ultrasound images confirm the presence of uterus and ovaries; (C) Intact urinary tract

Double Uterus

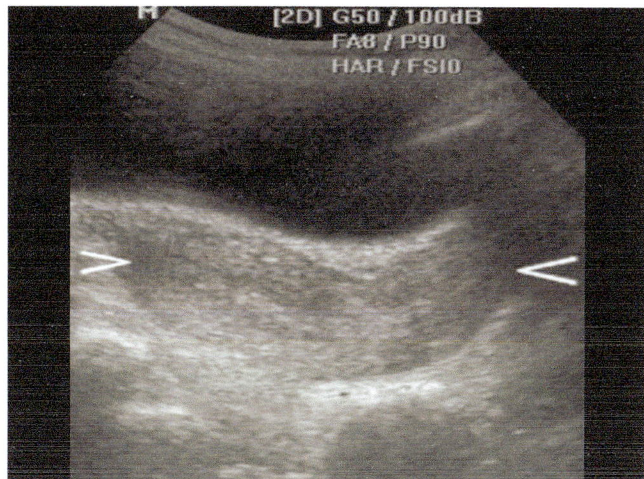

Fig. 2.39: Transabdominal sonography (TAS) 2D double uterus; 1>, 2<

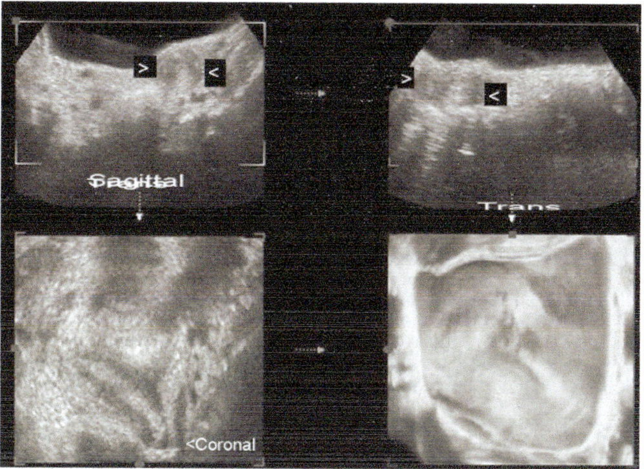

Fig. 2.40: Transrectal sonography (TRS) 3D bicornuate uterus; 1>, 2<. Coronal view clearly shows 2 uteri (>, <)

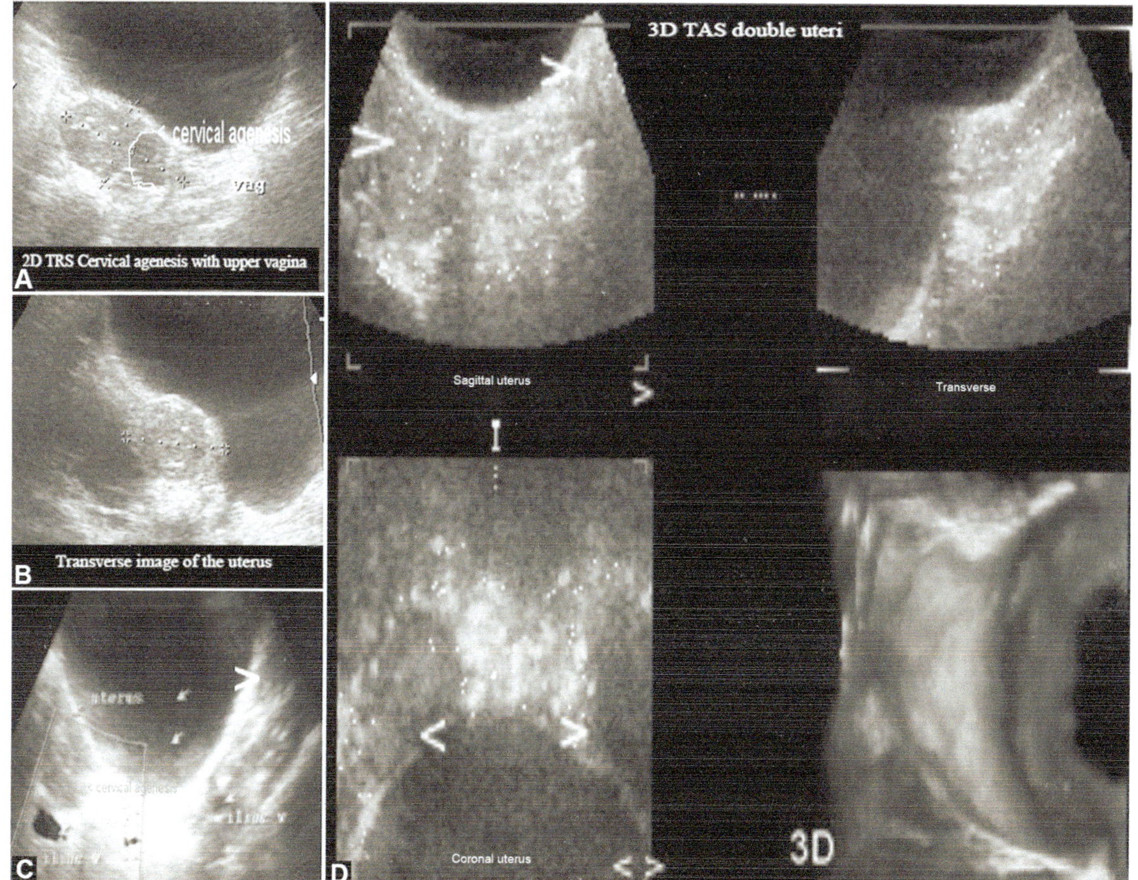

Figs 2.41A to D: Ultrasound examination of cervical agenesis, bicornuate uterus, rudimentary vagina. (A to C) 2D shows cervical agenesis and rudimentary upper vagina, thin lower vagina, 2 uteri; (D) 3D transabdominal sonography shows the 2 uteri without cervix (< >)

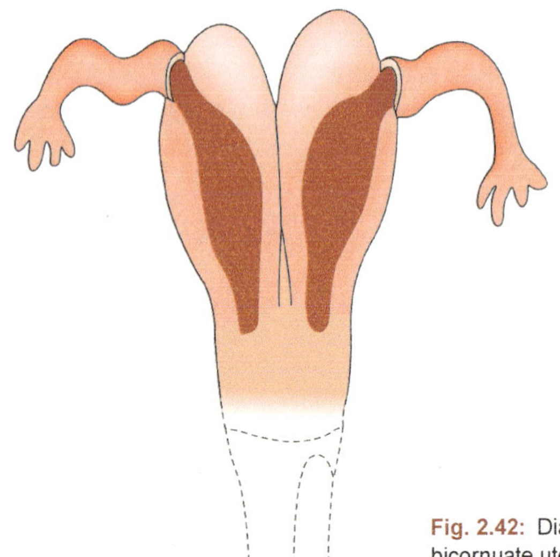

Fig. 2.42: Diagrammatic representation of the ultrasound findings of bicornuate uterus, cervical agenesis and rudimentary vagina

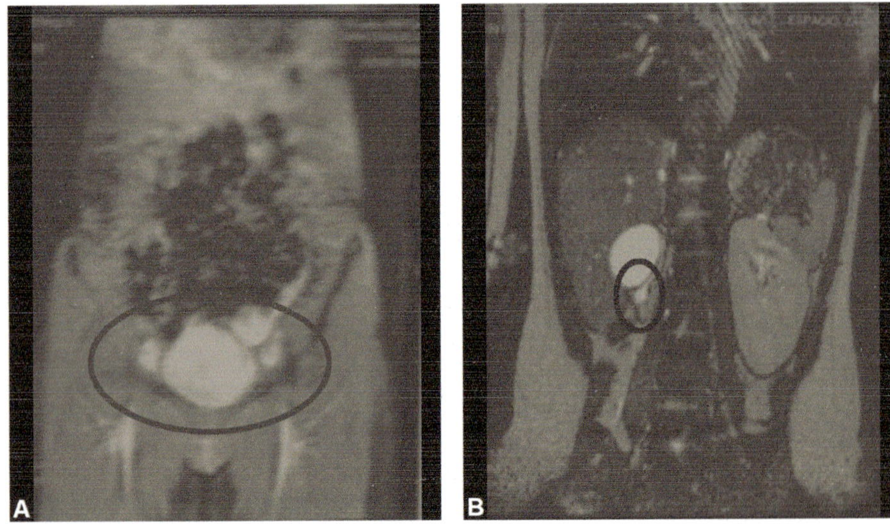

Figs 2.43A and B: (A) An MRI of same patient described in earlier figures showing double uterus with hematometra; (B) A hypoplastic right kidney

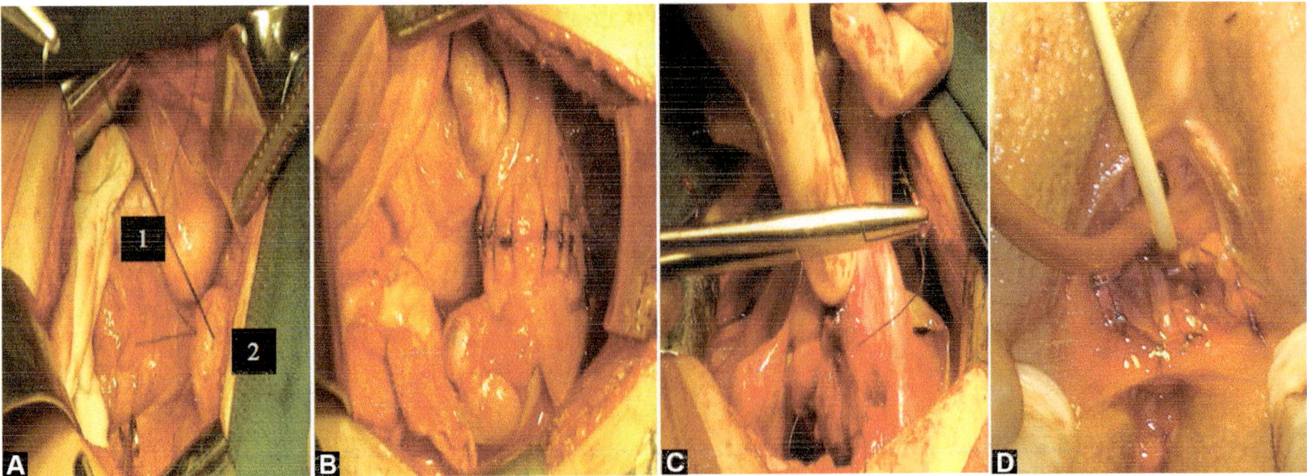

Figs 2.44A to D: (A) Intraoperative pictures showing 2 uteri; (B) Metroplasty; (C) Cervicoplasty; (D) Creation of neovagina

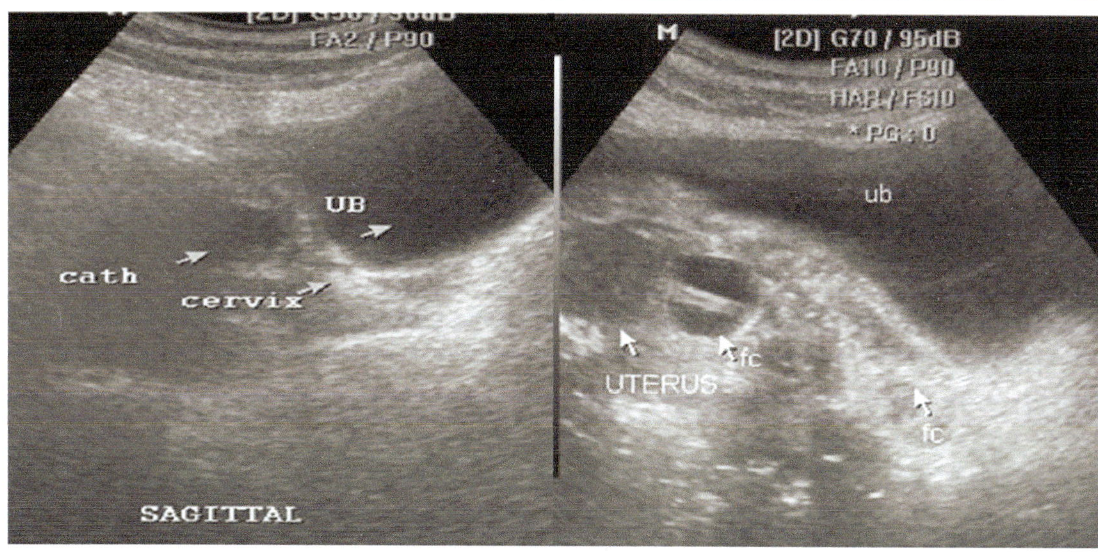

Fig. 2.45: Ultrasound images after the repair showing foley catheter balloon within the single uterine cavity, the cervix and the neovagina. One year after the surgery, the patient was menstruating regularly but still with vaginal mold in place

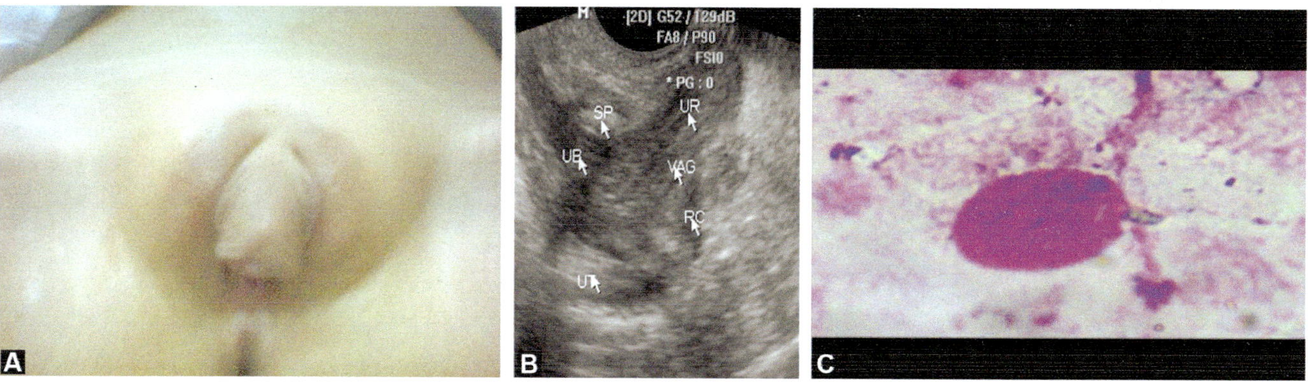

Figs 2.46A to C: (A) Clitoromegaly in a female infant; (B) Ultrasound images show presence of uterus and ovaries; (C) Examination of buccal smear demonstrates the presence of Barr bodies

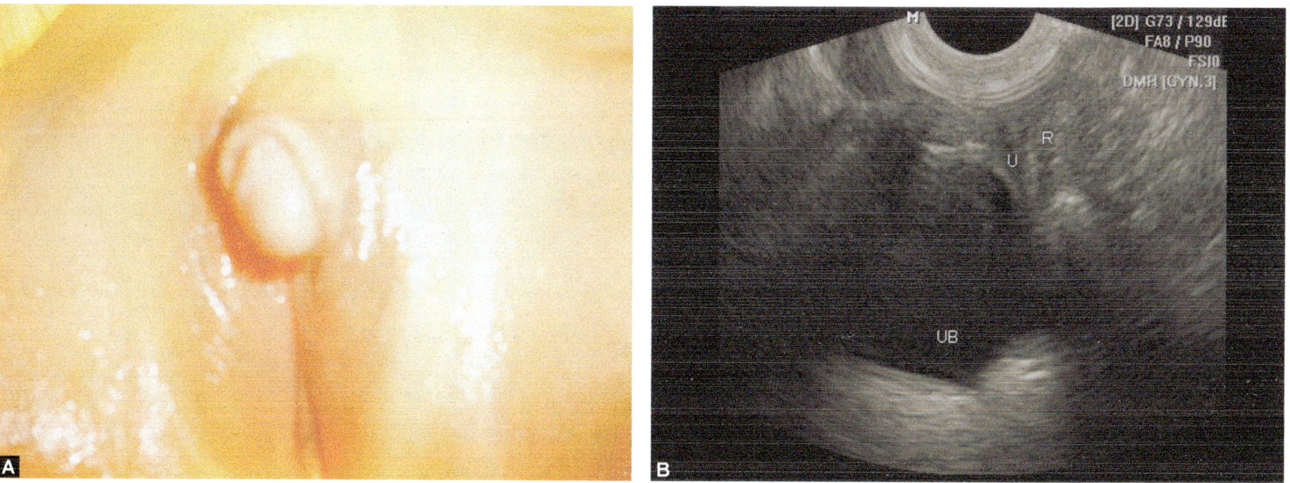

Figs 2.47A and B: (A) Ambiguous genitalia in a 4-year-old child patient. Karyotype shows 46XY; (B) Ultrasound examination demonstrates absence of uterus and ovaries

ULTRASOUND OF BREAST IN CHILDREN

Most of the children referred for breast ultrasound to the perinatal medical services co-operative ultrasound machine have a breast "mass", either at birth, during infancy or childhood. Breast asymmetry is also a common complaint especially during the early stages of breast development. Ultrasound is done to rule out a breast mass, cyst or abscess.

Newborn children normally have breast tissue and milk production, "witch milk", as a result of maternal hormonal stimulation. The breast bud is a criterion to estimate the gestational age at birth according to the Dubowitz Score where nipple, areola and breast tissue volume are evaluated and given points to assess maturity of the newborn. The more defined the nipple; the areola bigger than 0.75 cm and the palpable breast tissue more than 0.5 cm, the more mature the infant.

Tanner Stages

Breasts of children are classified according to the description for different Tanner stages. Generally, there are five different Tanner stages in the development of the breast.

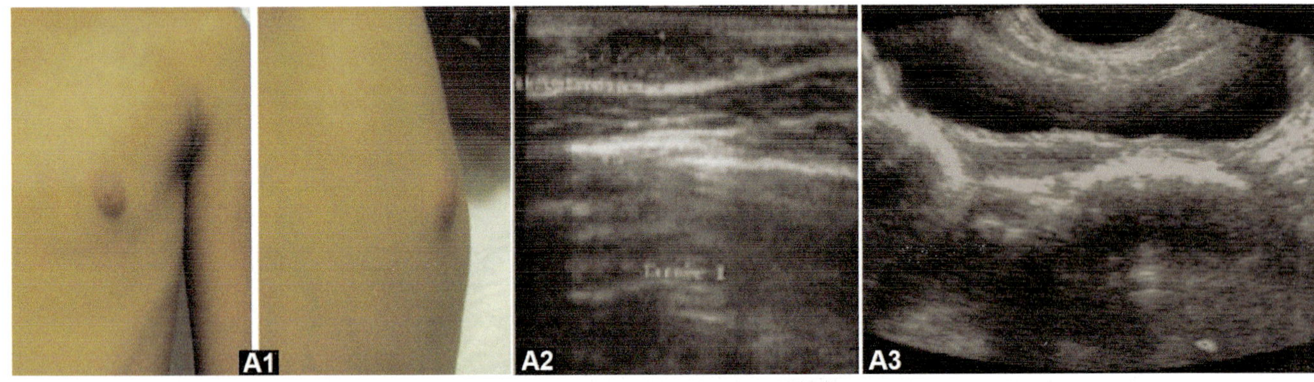

Fig. 2.48A

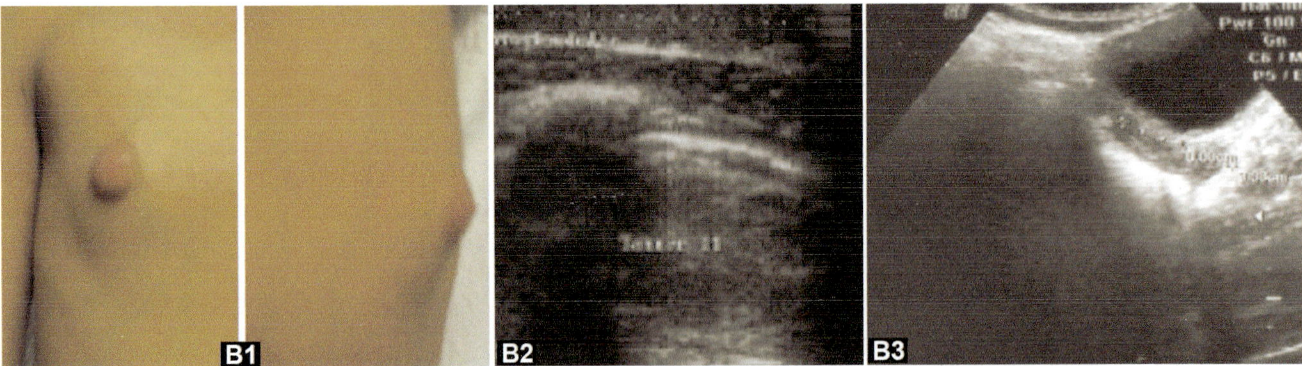

Fig. 2.48B

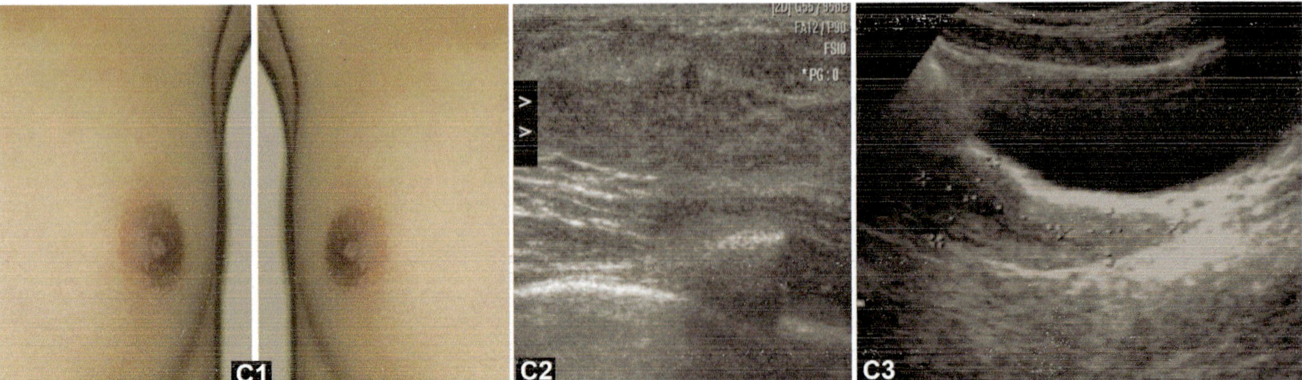

Fig. 2.48C

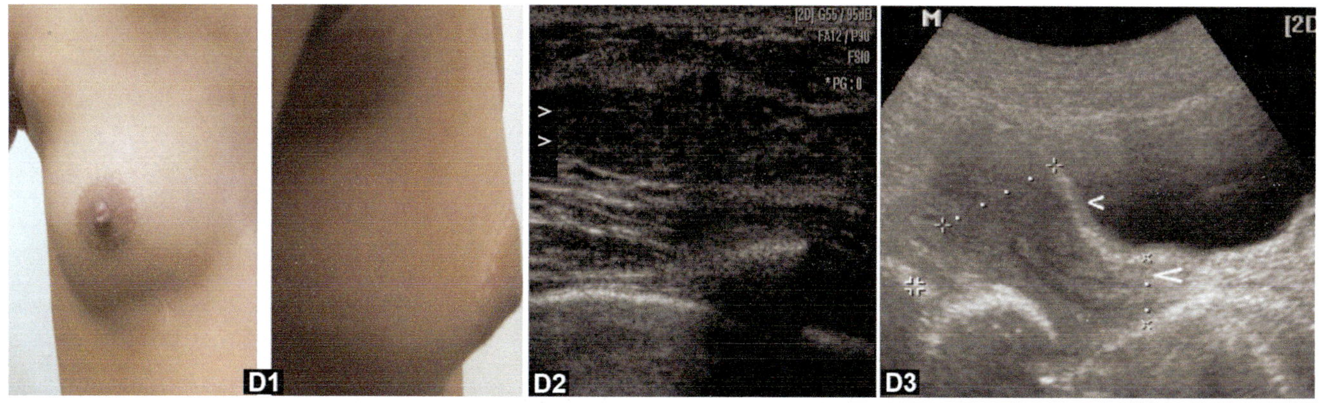

Fig. 2.48D

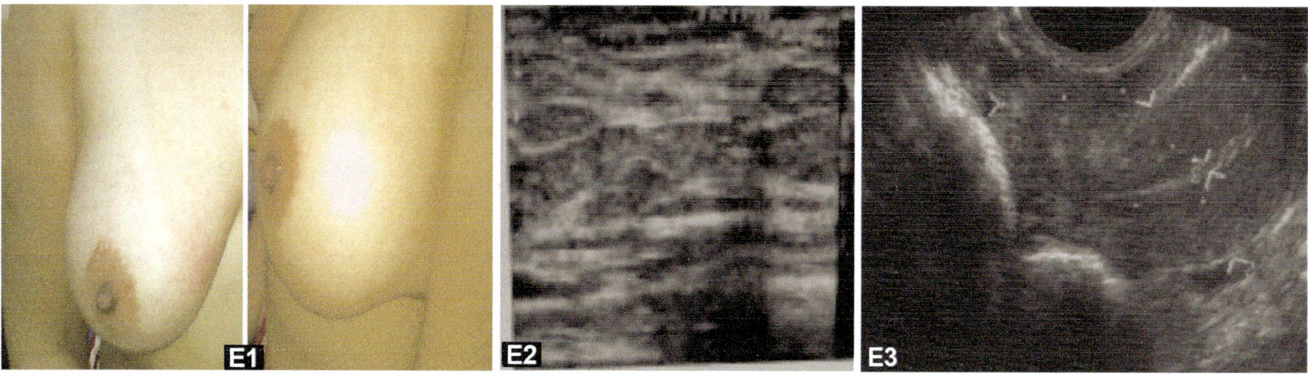

Fig. 2.48E

Figs 2.48A to E: Breast development at different Tanner stages: (A) Tanner stage I—(A1) Elevation of papilla only; (A2) Breast ultrasound shows fibroglandular tissue; (A3) Uterus is tubular in shape. Uterus to cervix ratio is 2:3. (B) Tanner stage II—(B1) Breast bud stage. Elevation of breast and papilla as small mound; (B2) Breast ultrasound shows bigger fibroglandular tissue; (B3) Uterus to cervix ratio is 3:1. (C) Tanner stage III—(C1) Enlargement. No separation of breast and areola; (C2) Breast ultrasound shows more defined fibroglandular tissues; (C3) Uterus is pear shaped, uterus to cervix ratio is 3:1. (D) Tanner stage IV—(D1) Projection of areola and papilla to form secondary mound; (D2) Ultrasound of the breast shows a developed fibroglandular layer >; (D3) Uterus to cervix ratio is 3:1<. (E) Tanner stage V—(E1) Mature stage. Projection of papilla only, caused by recession of areola to the general contour of the breast; (E2) Breast ultrasound shows fatty tissue in fibroglandular layer; (E3) TRS of a mature female. Uterus to cervix ratio is 3:1

Breast Budding in Neonates

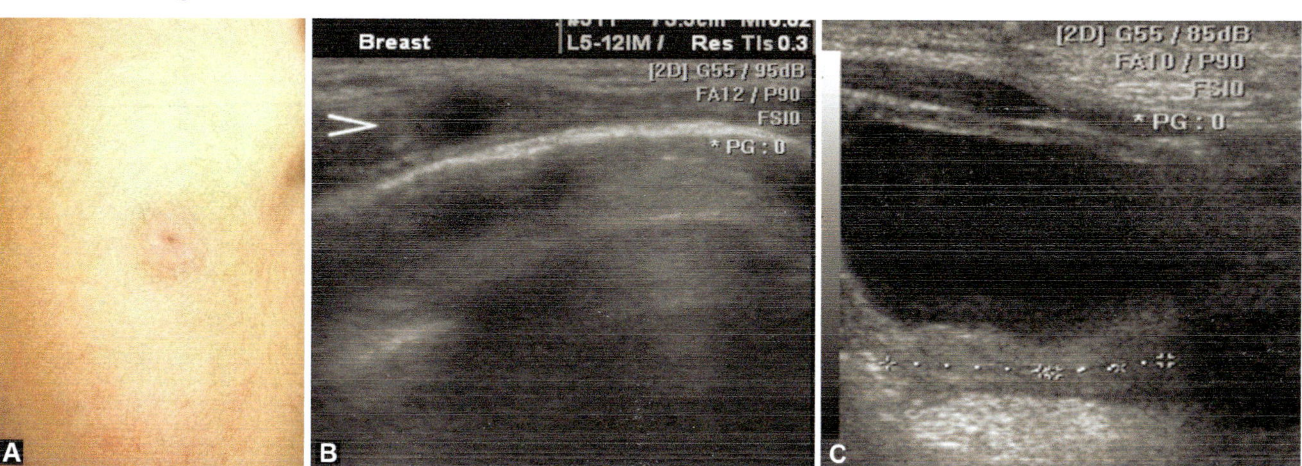

Figs 2.49A to C: (A) Breast of term neonate shows breast bud, a result of maternal hormonal stimulation; (B) Ultrasound of the breast; (C) Uterus and ovary are also shown, cervix to uterus ratio is 1:1

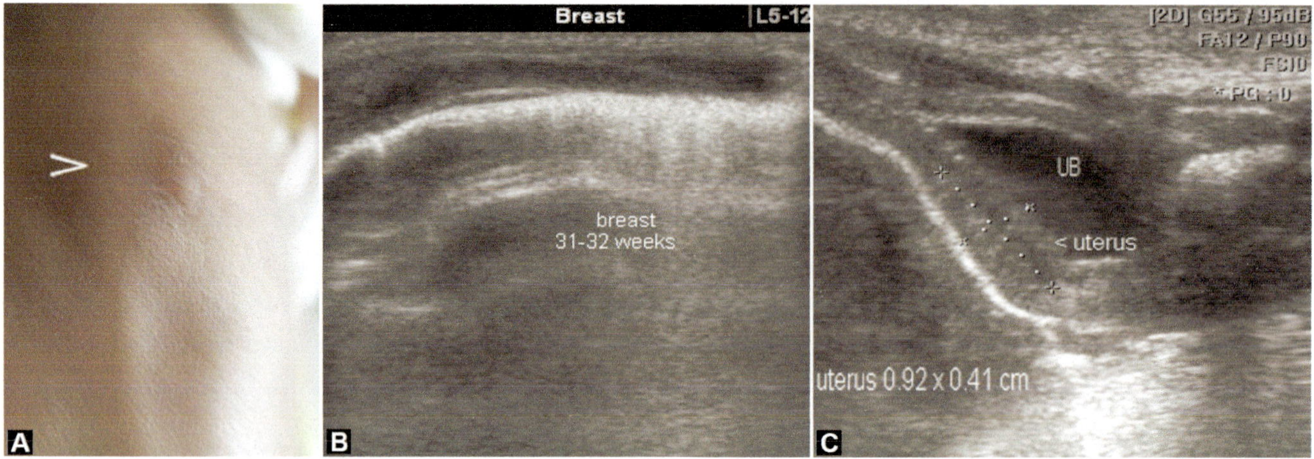

Figs 2.50A to C: (A) Breast of a preterm 32-week neonate by Dubowitz score; (B) Ultrasound images of the breast and the uterus of the preemie show less effects of maternal hormonal stimulation; (C) Tubular shaped uterus, cervix to uterus ratio is 1:1

Dubowitz Score

Dubowitz score = SUM (points for each parameter)

Interpretation

- Minimum score: 0
- Maximum score: 72 (neurological sign 35 external sign 37) - includes breast bud.

Estimated gestational age = 0.2642 x (total score) + 24.595.

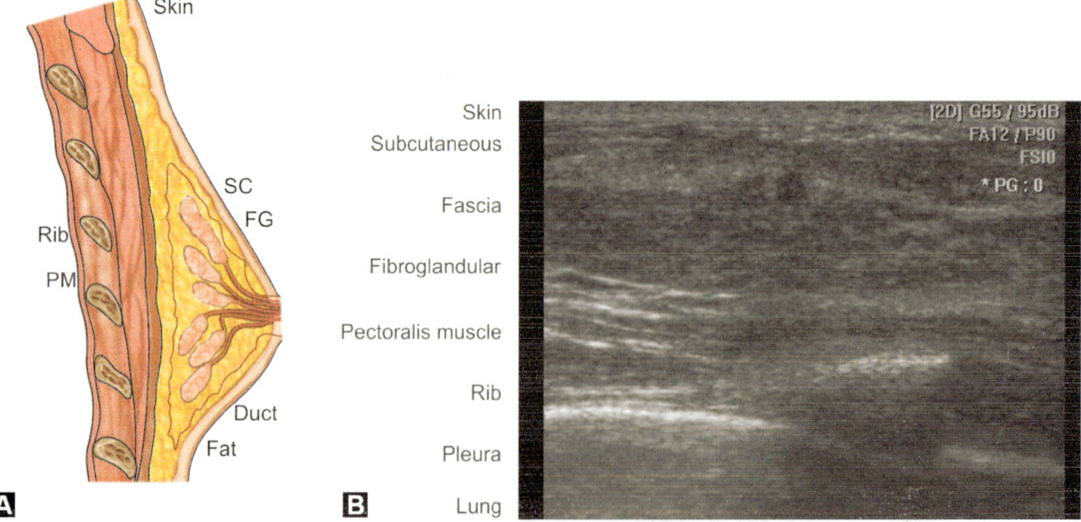

Figs 2.51A and B: (A) Parts of the breast; (B) Ultrasound picture with corresponding labels of the different tissue layers
Key: SC, subcutaneous; FG, fibroglandular; PM, pectoralis muscle

COMMON BREAST DISEASES AND CONDITIONS IN YOUNG FEMALES

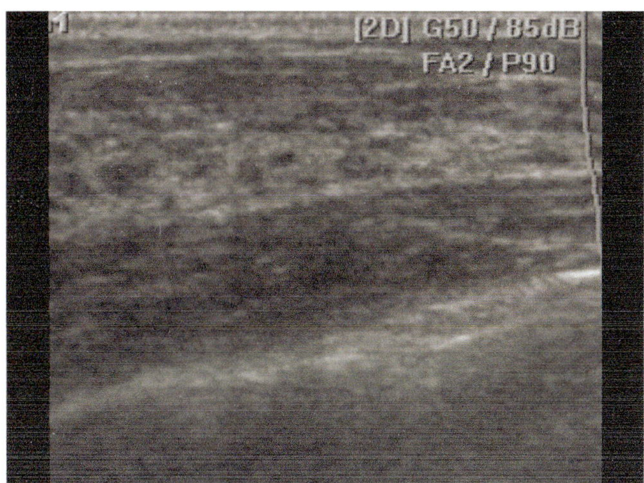

Fig. 2.52: Fibrocystic disease

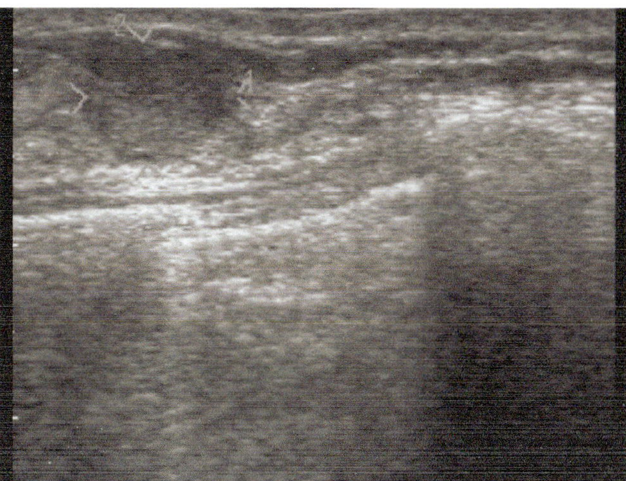

Fig. 2.53: Fibroadenoma

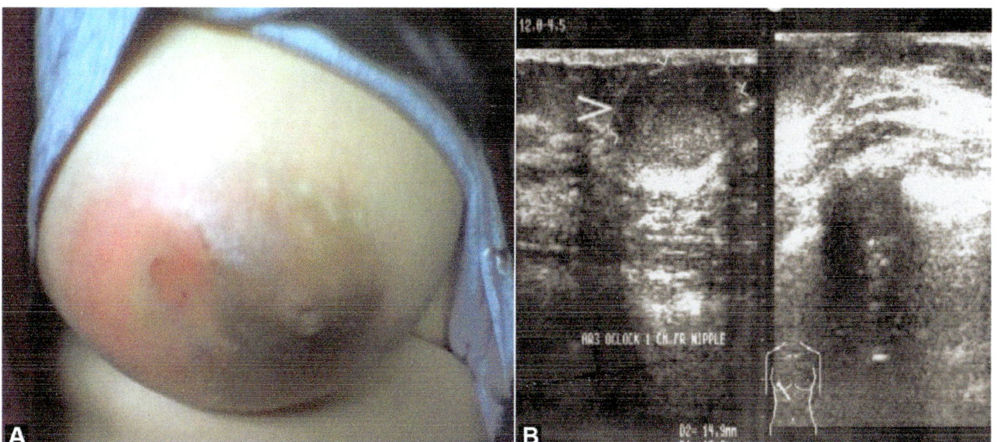

Figs 2.54A and B: (A) Breast abscess; (B) Ultrasound of breast showing mastitis and abscess

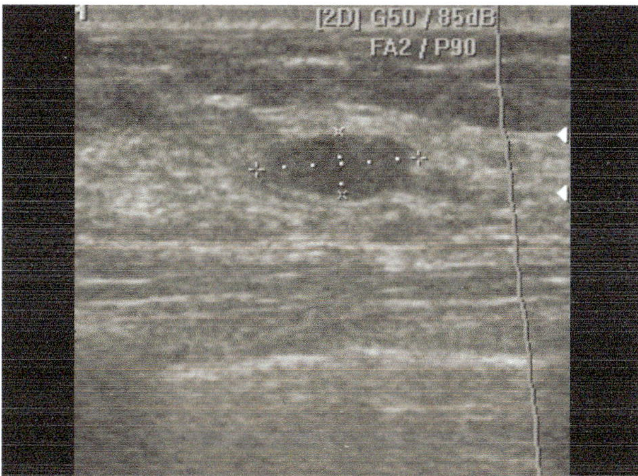

Fig. 2.55: Cyst

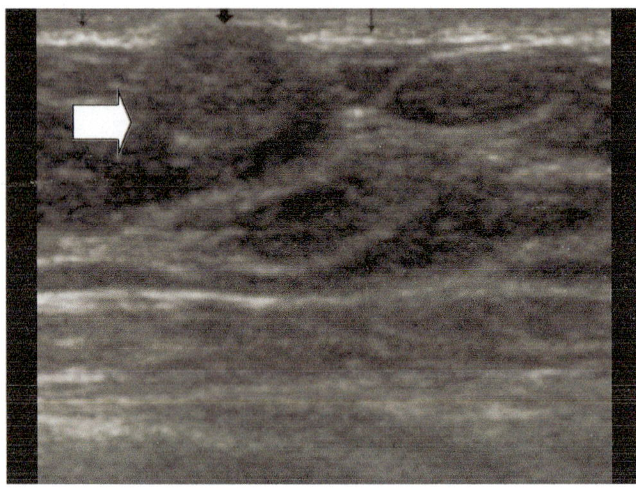

Fig. 2.56: Fat necrosis. Ultrasound shows a hypoechoic round area with fuzzy borders (with arrow) in the subcutaneous tissue that extends into the dermis

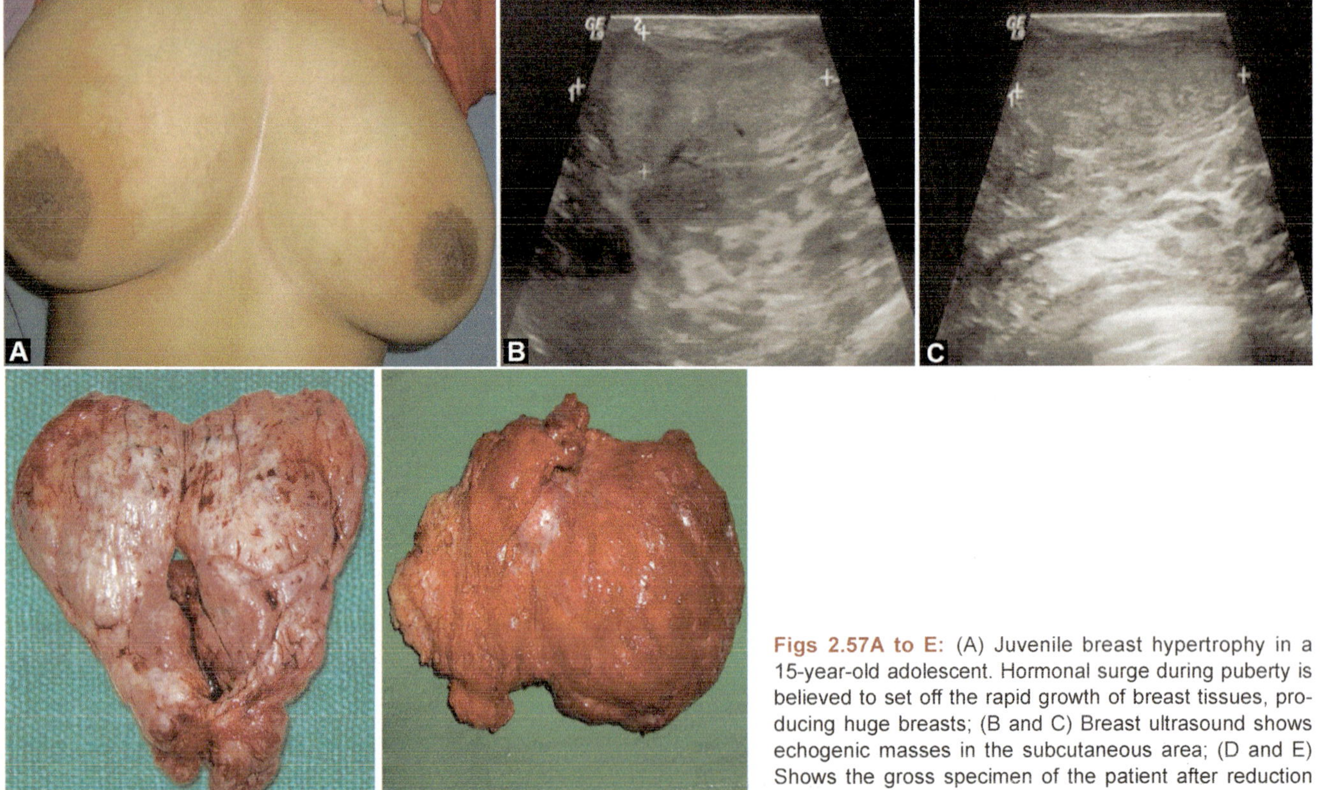

Figs 2.57A to E: (A) Juvenile breast hypertrophy in a 15-year-old adolescent. Hormonal surge during puberty is believed to set off the rapid growth of breast tissues, producing huge breasts; (B and C) Breast ultrasound shows echogenic masses in the subcutaneous area; (D and E) Shows the gross specimen of the patient after reduction mammoplasty

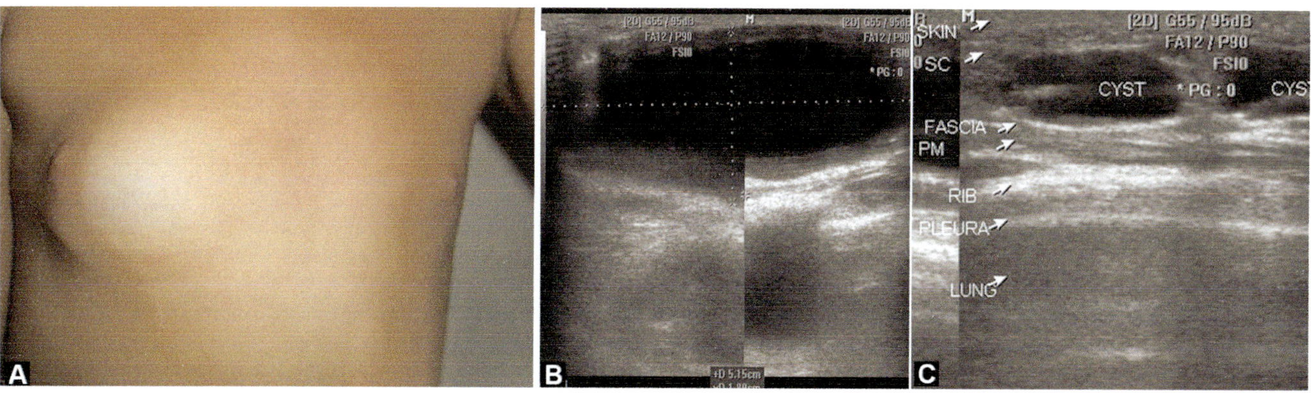

Figs 2.58A to C: (A) Unilateral breast mass; (B and C) Breast ultrasound reveals a huge cyst occupying the subcutaneous layer of the breast

CENTRAL PRECOCIOUS PUBERTY

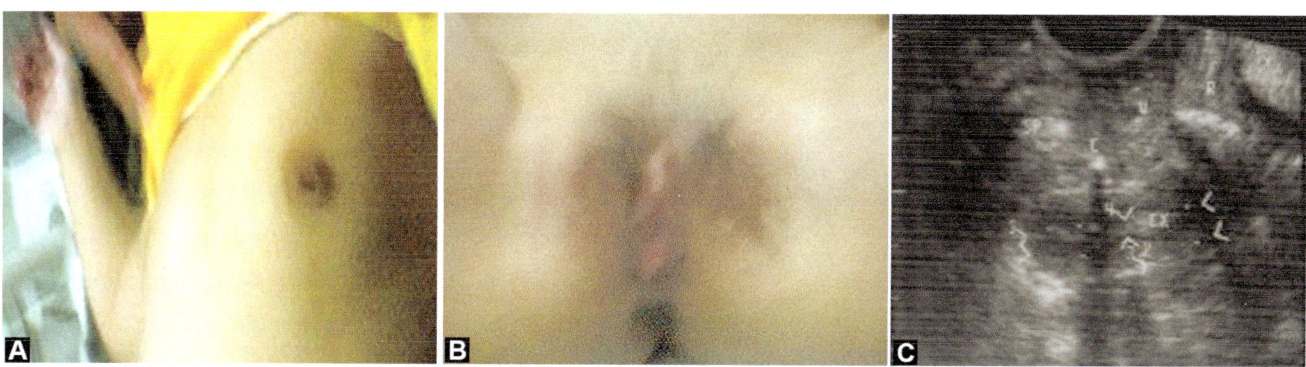

Figs 2.59A to C: (A) Three-year-old patient with epilepsy and Tanner 2 breast; (B) Pubis and enlarged uterus; (C) Ultrasound shows uterus which measures 3.4 x 1.18 x 1.38 cm

BIBLIOGRAPHY

1. Acien P, Acien M, Sánchez-Ferrer M, et al. Complex malformations of the female genital tract: new types and revision of classification. Human Reproduction 2004;19:2377-84.
2. Annual Reports (2002-2008). Pediatric and Adolescent Gynecology Unit, Philippine Children's Medical Center, Quezon City.
3. Bridges NA, Cooke A, Healy MJ, et al. Growth of the uterus. Arch Dis Child 1996;75(4):330-1.
4. Butaran M. Normal pelvic sonographic findings of patients seen at the Pediatric and Adolescent Gynecology Unit of the Philippine Children's Medical Center: a 6-year experience (to be published).
5. Digital Archives, Perinatal Medical Services Co-operative Ultrasound Machine 2002-2008.
6. Dubowitz LMS, Dubowitz V, Goldberg C. Clinical assessment of gestational age in the newborn infant. J Pediatr 1970;77(1):1-10.
7. Herter LD, Gelendziner E, Flores JA, et al. Ovarian and uterine sonography in girls between 1 and 13 years old: correlation of findings with age and pubertal status. AJR Am Roentgenol 2002;178(6):1531-6.
8. Ivarsson SA, Nilsson KO, Persson PH, et al. Ultrasonography of the pelvic organs in prepubertal and postpubertal girls. Arch Dis Child 1983;58(5):352-4.
9. Kass-Wolff J, Wilson E. Pediatric gynecology assessment strategies and common problems. Semin Reprod Med 2003;21(4):329-38.
10. Nussbaum AR, Sanders RC, Jones MD, et al. Neonatal uterine morphology as seen on real-time ultrasound. Radiology 1986;160(3):641-3.
11. Parsons L, Sommers S. Gynecology. Philadelphia: WB Saunders Co 1978; p. 16.
12. Sanfilippo JS, Muram D, DeWhurst J, et al. Pediatric and Adolescent Gynecology. New York: WB Saunders Co 2001; pp. 237-47.

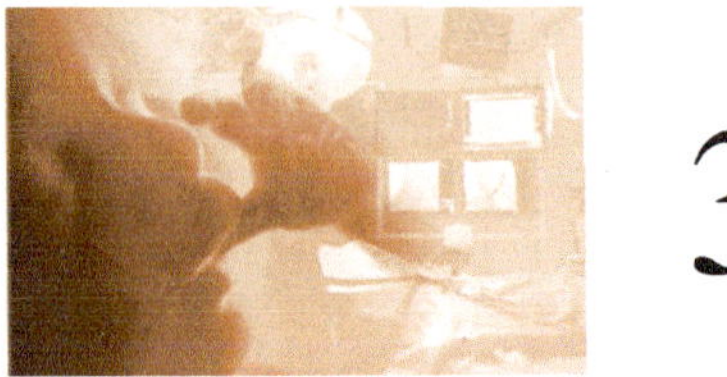

3 Abnormalities in Development

Franklin P Atencio

EMBRYOLOGY OF THE FEMALE REPRODUCTIVE SYSTEM

Ovarian Migration and Embryology

The primordial germ cells, from which the gonads are derived, start their migration (Fig. 3.1) from the yolk sac to the urogenital ridge at week 4 or 5 after conception. Bilateral urogenital ridges arise from the coelomic epithelium and underlying mesenchyme. Gonadal ridges are colonized by germ cells and produce the bipotential gonad primordium. Prior to six weeks of development, the male and female reproductive tracts are similar in appearance.

Differentiation of the Female Genital Tract

Differentiation of the female genital tract is shown in the Figures 3.2 to 3.4. The presence of testes-determining factor on a gene that is found in the Y chromosome determines the developing gonads to develop into testes or ovaries. Two sets of paired ducts—the paramesonephric (Müllerian) duct and mesonephric (Wolffian) duct—are initially present along the lateral aspects of the gonads. In females, the Müllerian ducts develop as an invagination of the coelomic epithelium. The caudal end of the duct lengthens and acquires a lumen in the process. The proximal segments remain unfused and eventually form the fallopian tubes, which opens into the peritoneal cavity. The caudal segments fuse to form the uterovaginal primordium that eventually becomes the lower uterine segment.

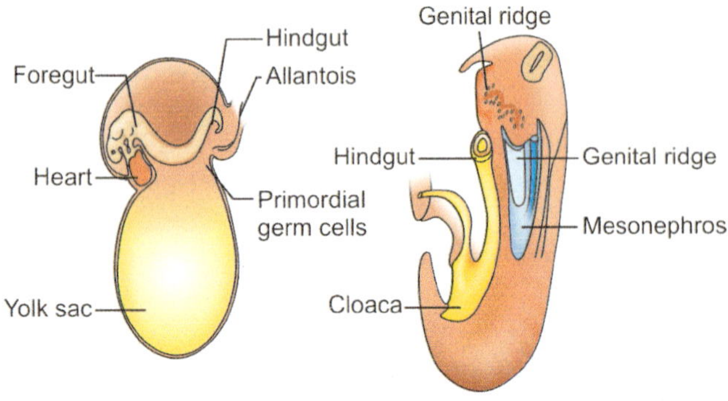

Fig. 3.1: Ovarian migration and embryology

OVARIES

As shown in the Figure 3.3, the following points can be mentioned about the ovary:

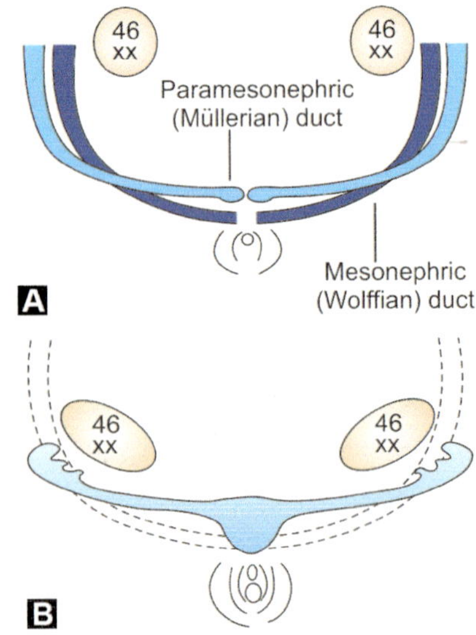

Figs 3.2A and B: Differentiation of the female genital tract: (A) Müllerian and Wolffian ducts present along the lateral aspect of the gonads; (B) regression of the Wolffian ducts and differentiation of the Müllerian duct into the uterus and upper portion of the vagina
Source: Illustration courtesy Lottman H and Thomas DFM, Disorder of sex Development in Essentials of Pediatric Urology

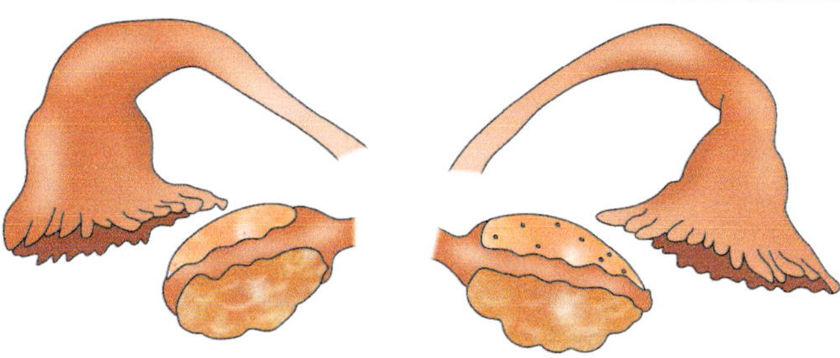

Fig. 3.3: Development of ovaries

- The ovary arises from the dorsal mesenchyme of the gonadal ridge
- The primordial germ cells that give rise to female oocytes are originally from the yolk sac
- Germ cells induce the mesonephros to form genital ridges which become the primitive sex cords
- If the germ cells fail to migrate, gonads do not form in the region.

DEVELOPMENT OF UTERUS

The fused Müllerian ducts are initially separated by a septum. Septal regression is believed to be due to apoptosis, mediated by the Bcl2 gene, the absence of which has been implicated in anomalies like septate or bicornuate uterus. The classical theory of septal regression hypothesizes a unidirectional pattern, which commences from the caudal to the cranial aspect of the uterovaginal canal, with the uterus initially bicornuate in configuration. An alternative bidirectional theory has been proposed wherein regression proceeds simultaneously in both the cranial and caudal directions. This would explain anomalies such as a complete septum with duplicated cervix or isolated vertical upper vaginal septum in an otherwise unremarkable uterus. Figure 3.5 shows the different stages of the development of uterus.

FORMATION OF VAGINAL CANAL

The sinusal tubercle forms the sinovaginal bulbs of the urogenital sinus during the formation of the uterovaginal canal. The urogenital sinus gives rise to the lower 20% of the vagina. A horizontal vaginal plate separates the sinovaginal bulb from the uterovaginal canal. Elongation of the vaginal plate occurs at third to fifth month. Its interface with the urogenital sinus forms the hymen which ruptures during the

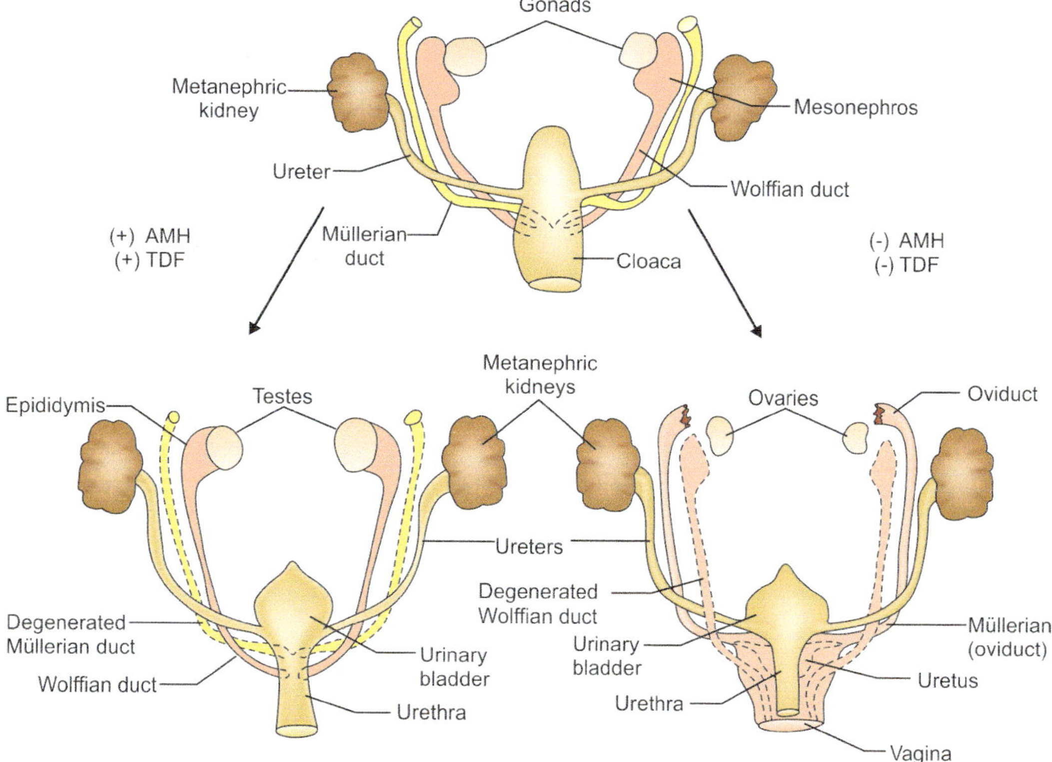

Fig. 3.4: In the presence of testes determining factor (TDF), the indifferent gonad develops into the testis. In its absence, the ovaries develop instead. The Sertoli cells produce anti müllerian hormone (AMH) which induces the regression of the paramesonephric (Müllerian) ducts; while Leydig cells produce testosterone which mediates the development of the vas deferens, epididymis and scrotum
Source: Illustration courtesy: In: Emans SJ, Laufer MR, Goldstein DP (Eds). Pediatric & Adolescent Gynecology

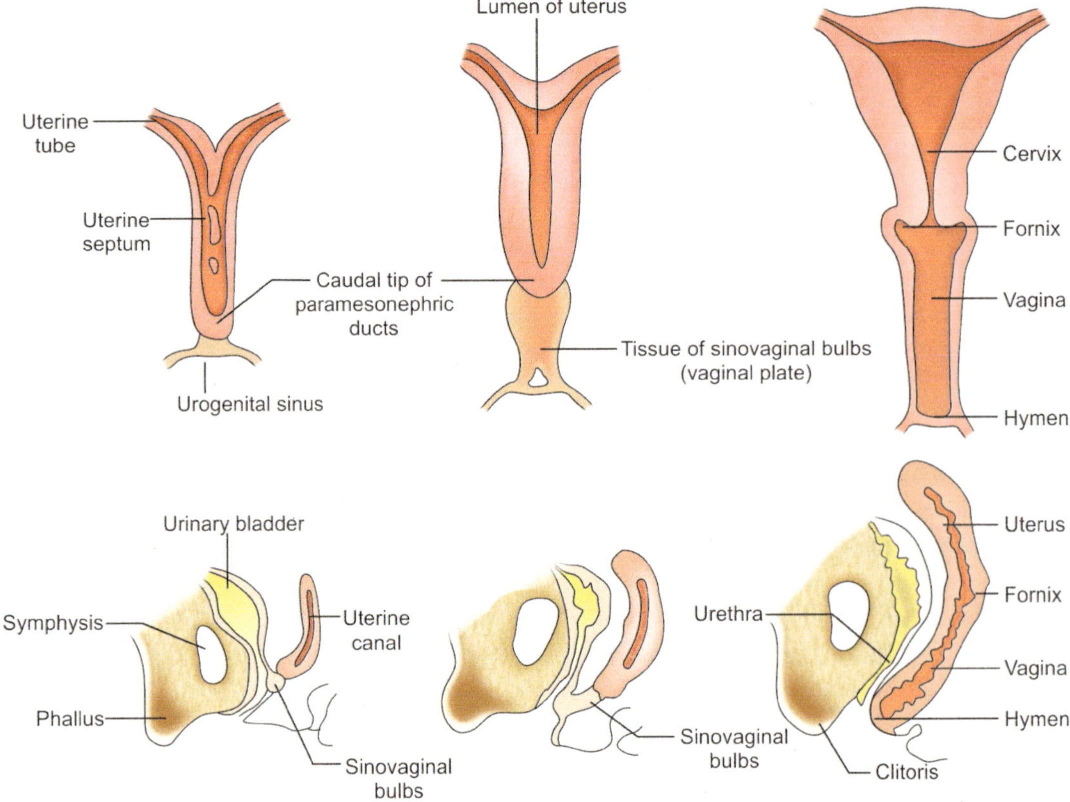

Fig. 3.5: Stages of development of the uterus
Source: Illustration courtesy In: Emans SJ, Laufer MR, Goldstein DP (Eds). Pediatric & Adolescent Gynecology

perinatal period; failure to do so gives rise to an imperforate hymen (Figs 3.6A and B).

Due to the common embryological origin for the genital and urinary systems, abnormalities in the differentiation of one may have associated defects in the other system.

The mesonephric duct gives rise to the uretral bud, from which the ureter, renal calyces and collecting tubules are formed.

Müllerian anomalies are often accompanied by anomalies in the kidney such as renal agenesis (Fig. 3.7), renal ectopy, cystic renal dysplasia and double collecting systems.

MÜLLERIAN ANOMALIES

Clinicians may find Müllerian anomalies as incidental findings (Tables 3.1 and 3.2) in asymptomatic patients, or patients may come in with complaints directly related to problems in Müllerian development. The diagnosis and management of these conditions rely not only on the knowledge of embryology, but also on awareness of their associated congenital defects which guide the physician

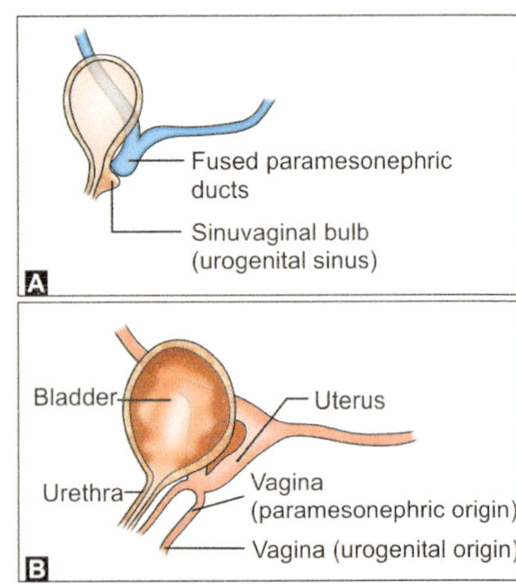

Figs 3.6A and B: Formation of vaginal canal
Source: Illustration courtesy In: Thomas DFM (Ed). Disorder of sex development in essentials of Pediatric Urology

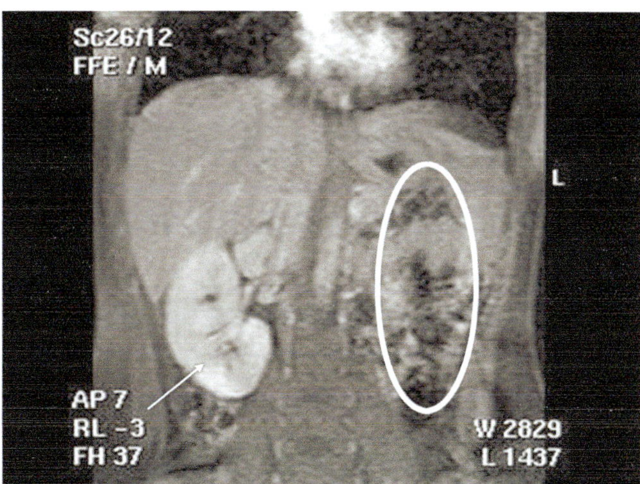

Fig. 3.7: MRI picture of a patient with renal agenesis with double uterus and obstructed hemivagina. The absence of kidney which is marked by circle is on the same side as the vaginal obstruction. Note the presence of a kidney on the contralateral side marked by an arrow

Table 3.1

Incidence of Müllerian anomalies

Anomaly	*Incidence*
Imperforate hymen	1/1000[3]
Strictly speaking, the imperforate hymen is not a Müllerian anomaly since the hymen is derived from the urogenital sinus and not the Müllerian ducts.	
Utero-cervico-vaginal agenesis (MRKH syndrome)	1/5000
Transverse vaginal septum	1/80,000[3]
Longitudinal vaginal septum	Not known

Table 3.2

Prevalance of Müllerian anomalies

Anomaly	*Prevalence*[17]
Müllerian duct anomalies (in general)	0.6–10%
Bicornuate uterus	10% of Müllerian duct anomalies
Septate uterus	55% of Müllerian duct anomalies
Uterus didelphys	5% of Müllerian duct anomalies
Unicornuate uterus	20% of Müllerian duct anomalies

on appropriate diagnostic evaluation and counseling for the patient.

American Fertility Society Classification of Müllerian Anomalies

The American Fertility Society classifies the Müllerian anomalies in seven different categories (Figs 3.8A to G). The classification is based on the degree of failure of normal development. It separates the anomalies into groups with similar clinical manifestations and prognoses for fertility. These subtypes are formulated to maintain a standard nomenclature for long-term studies of the reproductive outcomes of each type of anomaly. This classification does not include vaginal anomalies (i.e. vaginal septum, vaginal stenosis).

Non-Obstructive Müllerian Anomalies

Uterine duplication may be secondary to failure of fusion of the two Müllerian ducts (giving rise to a uterine didelphys) or failure of resorption of the septum between the fused Müllerian cavities [giving rise to a septate uterus or a bicornuate uterus (Figs 3.9 to 3.11A and B)].

In the case of a uterine septum, the external surface of the uterus appears to have a normal configuration, but there are two endometrial cavities. In the patients with bicornuate uterus, the uterine fundus is deeply indented. The level of indentation may be complete, partial or arcuate.

For patients with non-obstructed anomalies, therapy is not warranted. However, studies have shown that patients with septate uterus have a high risk of miscarriage in their reproductive life. This has to be kept in mind during counseling of teenagers or parents of children with this anomaly.

Correction may be necessary in women who are present with septate uterus and a history of infertility or recurrent miscarriage.

Different approaches have been described in removing the uterine septum. Strassman metroplasty involves a wedge incision and the reunification of the two cavities during laparotomy. Hysteroscopic resection has also been described, in conjunction with laparoscopy, to visualize the uterus during the procedure.

MAYER-ROKITANSKY-KUSTER-HAUSER SYNDROME

Mayer-Rokitansky-Kuster-Hauser (MRKH) syndrome is a syndrome consisting of the congenital absence of the vagina, cervix and uterus. It occurs in 1 out of 5,000 women. The vast majority of MRKH is sporadic, but familial aggregates have been reported. There are two subtypes of MRKH:

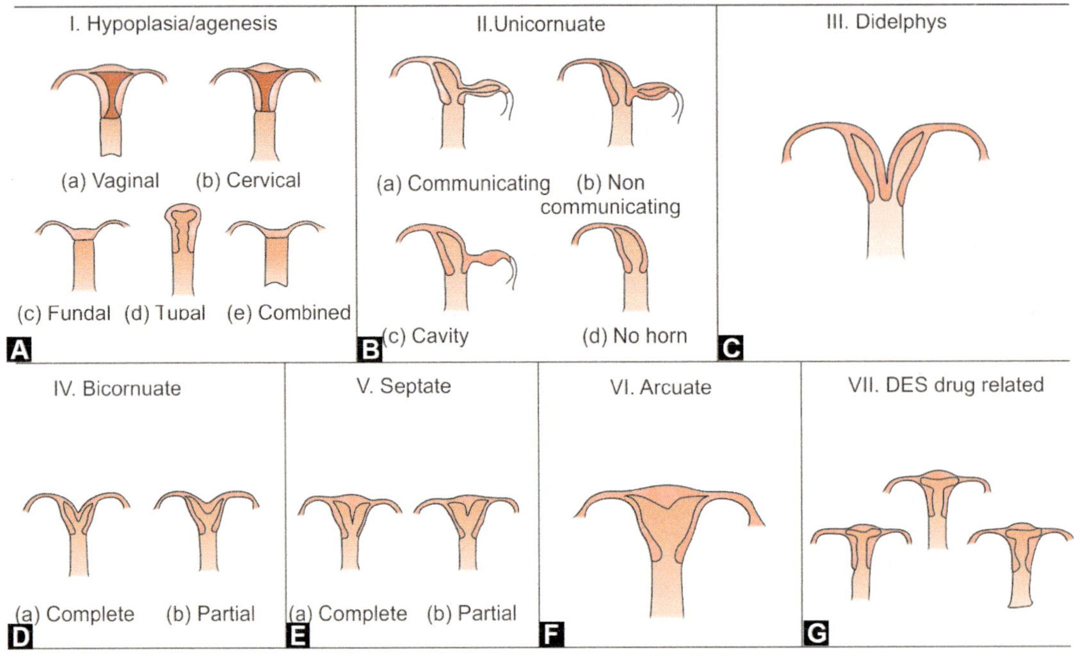

Figs 3.8A to G: The American Fertility Society (AFS) classification of Müllerian anomalies: (A) Hypoplasia or agenesis; (B) Unicornuate; (C) Didelphys; (D) Bicornuate; (E) Septate; (F) Arcuate; (G) DES drug related

Typical or Type I or Isolated

- Agenesis of the vagina, cervix and uterus
- Fallopian tubes and ovaries are present and normal.

Atypical or Type II

In addition to type I, type II may be associated with other anomalies including:

- Renal defects (unilateral agenesis or ectopia of one or both kidneys in 40–60% of patients)
- Cervicothoracic anomalies (asymmetric, fused or wedged vertebrae, scoliosis and Klippel-Feil anomaly in about 20% of patients)
- Digital anomalies
- Hearing defects.

Clinical Presentation

- Primary amenorrhea
- Presence of secondary sexual characteristics
- A 46 XX karyotype

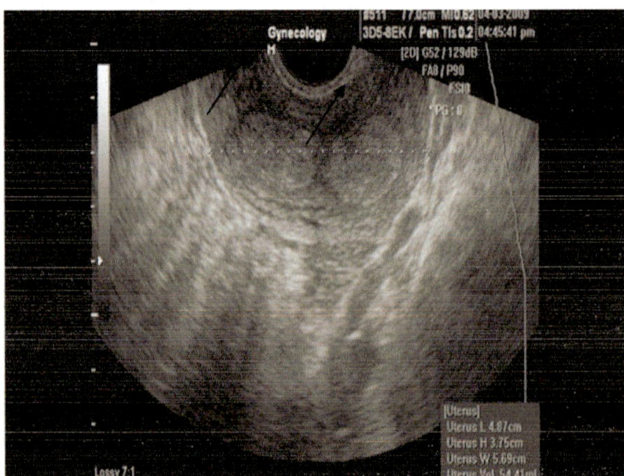

Fig. 3.9: Septate uterus; this is the case of an 18-year-old girl with an incidental finding of a septate uterus on ultrasound. Note the presence of two endometrial cavities shown by arrows

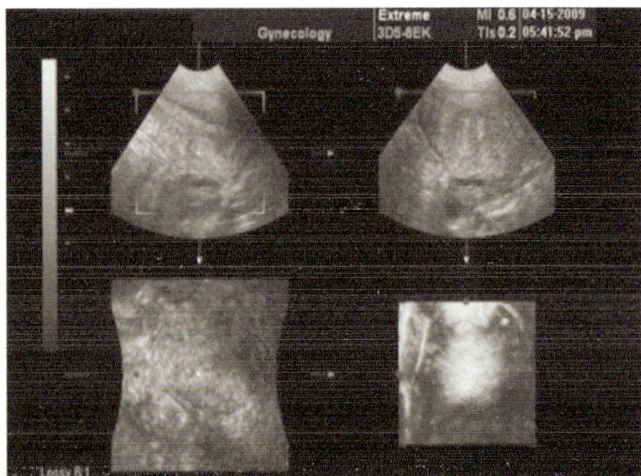

Fig. 3.10: The septate uterus in 3D ultrasound

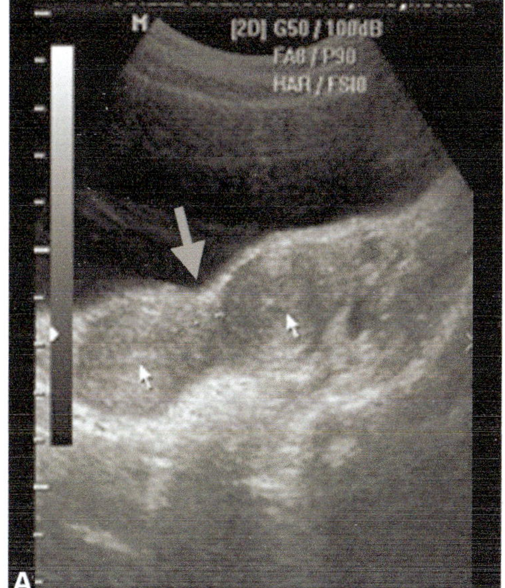

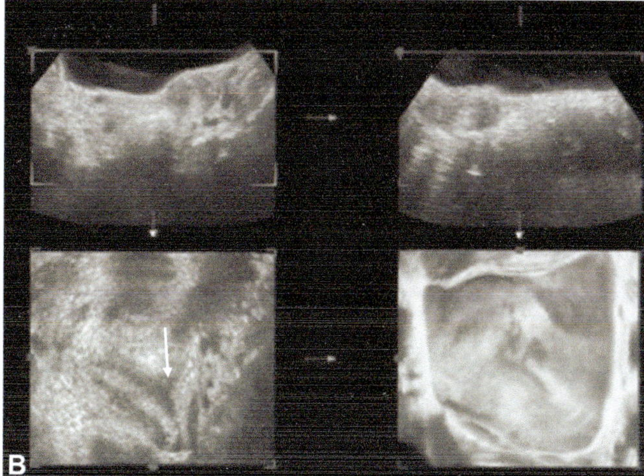

Figs 3.11A and B: Bicornuate uterus—a 13-year-old girl with incidental finding of bicornuate uterus: (A) Deep indentation on the uterine fundus is shown by gray arrow; (B) Wide angle between the two endometrial cavities are shown by white arrow

- Absence or hypoplasia the upper vagina and cervix
- Uterine agenesis diagnosed by ultrasound and other imaging modalities
- May be associated with skeletal, renal and hearing problems.

The patient shown in the Figure 3.12 is a 24-year-old woman with primary amenorrhea. At 14 years of age, she underwent diagnostic work up including an ultrasound and karyotyping and she was diagnosed to have Mayer-Rokitansky-Kuster-Hauser (MRKH) syndrome.

CREATION OF NEOVAGINA BY LABIAL FLAP VAGINOPLASTY

The different steps for the creation of neovagina by labial flap vaginoplasty are shown in the Figures 3.13 to 3.18.

VAGINOPLASTY: DIFFERENT TECHNIQUES AND APPROACHES

The diagnosis of MRKH or uterovaginal agenesis is emotionally traumatic for a young woman. The patient is confronted

Fig. 3.12: The patient has a shallow blind ending vaginal pouch. Only 1.5 cm of a cotton pledget could be inserted. MRI revealed the absence of cervix and uterus with normal-looking ovaries

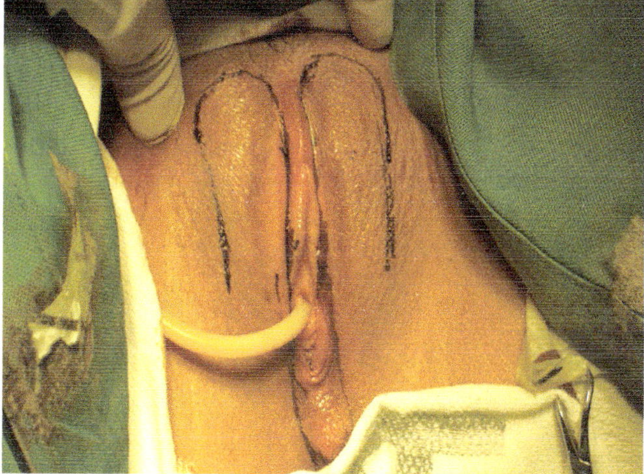

Fig. 3.13: The patient wanted to have a neovagina for the purpose of sexual intercourse. The picture shows the preparation for labial-flap vaginoplasty

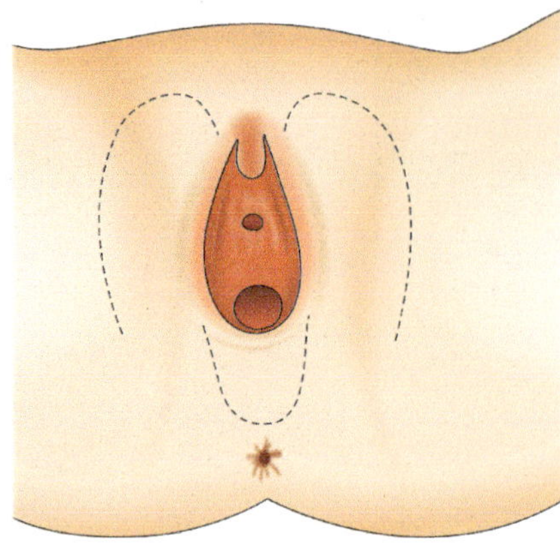

Fig. 3.14: Areas where the labial flaps are to be harvested are marked

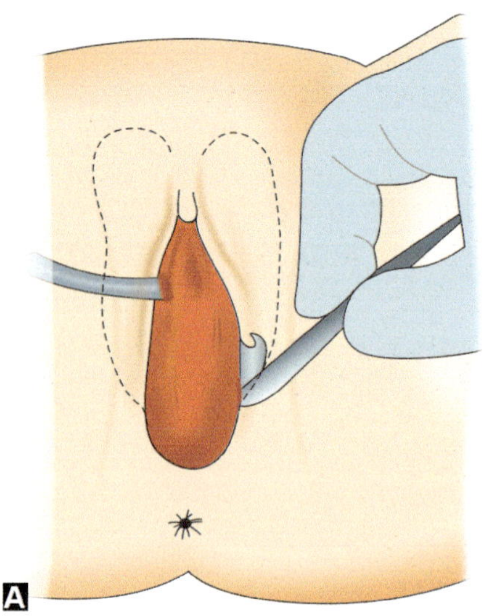

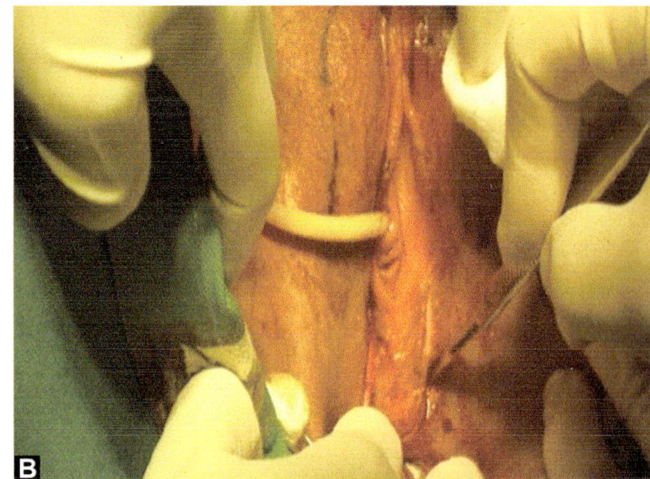

Figs 3.15A and B: The labial flaps are incised as shown in the picture

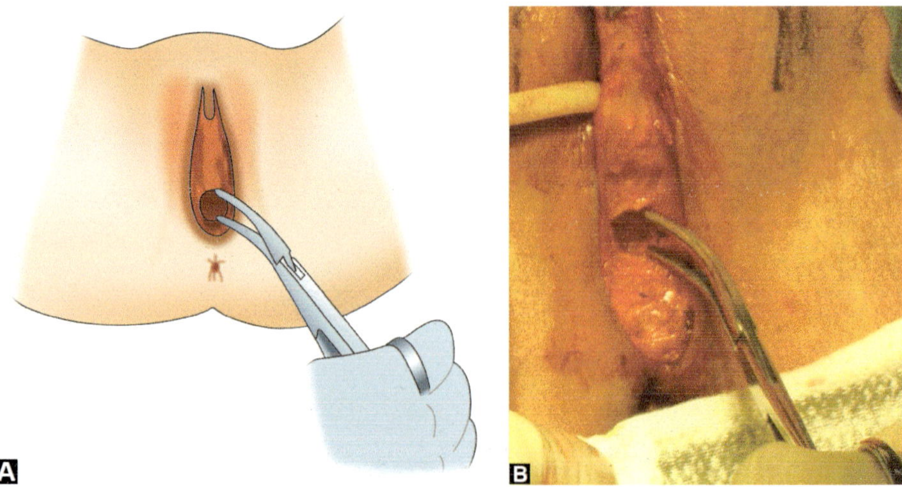

Figs 3.16A and B: Dissection of a space for a neovagina in the area of the perineal body

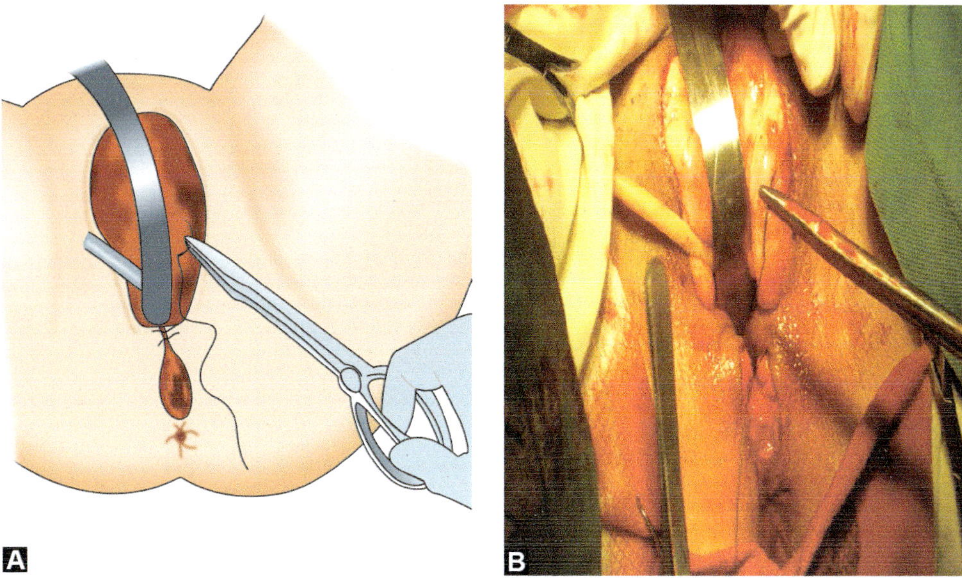

Figs 3.17A and B: The flaps are sutured to line the dissected—vaginal space

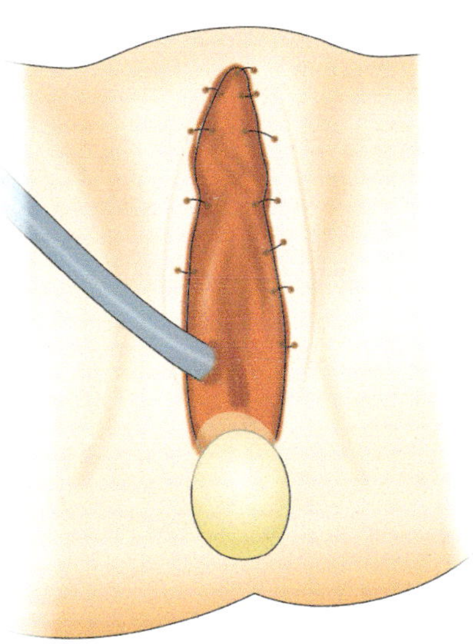

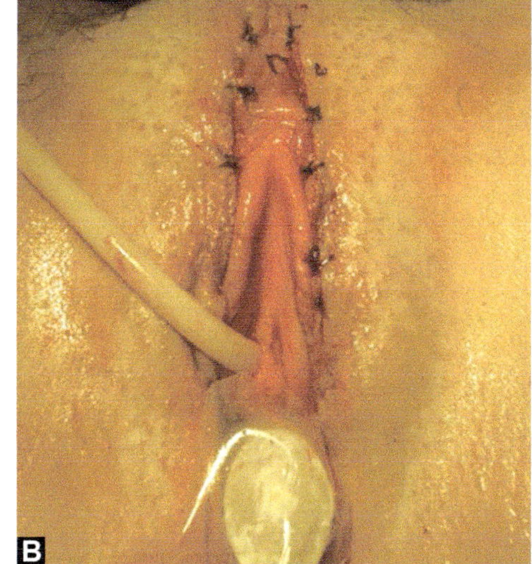

Figs 3.18A and B: Postoperative with vaginal mold inserted

with the loss of fertility and the fact that their vagina may not be adequate for sexual intercourse. The physician's approach is very important for patients' psychological well-being and future medical management.

At present, there is no consensus regarding the best management option. As stated by the American College of Obstetrics and Gynecology (ACOG Committee Opinion, 2002), nonsurgical treatment is the first choice. In patients who refuse or fail to achieve a functional vagina with passive dilatation, a surgical approach may be required, but the surgical reconstruction has to be postponed until such time as the patient is emotionally mature and motivated to maintain a neovagina once it has been created.

Non-surgical Methods for Vaginal Dilation

1. Frank's method: Insertion of cylindrical shaped gradually enlarging vaginal dilators on the vaginal dimple
2. Modification of Frank's method using a bicycle

Surgical Method for Creating a Neovagina

1. McIndoe procedure: Use of a split-thickness skin graft to line the neovagina. The graft is commonly harvested from the buttocks; some report the use of cultured autologous vaginal tissue or cultured buccal mucosa.
2. Full thickness skin grafts from the groin area.
3. Davydov procedure: Laparoscopic and perineal approach, abdominal peritoneum is harvested and brought down to the area between the bladder and rectum to line the neovagina.
4. Modified Wharton procedure: Incision is made in the vestibular part of the vagina; bladder and rectal lumen are detached bluntly, reaching the pouch of Douglas. An artificial dermis made of atelocollagen sponge is wrapped around a mold made up of acrylic resin. The mold is inserted into the newly created vaginal space, and the edge is sutured to the vaginal entrance in an interrupted fashion using 2-0 polyglactin 910. The labia are sutured together over the mold.[14]
5. William's operation: Use of the tissue of the labia to form an external pouch that could function as vagina.
6. Thigh flap vaginoplasty.
7. Use of the sigmoid colon or ileum as vaginal replacement.
8. Vecchietti operation: Combination of both surgical and non-surgical methods. It involves the dilatation with a traction device attached to the abdomen and sutures are placed subperitoneally by laparotomy or laparoscopy, a plastic olive is placed in the vaginal dimple.

OBSTRUCTIVE ANOMALIES

Imperforate Hymen

Imperforate hymen (Fig. 3.19) may be recognized as early as the neonatal period when significant amounts of mucus from the endocervical glands are secreted due to increased maternal estrogen; this may result in a bulging of translucent yellow-gray mass at the vaginal introitus. Unless thorough observation of the neonatal genitalia is done, this may go unrecognized since most of the hydrocolpos or mucocolpos may be asymptomatic and resolve as the mucus is reabsorbed and estrogen level decreases. Large mucocolpos may result in ureteral obstruction and hydronephrosis and even respiratory distress. Resection of the hymen is recommended in the symptomatic infant.

The optimal management for imperforate hymen is hymenal resection; definitive surgery should take place after appropriate evaluation which includes an examination of the external genitalia and a direct rectal examination. If indicated, radiographic imaging may be done to confirm the diagnosis.

Aspiration, without making a definitive hymenal opening for continued drainage, should be avoided, because of the risks of reaccumulation with recurrence of a mass or ascending infection. Asymptomatic girls with an imperforate hymen can be monitored throughout childhood and avoid the risks of surgery in infancy.

Most patients with imperforate hymen present in puberty (Fig. 3.20) with the complaint of hypogastric pain.

At the pediatric gynecology unit, a total of ten patients with imperforate hymen were seen from 2002 to 2009. Three of these patients presented with symptomatic mucocolpos in the neonatal period. The rest presented at puberty with age range of 8 to 13 years. All of them had cyclic abdominal pain as reason for consult. On physical examination, a bluish-tinged, bulging mass was seen at the introitus, clinching the diagnosis. Some patients were also presented with urinary retention due to mass effect of the large hematocolpos.

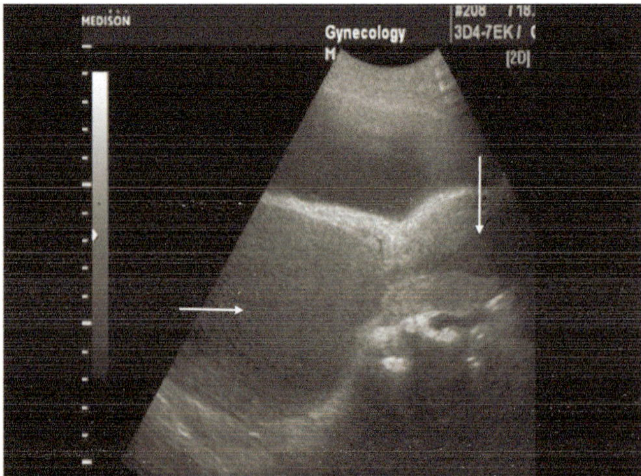

Fig. 3.19: Ultrasound of a patient with imperforate hymen. The large hematocolpos is marked with thick arrow in comparison with the smaller hematometra marked with thin arrow. Hematocolpos may become quite large because the vagina is distensible and the obstruction is so distal

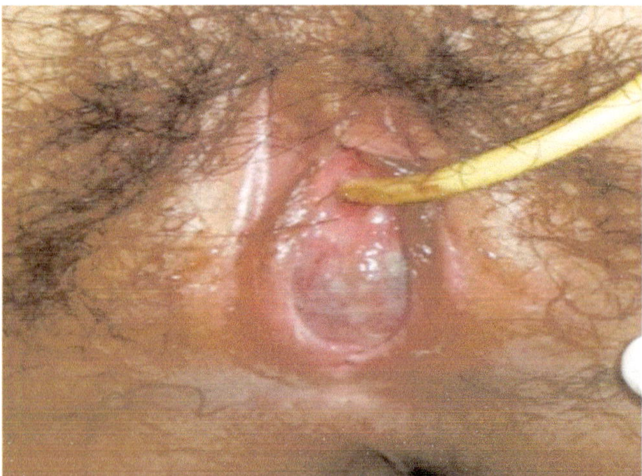

Fig. 3.20: Imperforate hymen in a 14-year-old girl presenting with cryptomenorrhea. Note the bulging bluish-hued membrane at the introitus

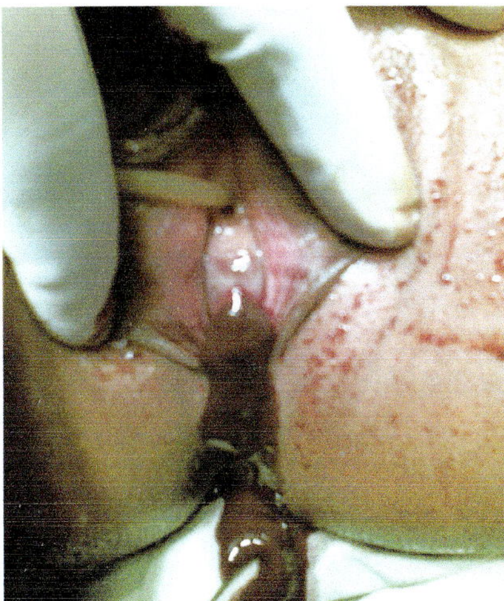

Fig. 3.21: Cruciate incision is done on the hymenal membrane. Evacuation of hematocolpos

The distal vagina is very distensible and as it enlarges, it may impinge the urethra, bladder and even the ureter, thus causing urinary problems. In some instances, it may obstruct the rectum, causing constipation.

The goal of hymenotomy or hymenectomy is to open the hymenal membrane (Figs 3.21 and 3.22). The opening should be big enough to allow the egress of menstrual flow, tampon use and eventually comfortable sexual intercourse. Small punctures should be avoided. There is risk that the viscous fluid may not drain adequately, which would result in the ascension of bacteria and the possibility of infection, such as pelvic inflammatory disease or tubo-ovarian abscess.

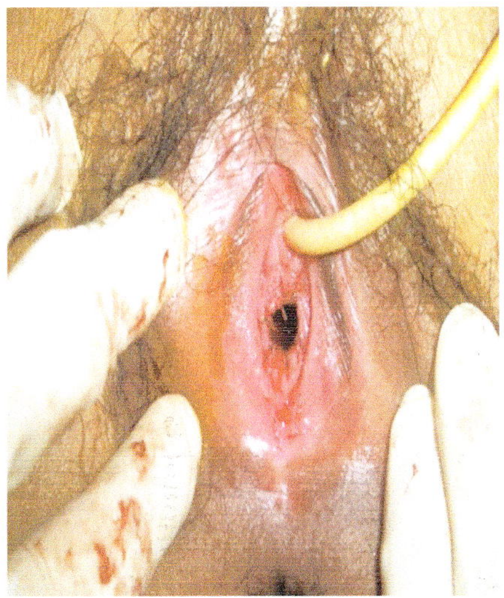

Fig. 3.22: Posthymenectomy

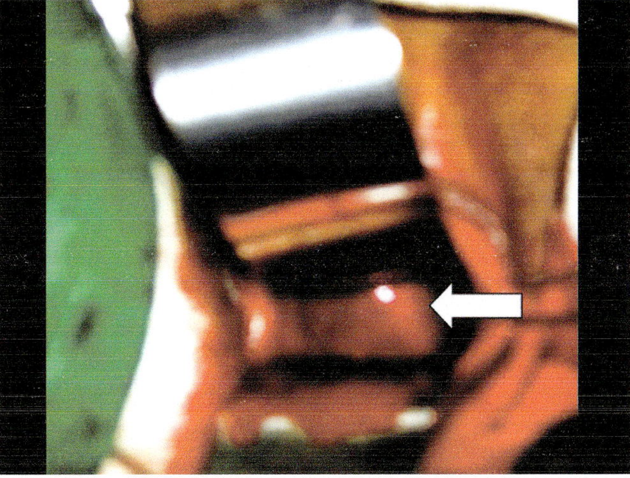

Fig. 3.23: Transverse vaginal septum (arrow) in a 12-year-old girl presenting with cyclic abdominal pain. Behind the septum is old menstrual blood (hematocolpometra) of which 500 cc is evacuated

Hymenectomy is usually performed under regional anesthesia with the patient in dorsal lithotomy position. Sterile prepping and draping are done, after which a straight or Foley's catheter is inserted to drain the bladder and properly delineate the urethra. A cruciate incision is made on the hymen. After suctioning of the hematocolpos, the vagina is left to drain. The edges of the cruciate incision are excised and interrupted sutures are placed on the hymenal edges for hemostasis.

TRANSVERSE VAGINAL SEPTUM

As shown in the Figures 3.23 to 3.25; the transverse vaginal septum may show the following features:

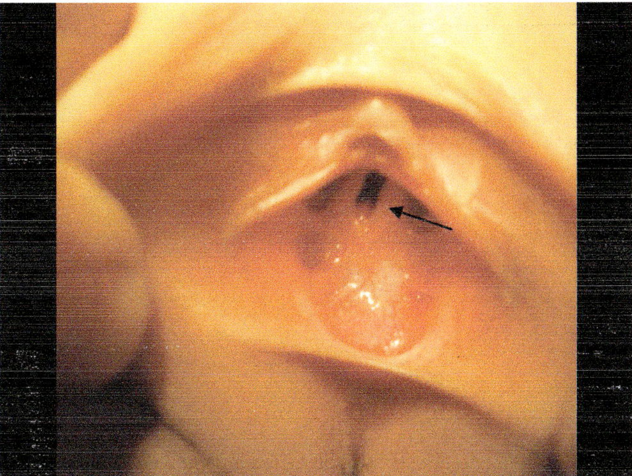

Fig. 3.24: Lack of vaginal opening. Note the dilated urethra (arrow) which can be misconstrued for the vagina

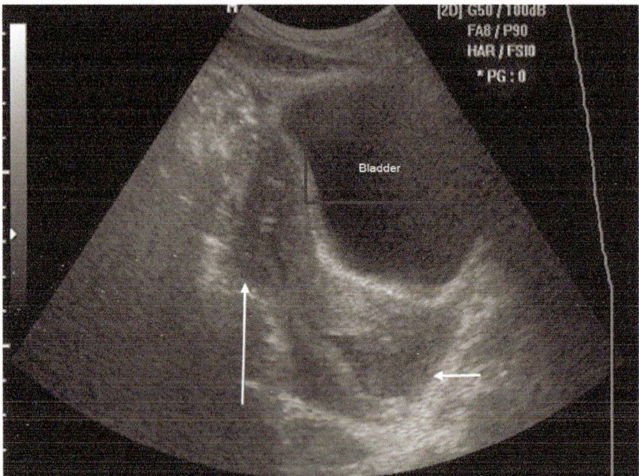

Fig. 3.25: Ultrasound shows accumulated blood in the uterus (small arrow) and vagina (big arrow) due to obstruction

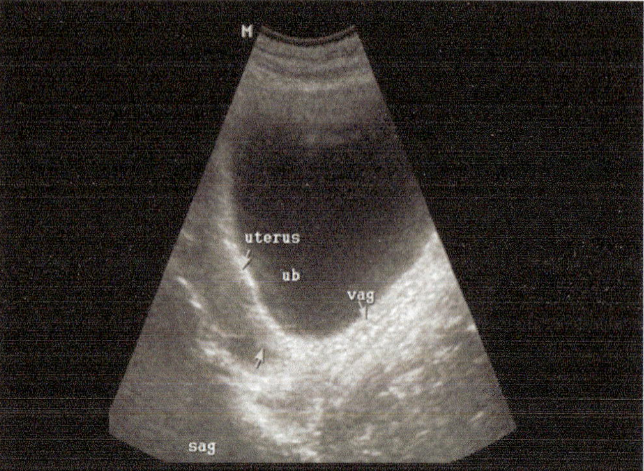

Fig. 3.26: Shallow vaginal canal. Absence of cervix

- More rare than vaginal, cervical or uterine agenesis
- Secondary to incomplete fusion of the paired Müllerian ducts and urogenital sinus
- Presenting symptoms and physical examination findings are due to obstructive nature of this anomaly
  - Amenorrhea
  - Cyclic abdominal pain
  - Urinary retention
  - Tender hypogastric mass
- According to location, there are three types of vaginal septum:
  - Upper vaginal septum (46%)
  - Middle vaginal septum (35–40%)
  - Lower vaginal septum (15–20%)

Cervicovaginal Agenesis and Uterine Didelphys in a Teenager with Hypogastric Pain and Primary Amenorrhea

The exact cause of vaginal agenesis is unknown, but is hypothesized to be due to the failure of the caudal migration of the paramesonephric duct. It is often associated with abnormalities of the kidneys, rectum or anus. It has also been associated with skeletal deformities.

Vaginal atresia is clinically indistinguishable from vaginal agenesis, but is said to be due to failure of recanalization of the vaginal cord at the 150 mm crown-rump stage. The atresia may take the form of a septum—in any plane and at any level, including the site of the hymen—or it may take the form of stenosis.

In cases where vaginal agenesis coexists with uterine agenesis, there is no urgency to institute surgical treatment because lack of menstrual products would not cause obstructive symptoms.

In the following case, however, the patient presented with cervicovaginal agenesis and uterine didelphys with functioning endometrium. The reason for consult and subsequent surgery was the presence of obstructive symptoms.

A case of a 17-year-old girl (Figs 3.26 to 3.29) consulted for cyclic abdominal pain and primary amenorrhea. On physical examination, secondary sexual characteristics were at par with age; however, on the examination of external genitalia, there was only a shallow vaginal dimple which measured 1.5 cm in depth. Karyotyping was done which showed a normal female karyotype. Ultrasound revealed the two endometrial cavities and the lack of a cervix.

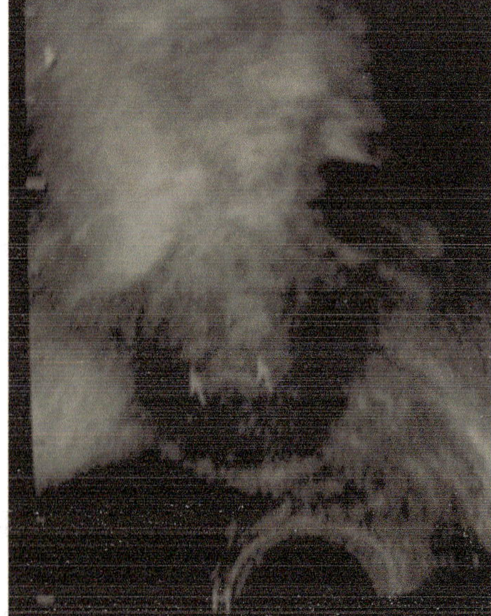

Fig. 3.27: Presence of two endometrial cavities (arrows)

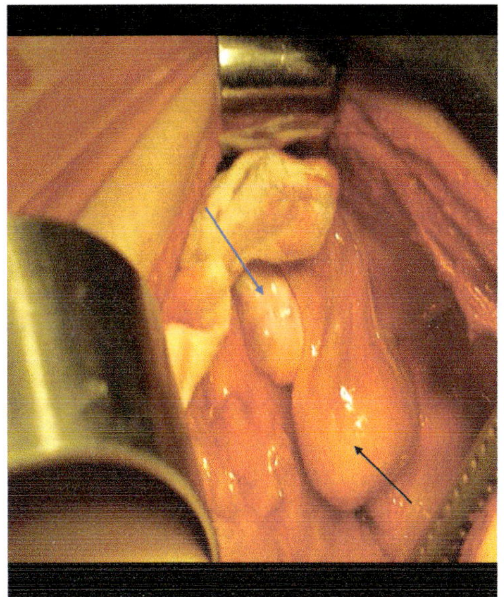

Fig. 3.28: Left uterine body (black arrow) and left ovary (blue arrow)

Cervicoplasty and meteroplasty is done on the patient as shown in the Figures 3.30 to 3.33. A neovagina is created using a flap from the bladder peritoneum (Figs 3.34 to 3.37).

A neovagina is created (Figs 3.34 to 3.37) by dissecting the space between the bladder and the rectum. It is then lined with peritoneum harvested from the bladder. A condom-covered mold is inserted postoperatively to prevent stenosis.

DOUBLE UTERUS WITH VAGINAL SEPTUM AND OBSTRUCTED HEMIVAGINA

A case of 12-year-old girl patient consulted for dysmenorrhea. She had her menarche three months before and since

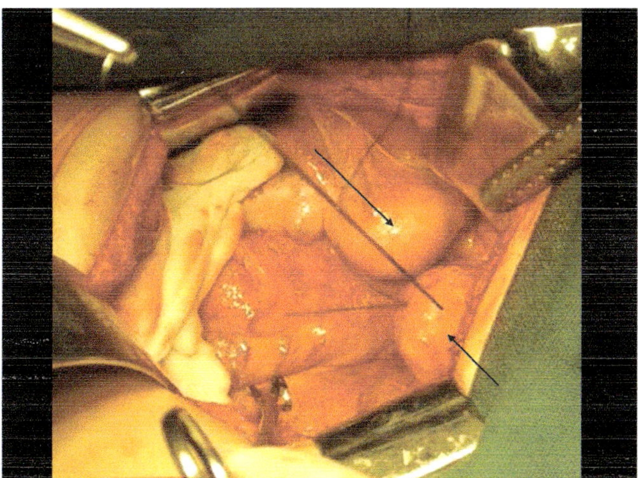

Fig. 3.29: Two uterine bodies (arrows)

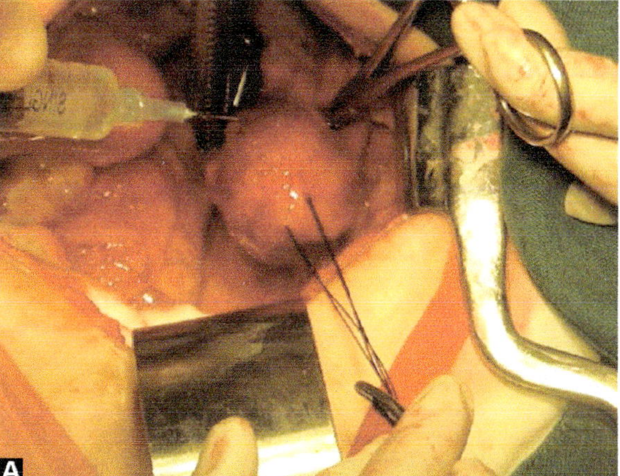

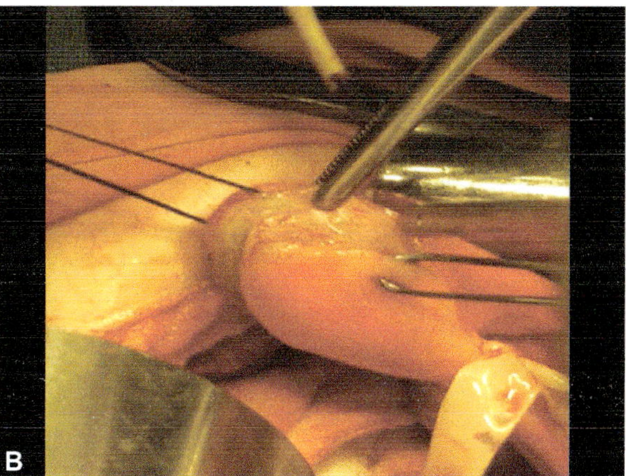

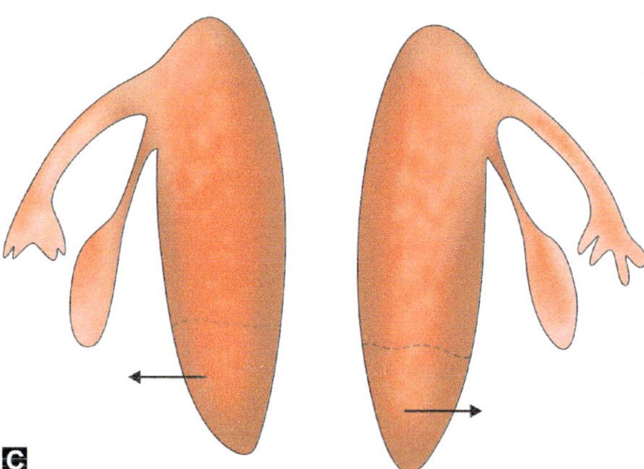

Figs 3.30A to C: Preparation; instillation of epinephrine and placing of tourniquet. The lower one-third of each of the two uterine bodies is excised (arrows)

then her dysmenorrhea had been worsening. Increased severity of the hypogastric pain with radiation to the right thigh eventually prompted her to consult. On rectal examination, a bulging of right paravaginal mass was noted. Ultrasound showed a hematocolpos and two endometrial cavities (Figs 3.38 and 3.39). Magnetic resonance imaging

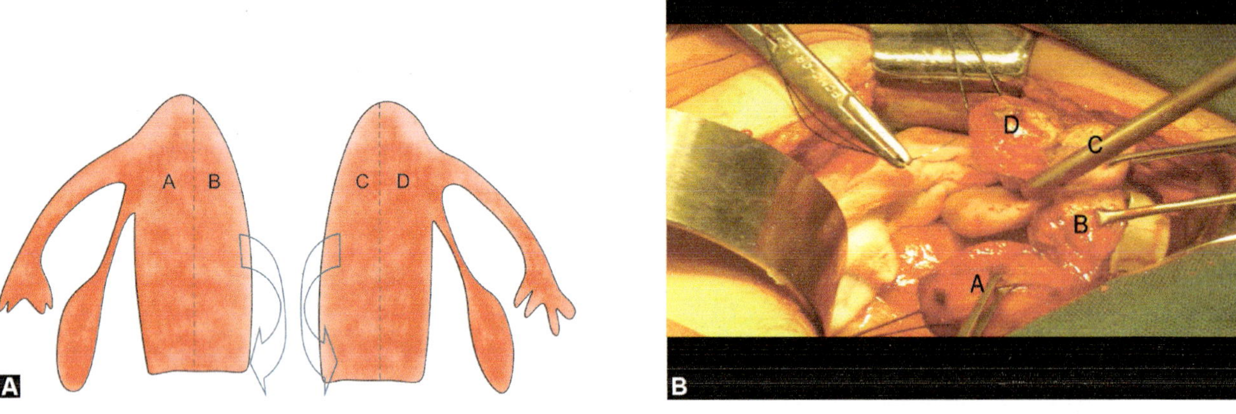

Figs 3.31A and B: Vertical incision is done on the uterine bodies. Segments B and C shown in the figure is brought down

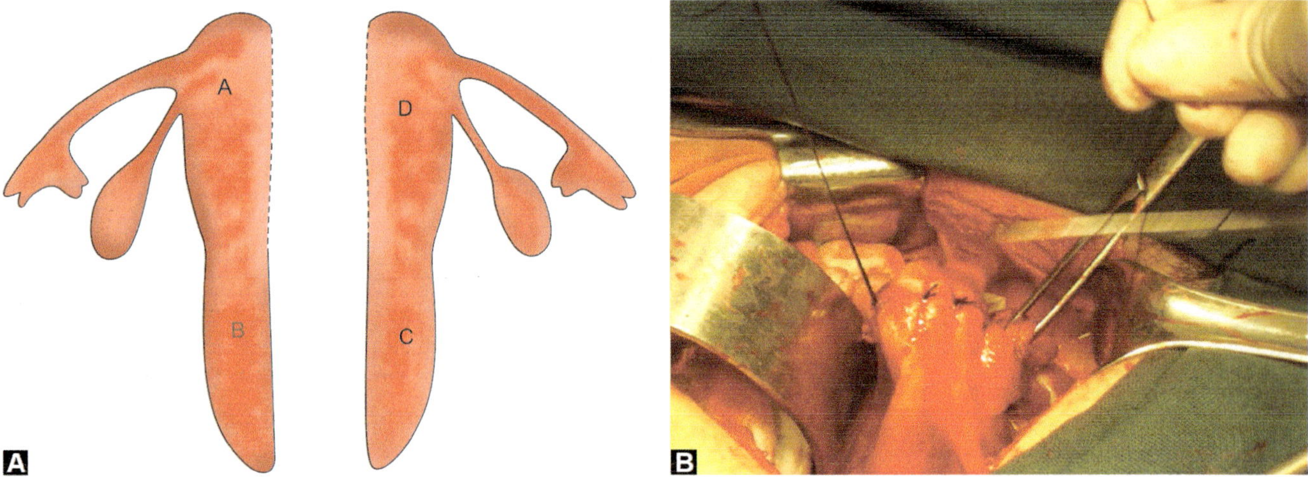

Figs 3.32A and B: Segment B and C are flaps which are converted into the cervix

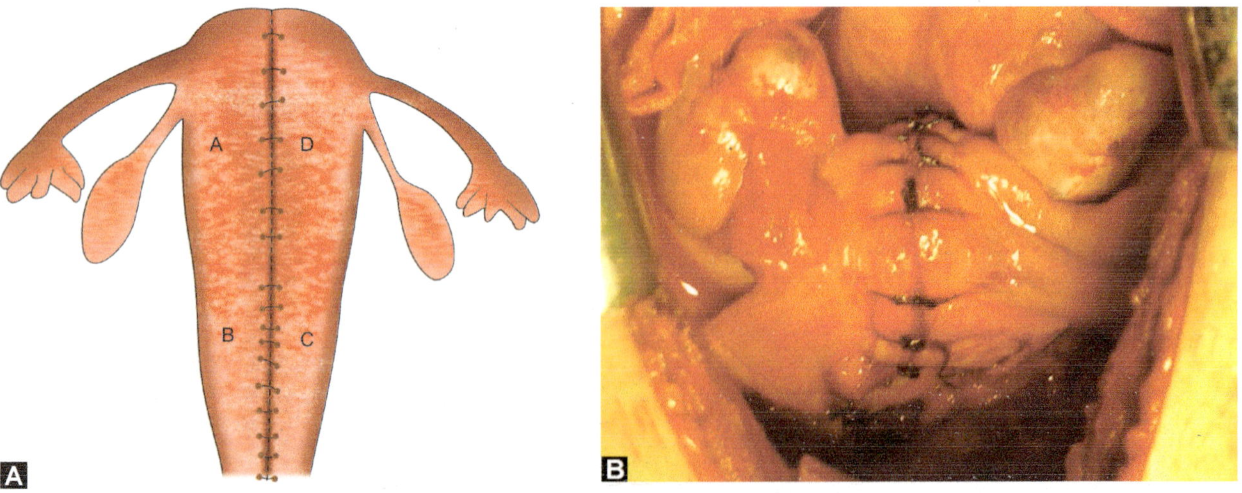

Figs 3.33A and B: Metroplasty and cervicoplasty completed

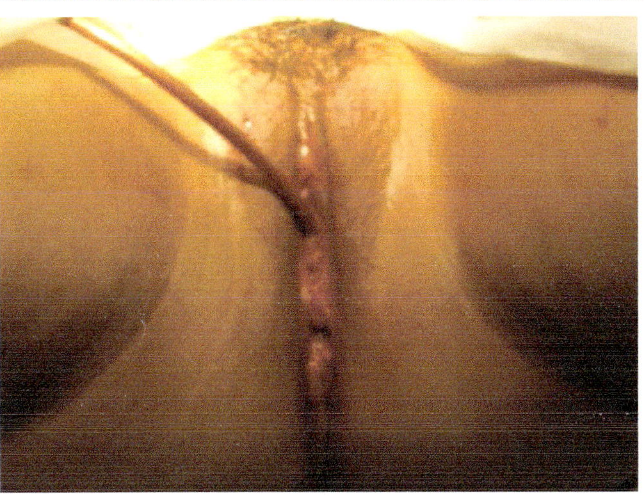

Fig. 3.34: Preoperative picture showing the presence of a 1.5 cm vaginal dimple

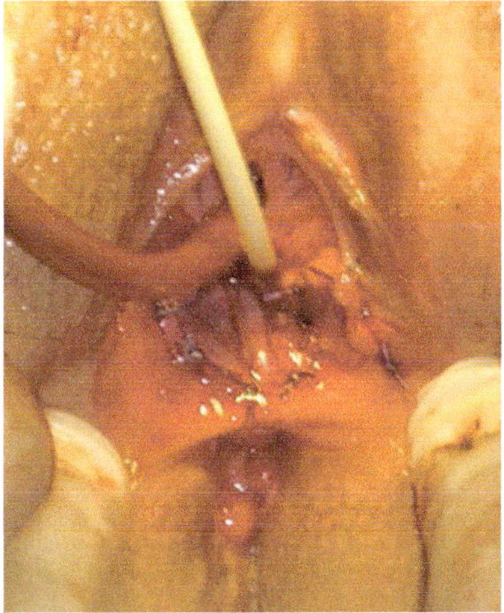

Fig. 3.37: Harvested bladder peritoneum sutured to the vaginal wall

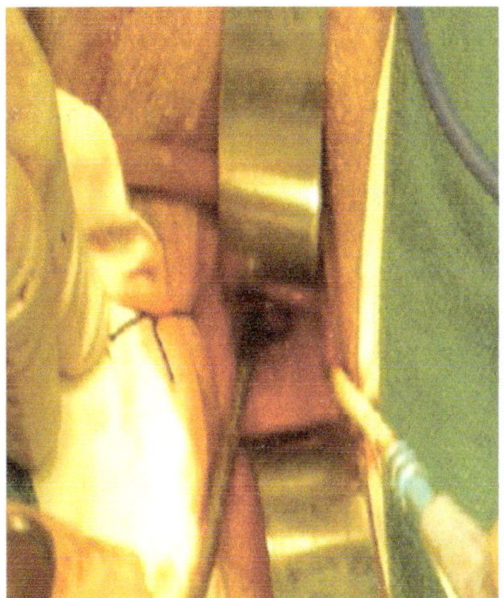

Fig. 3.35: Vagina dilatation

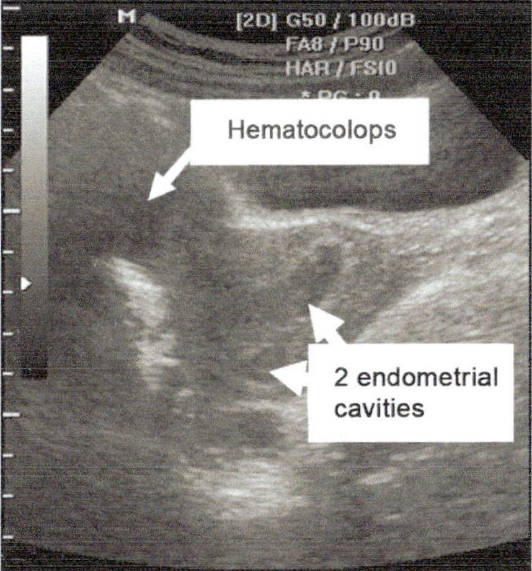

Fig. 3.38: Ultrasound image showing the presence of hematocolpos and two endometrial cavities

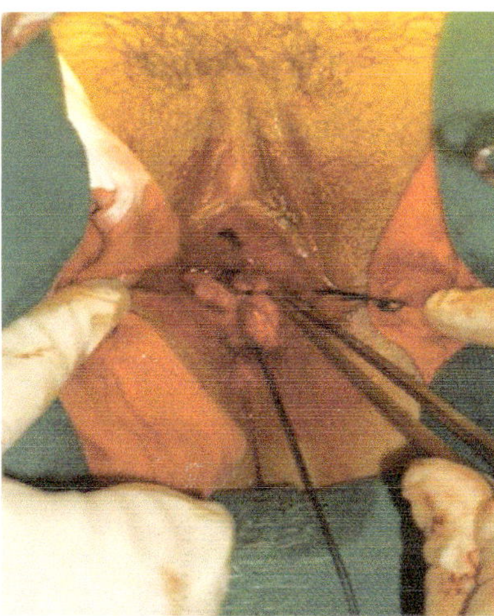

Fig. 3.36: Bladder peritoneum is pulled down through the vaginal canal to serve as its epithelial lining

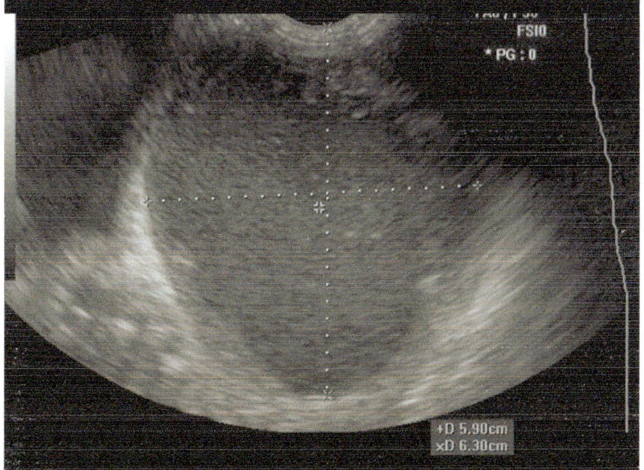

Fig. 3.39: Hematocolpos may get so big that on ultrasound, it could be misconstrued for an ovarian mass

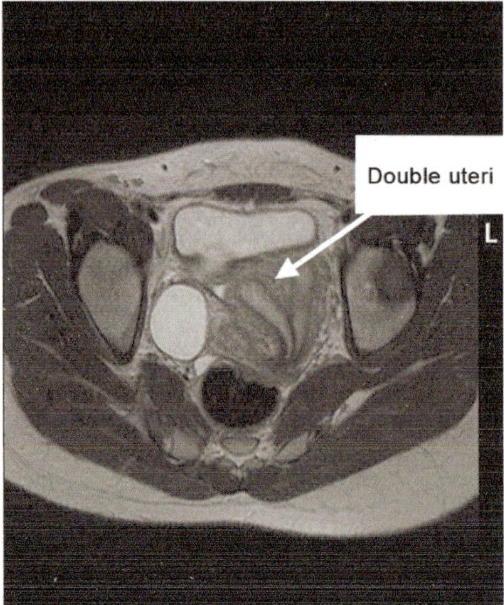

Fig. 3.40: MRI confirming the presence of double uteri

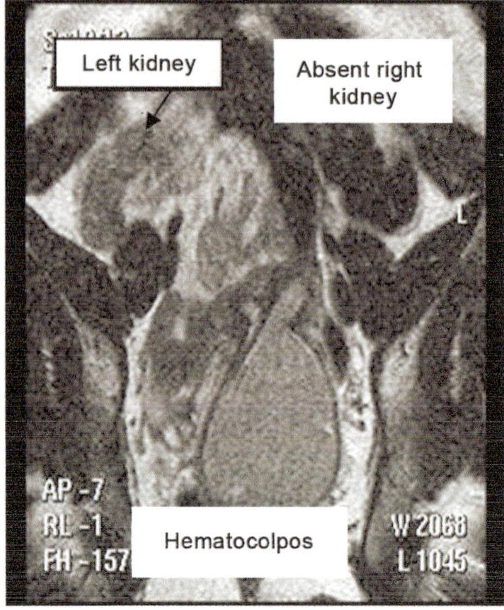

Fig. 3.42: MRI revealing the presence of a kidney on the side of the hematocolpos (ipsilateral renal agenesis)

(Figs 3.40 to 3.42) also confirmed the presence of double uteri and hematocolpos.

A patient presents with a syndrome of uterine didelphys, obstructing hemivaginal septum [Fig. 3.43 (resulting in a hematocolpos)] and renal agenesis on the side of the hematocolpos. It is considered to be extremely rare; however, the pediatric gynecology unit has seen in five cases in its seven years of existence.

These patients present later with other obstructing vaginal anomalies (like the transverse vaginal septum and imperforate hymen), presumably because menstrual flow occurs normally from the non-obstructed hemiuterus.

It is under-reported because of difficulty in diagnosis; the lack of a standard name makes it difficult to find in an index or a review of the literature.

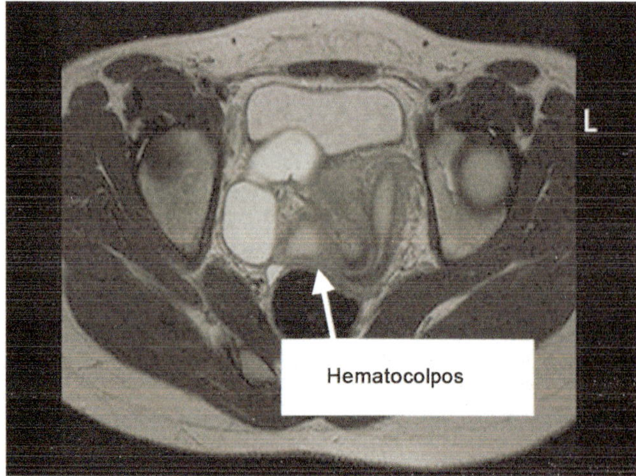

Fig. 3.41: MRI confirming the presence of hematocolpos

There are relatively few case reports each of which uses different descriptions. An acronym has been proposed, OHVIRA (obstructed hemivagina and ipsilateral renal anomaly), to describe the syndrome. Some authors also refer to this anomaly as the Herlyn-Werner-Wunderlich syndrome.

Patients would complain of progressive dysmenorrhea or unilateral cyclic pain which may radiate to the thigh. In

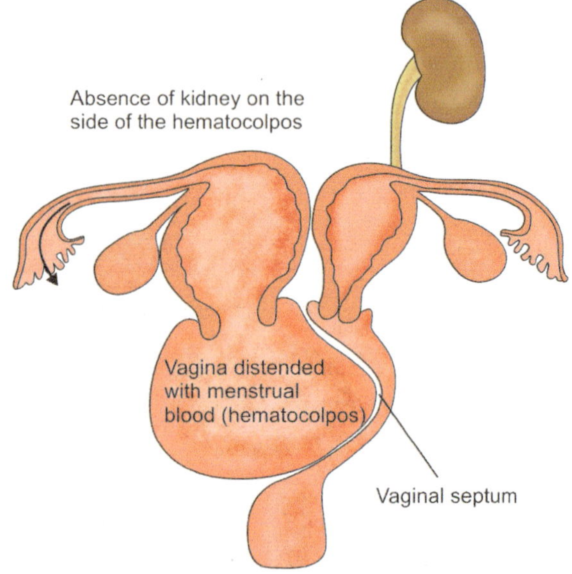

Fig. 3.43: Obstructed hemivagina with ipsilateral renal anomaly (OHVIRA)

Courtesy: Illustration In: Altchek A (Ed). Congenital gynecologic anomalies in pediatric, adolescent and young adult gynecology

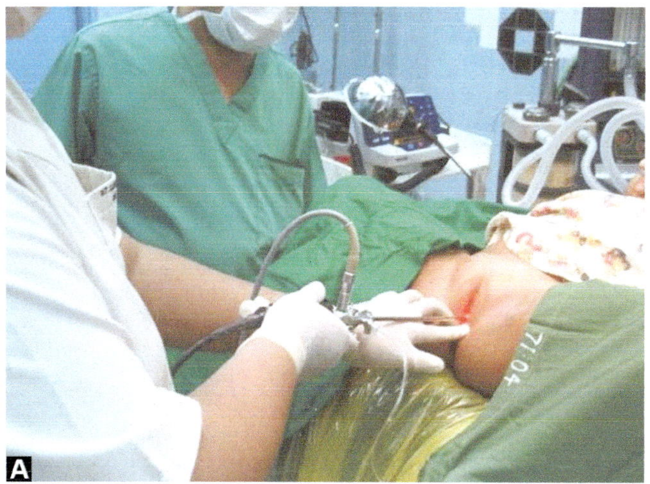

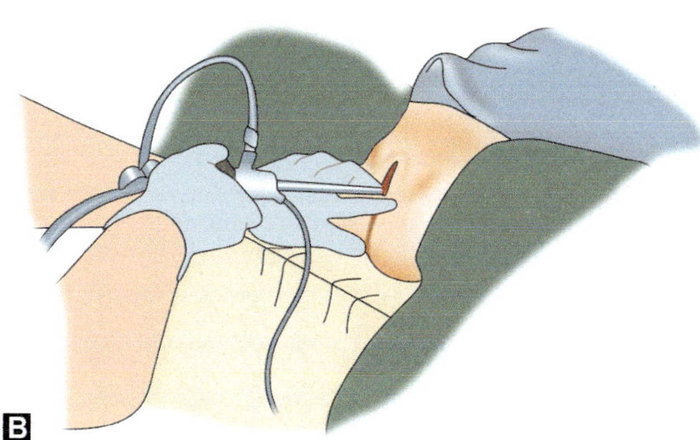

Figs 3.44A and B: (A) For the patient, vaginoscopy with the excision of vaginal septum was done; (B) Vaginoscopy

a few cases, there may be a microperforation allowing for communication from the obstructed to the non-obstructed side resulting in prolonged or intermenstrual discharge, or very rarely, even pyocolpos.

On physical examination, a mass is felt to bulge from the lateral wall of the vagina toward the midline. Ancilliary diagnostic procedures include: ultrasound, MRI and diagnostic laparoscopy.

Most patients with this anomaly undergo excision of the obstructing septum (the common wall of the hemivaginas). The septal wall is resected (Figs 3.44 and 3.45) to create a single vaginal vault.

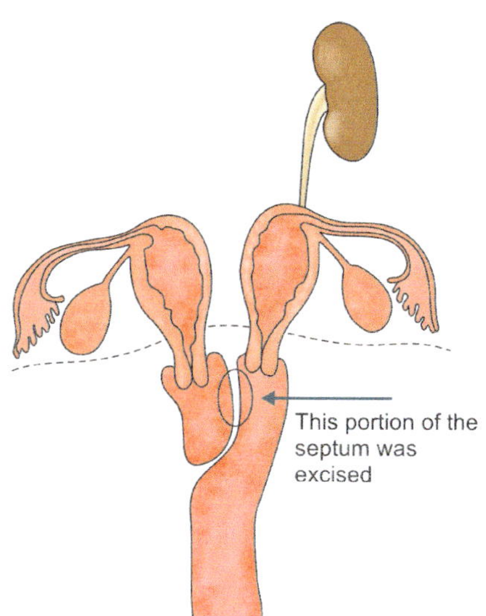

Fig. 3.45: Excision of septum
Courtesy: Illustration In: Altchek A (Ed). Congenital gynecologic anomalies in pediatric, adolescent and young adult gynecology

After resection of the septal wall of the obstructed hemivagina, the patient has normal function with a single vagina, two cervices and two hemiuteri (uterus didelphys).

Reasons for Misdiagnosing the Syndrome of Double Uterus with Obstructed Hemivagina

- There is a regular menstrual period from the non-obstructive side
- Previous physicians may treat the dysmenorrhea with pain relievers (NSAIDs) and hormones, which diminishes or eliminates menstruation thus delaying the diagnosis
- The lower abdominal pain may be misdiagnosed as pelvic inflammatory disease.

GOALS OF THERAPY IN YOUNG WOMEN WITH THE MÜLLERIAN ANOMALIES

- Relieve obstructive symptoms
- Facilitate normal egress of menstrual blood
- Establish sexual function
- Preserve future fertility
- Girls with non-obstructive Müllerian anomalies may not need surgical correction.

URORECTAL MALFORMATION ANOMALY

Cloacal Malformation

Cloacal malformation or persistent cloaca (Figs 3.46 to 3.51) is marked by the presence of a common abnormal termination of the urinary, genital and alimentary tract. There is usually a common chamber (the cloaca) with a single exterior opening.

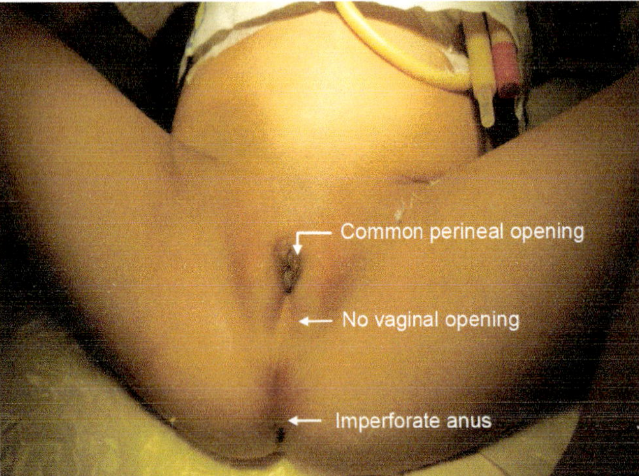

Fig. 3.46: This child was referred for lack of vaginal opening. A few days after birth, she underwent emergency colostomy and gastrostomy. She had multiple congenital anomalies which included tracheoesophageal fistula, imperforate anus, vaginal agenesis and a persistent cloaca. At 2 years of age, she was admitted to the hospital for recurrent urinary tract infection. A voiding cystogram (VCUG) was done which showed severe vesico-ureteral reflux and cystolithiasis. There was also note of a bicornuate uterus with hystero-vesical fistula and opacities within the uterine cavity

This is a rare condition, occurring 1 in 50,000 of births. Congenital anomalies in other parts of the body would coexist in these patients, such as, vertebral defects, tracheoesophageal fistula and renal abnormalities. Children with cloacal malformations present at birth with abdominal distention presumably because of obstruction in the urinary or gastrointestinal tract. Decompressive colostomy is usually warranted.

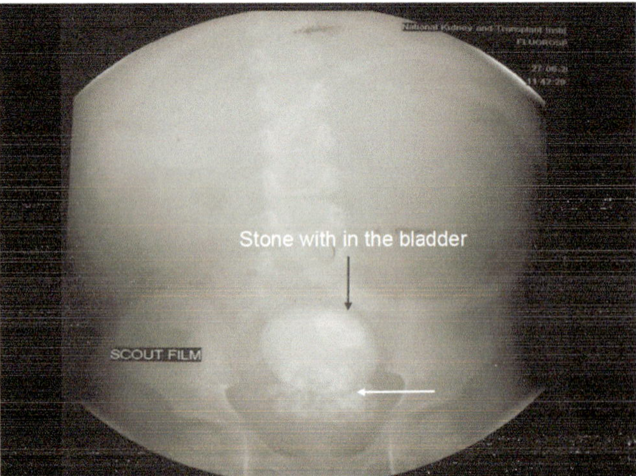

Fig. 3.47: Opacities within the uterine cavity (white arrow). These would prove to be stones that formed due to the severe vesico-ureteral reflux and common opening between the bladder and uterus

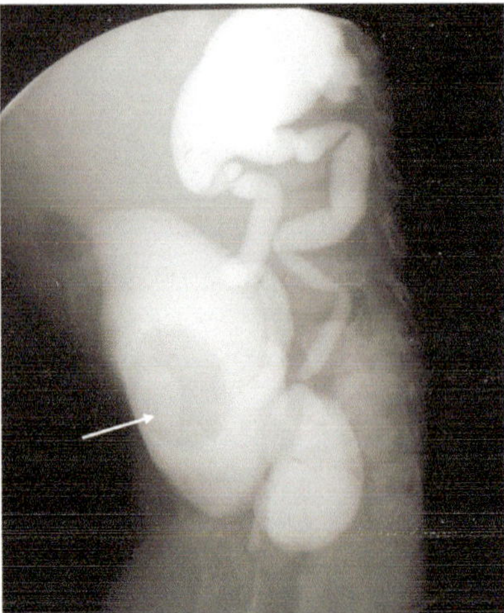

Fig. 3.48: VCUG; severe vesico-ureteral reflux. The filling defect (arrow) indicates the presence of cystolithiasis

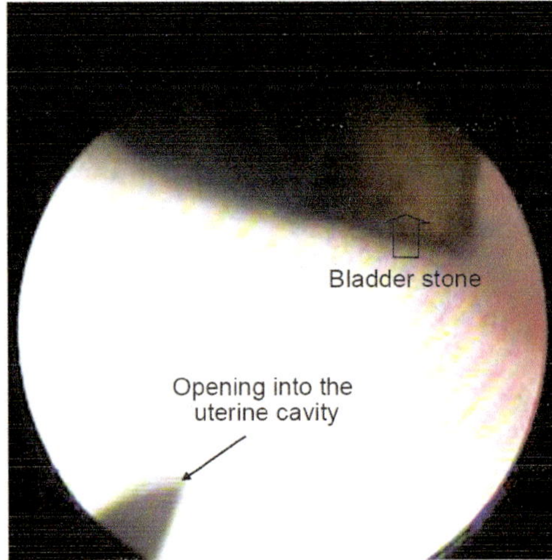

Fig. 3.49: Endoscopy; a cystoscope passes into the common perineal opening. A channel going into the uterine cavity is found

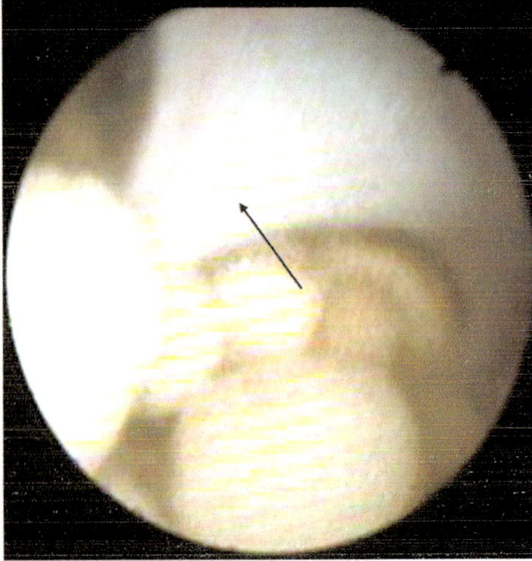

Fig. 3.50: Stones within the uterine cavity. Note the presence of a partial uterine septum (arrow) consistent with a bicornuate uterus

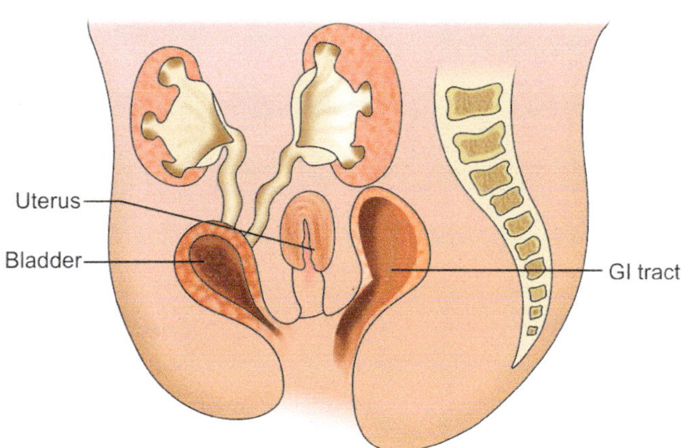

Fig. 3.51: Cloacal malformation

Definitive surgical correction may be done between 6 and 24 months. The posterior sagittal approach has been advocated. A multidisciplinary team of pediatric surgeons, pediatric urologists and pediatric gynecologists has to be involved in the operation to ensure maximum restoration of anatomy and function in these children.

BIBLIOGRAPHY

1. Altchek A. Congenital Gynecologic Anomalies. In: Altchek A, Deligdisch L (Eds). Pediatric, adolescent and young adult gynecology. West Sussex, UK: Blackwell Publishing 2009; pp. 159-70.
2. Annual Reports 2002-2008. Pediatric and Adolescent Gynecology Unit. Philippine Children's Medical Center.
3. Breech L, Laufer M. Müllerian Anomalies. In: Rayburn W, Hertwick SP (Eds). Obstet Gynecol Clin N Am. Elsevier Inc 2009; pp. 47-67.
4. Burgis J. Obstructive Müllerian Anomalies: Case report, diagnosis, and management. Am J Obstet Gynecol 2001;185:338-44.
5. Capitulo RB, Almirante CY, De Guia B. Persistent Cloaca: An Eleven Year Review at the Philippine Children's Medical Center, 2006. (Unpublished)
6. Defarges JV, Haddad B, Musset R, et al. Utero-vaginal anastomosis in women with uterine cervix atresia: long term follow-up and reproductive performance. A study of 18 cases. Human Reproduction 2001;16:1722-5.
7. Foley, Sallie, George W. Morley. Care and counseling of the patient with vaginal agenesis. The Female Patient 1992;17:73-80.
8. Guerrier D, Mouchel T, Pasquier L, et al. The Mayer-Rokitansky-Kuster-Hauser syndrome (congenital absence of uterus and vagina)- phenotypic manifestations and genetic approaches. Journal of Negative Results in Biomedicine 2006;5:1.
9. Haddad B, Barranger E, Paniel BJ. Blind hemivagina: long term follow-up and reproductive performance in 42 cases. Human Reproduction 1999;14:1962-4.
10. Hendren WH. Cloaca, the most severe degree of imperforate anus: experience with 195 Cases. Annals of Surgery 1998;3:331-46.
11. Madureira AJ, Mariz CM, Bernardes JC, et al. Uterus didelphys with obstructing hemivaginal septum and ipsilateral renal agenesis. Radiology 2006;239:602-6.
12. Morcel K, Camborieux L, Guerrier D, et al. Mayer-Rokitansky-Kuster-Hauser (MRKH) syndrome. Orphanet Journal of Rare Diseases 2007;2:13.
13. Shaw LM, Jones WA, Brereton RJ. Imperforate hymen and vaginal atresia and their associated anomalies. Journal of the Royal Society of Medicine 1983;76:560-6.
14. Soichi N, Nakatsuka M, Sugiyama Y, et al. Use of artificial dermis and recombinant basic fibroblast growth factor for creating a neovagina in a patient with Mayer-Rokitansky-Kuester-Hauser syndrome. Human Reproduction 2004;19:1629-32.
15. Tan EK, Lee GH, Choi YM, et al. Hysteroscopic resection of the vaginal septum in uterus didelphys with obstructed hemivagina: a case report. J Korean Medical Sci 2007;22:766-9.
16. Tsai CH, Chen CP, Chang MDT, et al. Hematometrocolpos secondary to didelphic uterus and unilateral imperforated double vagina as an unusual cause of acute abdomen. Taiwan J of Obstet Gynecol 2007;46:448-52.
17. Trojano RN, McCarthy SM. Müllerian duct anomalies: imaging and clinical issues. Radiology 2004;233:19-34.
18. Wu WC, Chang WC, Yeh LS, et al. Didelphic uterus and obstructive hemivagina with ipsilateral renal agenesis complicated by pyocolpos. Taiwan J Obstet Gynecol 2007;46:295-8.
19. Emans SJ, Laufer MR, Goldstein DP (Eds). Pediatric & Adolescent Gynecology, 5th edn. USA: Lippincott Williams & Wilkins, 2005.
20. Thomas DFM, Duffy PG, Rickwood AMK (Eds). Essentials of Pediatric Urology, 2nd edn. UK: Informa Healthcare, 2008.

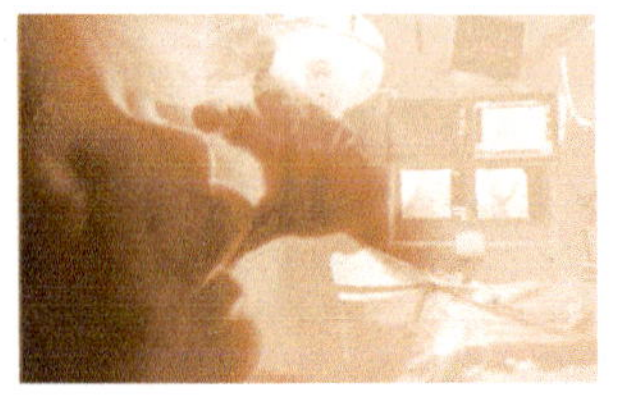

4 Abnormalities in Sexual Differentiation

Eva Maria Cutiongco-Dela Paz

NORMAL DEVELOPMENT OF THE GENITAL SYSTEM

An appreciation of normal genital development (Flow chart 4.1) is important in understanding sexual ambiguity and abnormal sexual differentiation. Chromosomal and genetic sex is clearly established at fertilization. However, sexual determination occurs only during gonadal development. The initial stage of development consists of the gonads of both sexes being identical and indifferent before the 7th week of gestation. Development into male gonads is largely dependent on the presence of the Y chromosome that bears the sex determining region Y (SRY). Gene for a testis-determining factor (TDF) is present on the short arm of Y chromosome, which determines the differentiation of the medulla into the testis and causes the cortex to regress. The absence of Y chromosome, having two copies of the X chromosome, leads to the development of ovaries and the regression of medulla takes place later, at around 12 weeks of gestation.

Flow chart 4.1: Normal genital development

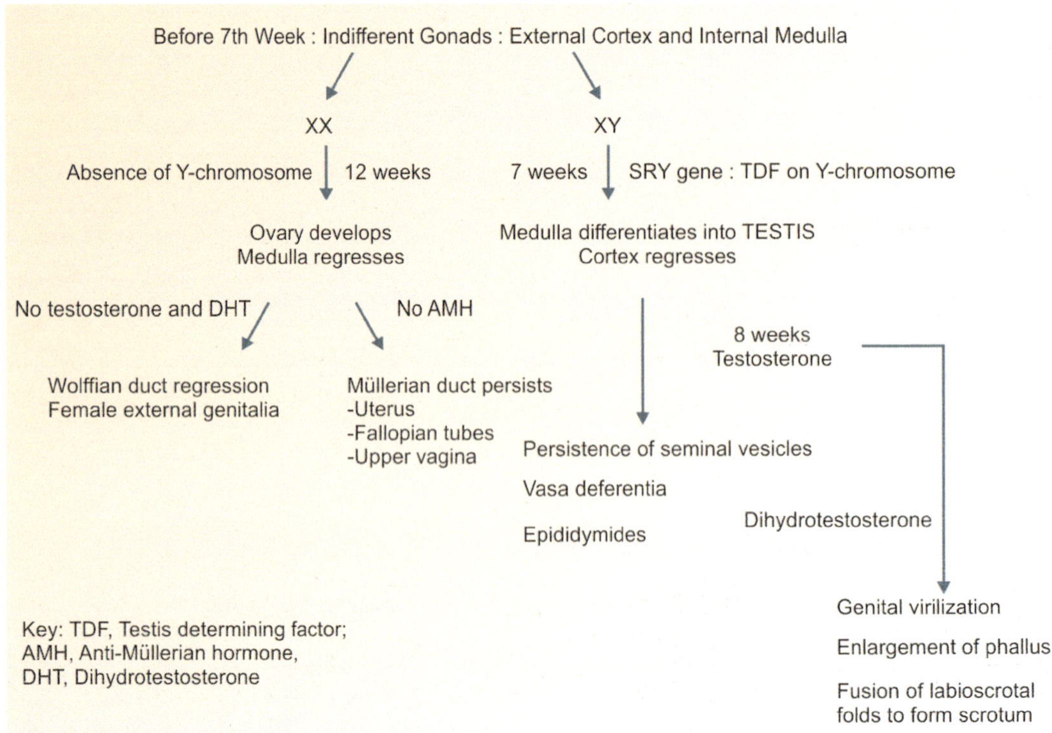

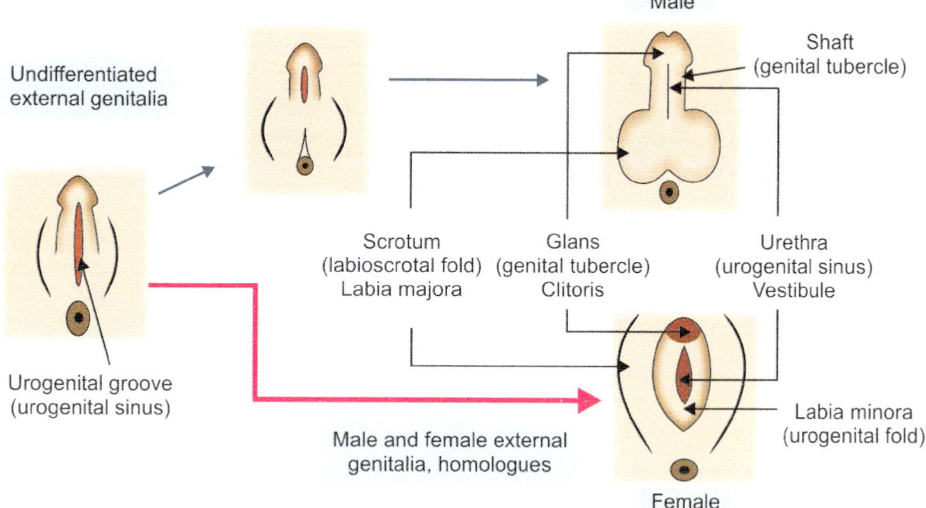

Fig. 4.1: Differentiation of the male and female external genitalia

The subsequent events in the development of the internal reproductive organs and the external genitalia are largely determined by hormones produced by gonads (ovaries or testes) and the response of the target cells. The secretion of testosterone by the Leydig cells causes the Wolffian ducts to develop into vasa deferentia and epididymis as well as for the seminal vesicles to persist. The Sertoli cells produce the anti-Müllerian hormone, which induces the involution of the Müllerian structures.

Dihydrotestosterone facilitates the formation of the male external genitalia, mainly the penis and the scrotum, through the process of growth and fusion. The absence of androgen, on the other hand, allows the Müllerian ducts to develop into the fallopian tubes, the uterus and the upper vagina while, the Wolffian ducts degenerate. Externally, the tubercle becomes the clitoris and the folds and swellings become the labia giving rise to the female external genitalia as shown in the Figure 4.1.

In recent years, many autosomal and X-linked genes have been identified which are important in sexual differentiation and determination. On the short arm of X chromosome, is the DAX1 gene, which encodes a transcription factor that plays a role in determination of the gonadal sex and closely interacts with the SRY gene. It is one of those linked gene in the conversion of an indifferent gonad into a testis. Another gene which appears to be required for normal testis formation is the SOX9 gene on the long arm of chromosome 17, which has been implicated as a primary testes determinant.

With normal sexual differentiation, appearance of the external and internal genitalia is consistent with the sex chromosome complement. Genital ambiguity arises when determination of sex is difficult because the genitalia resemble those of the opposite chromosomal sex with anomalies ranging from hypospadia, bilateral cryptorchidism and mircopenis in males and clitoromegaly and labial fusion in females as shown in Figure 4.2.

It is critical to determine whether the ambiguous genitalia during the newborn period is an overvirilized female or an undervirilized male. Individuals with an XX chromosomal constitution who are virilized have either been exposed to exogenous androgens or have large amounts of endogenous androgens resulting from defects in the biosynthesis of adrenal steroids. XY individuals with inadequate

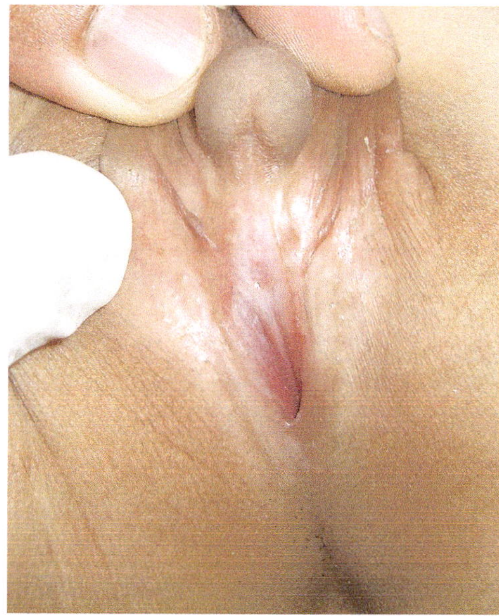

Fig. 4.2: Severe perineoscrotal hypospadia. The patient had ambiguous genitalia at birth and was brought up as female. Karyotyping was done only when she was 9 years old which showed XY chromosomes

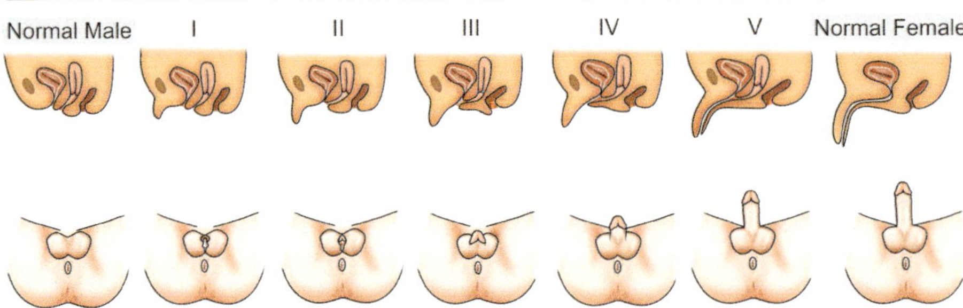

Fig. 4.3: Prader's classification of grade

virilization, on the other hand, may fall into the following categories: inadequate androgen production because of central (hypothalamic) or peripheral (testis) defects, inborn errors of testosterone biosynthesis and presence of androgen resistance. These various abnormalities of sexual differentiation (Fig. 4.3) can be caused by sex chromosome abnormalities as well as mutations in genes involved in sexual differentiation and determination.

Hermaphroditism occurs when a discrepancy exists between the morphology of the gonads, whether the testes or the ovaries, and the appearance of the external genitalia. True hermaphrodites have ovarian and testicular tissues either in the same or in opposite gonads. Although the majority of cases of true hermaphroditism have 46XX chromosomal complement, other chromosomal abnormalities which have been described include 46XX or 46XY, 46XY and 46XX or 47XXY.

Pseudohermaphroditism, on the other hand, refers to have a gonadal tissue of only one sex. Female pseudohermaphrodites have ambiguous genitalia or male external genitalia, but with 46XX karyotypes and normal ovarian tissue. In most instances, they are caused by congenital adrenal hyperplasia. Male pseudohermaphrodites are 46XY individuals who have abnormalities of gonadotropins, inborn errors of testosterone biosynthesis and metabolism, and abnormalities of androgen target cells. The best example of the latter is the androgen insensitivity syndrome.

A useful approach proposed by Jones to a child with ambiguous external genitalia would be to delineate the presence or absence of nongenital anomalies. A peripheral blood karyotype is mandatory in all cases of intersex problems and the analysis of cells should be extended to a sufficient number of about 100 cells to exclude mosaicism. In the absence of nongenital anomalies, and cytogenetic analysis shows that the chromosomal sex is XX, errors in sterol biosynthesis are the primary consideration because this produces endogenous androgens. A determination of 17-OH progesterone levels, if elevated, leads to the diagnosis of congenital adrenal hyperplasia or multiple defects in testosterone biosynthesis. When levels of 17-OH progesterone levels are normal, maternal androgen-secreting tumors and placental aromatase deficiency need to be ruled out. Interestingly, chromosomal studies may also show a mosaic karyotype of XX or XY in such a situation. When the karyotype reveals an XY chromosomal sex, complete or partial androgen insensitivity syndrome, hypothalamic or testicular defects and anomalies of the external genitalia are included in the differential diagnoses. The following are the examples of disorders in which ambiguous genitalia are not associated with nongenital anomalies.

CONGENITAL ADRENAL HYPERPLASIA

Congenital adrenal hyperplasia (CAH), an autosomal recessive group of disorders, is due to the deficiency of enzymes involved in adrenal steroidogenesis. Deficiency of 21-OH enzyme is the most common cause of CAH. Severe enzyme deficiency with prenatal onset characterizes the classic forms of the disorder, both salt wasting (SW) and simple virilizing (SV). Androgen excess produces prenatal masculinization [ambiguous genitalia, (Fig. 4.4)] in females and postnatal virilization in both the sexes.

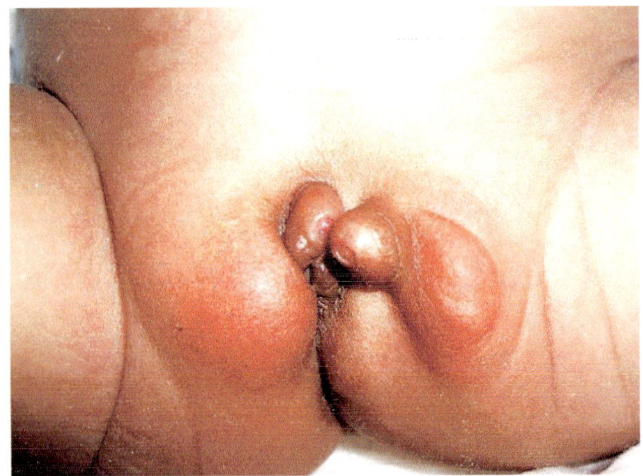

Fig. 4.4: Newborn infant with the ambiguous genitalia

Clinical diagnosis for 21-OH enzyme deficiency should be suspected in females who are virilized at birth, who become virilized postnatally, or who have contrasexual precocious puberty or premature adrenarche. The worldwide incidence of the classic forms of CAH (both SW- and SV-) is approximately 1 in 15000, with ethnic and racial variability. In the Filipino population, the newborn screening program reports an estimated crude incidence of classic CAH to be approximately 1 in 8,408 which is considered a bit higher compared to prevalence reports in most populations.

ANDROGEN INSENSITIVITY SYNDROME

Androgen insensitivity syndrome (Fig. 4.5), also known as testicular feminization syndrome, has a 46XY chromosome constitution with testes, but a normal female appearance.

Although the external genitalia are grossly female, the vagina ends blindly in a pouch and in addition, the uterus and fallopian tubes are absent. During the time of puberty, there is adequate development of the breast and female characteristics, but the pubic hair is scanty. Menstruation does not commence and may be the primary reason for consultation. The testicles can usually be found intra-abdominally or in the inguinal canals. These abnormalities are related to undervirilization that takes place, though the testes secrete normal amounts of androgens, androgen receptors in the cytosol of target cells are absent. Mutations in the androgen receptor (AR) gene on the X chromosome cause the androgen insensitivity syndrome.

For disorders in which the ambiguous external genitalia are associated with nongenital anomalies, these are further grouped into those which are a part of chromosomal anomaly syndromes such as those with mixed gonadal dysgenesis and those which are nonchromosomal anomaly syndromes such as the urorectal malformation sequence.

MIXED GONADAL DYSGENESIS

Mixed gonadal dysgenesis is a condition characterized by the presence of unilateral testis and a streak gonad on the contralateral side with the persistence of Müllerian structures. Oftentimes, the external genitalia are that of a normal male phenotype as a result of masculinization. Karyotyping reveals mosaicism which may have a 45X cell line and a 46XY cell line. The phenotype can range from a classic Turner syndrome with grossly normal female genitalia, may have a certain degree of ambiguity or may appear as normal male external genitalia. Mixed gonadal dysgenesis is attributed to mitotic nondisjunction.

URORECTAL MALFORMATION SEQUENCE

The urorectal malformation sequence is one example of the former caused by the incomplete migration and/or fusion with the cloacal membrane. This causes the persistence of the cloaca leading to a vesico-uretero-rectal fistula, complete or partial persistence of the cloacal membrane leading to the absence of urethral opening, no vaginal opening and imperforate anus and the failure of normal differentiation of the external genitalia leading to ambiguity in the genitalia and the presence of a phallic structure (Fig. 4.6). Most of these patients are stillborn or die during the neonatal period due to respiratory complications.

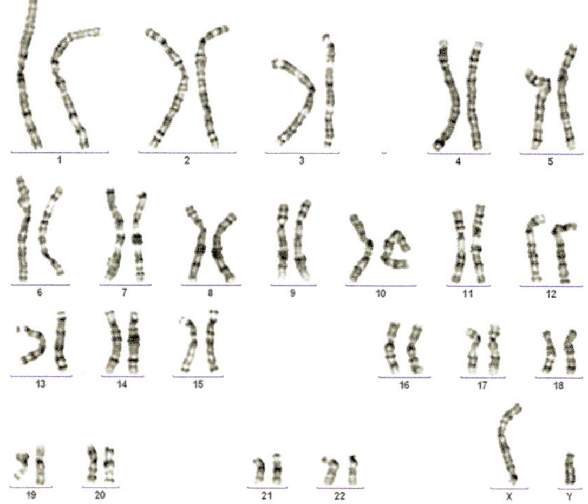

Fig. 4.5: Patients with androgen insensitivity syndrome have a normal male karyotype, although they are female in physical appearance *Courtesy*: Institute of Human Genetics, National Institute of Health, University of the Philippines-Manila

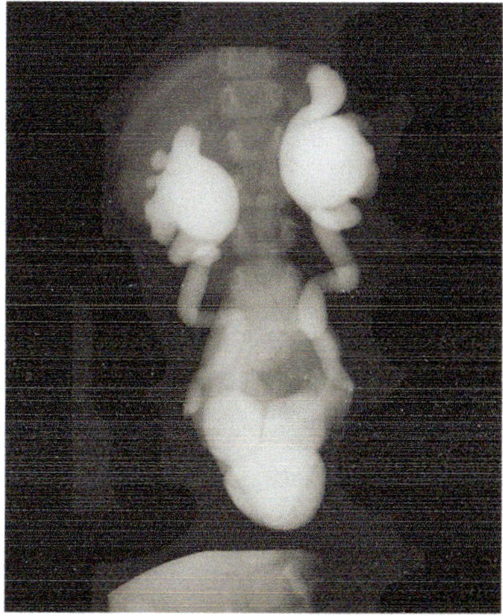

Fig. 4.6: Voiding cystourethrogram (VCUG) of patient with cloacal malformation shows hysterovesical fistula and severe vesicoureteral reflux. Cloacal malformation is a type of urorectal malformation sequence

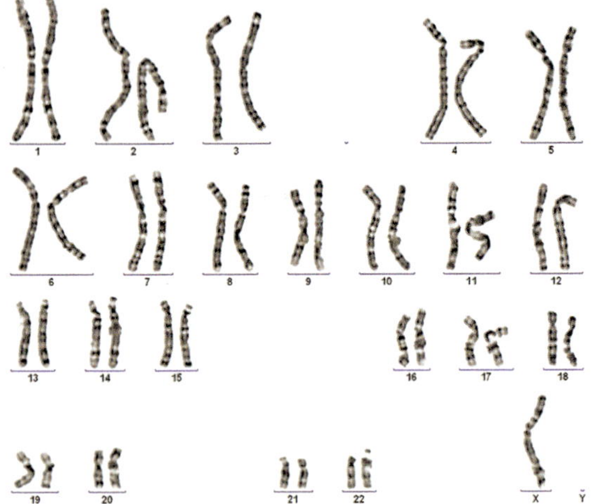

Fig. 4.7A: Karyotype of a patient with Turner syndrome
Courtesy: Institute of Human Genetics, National Institute of Health, University of the Philippines-Manila

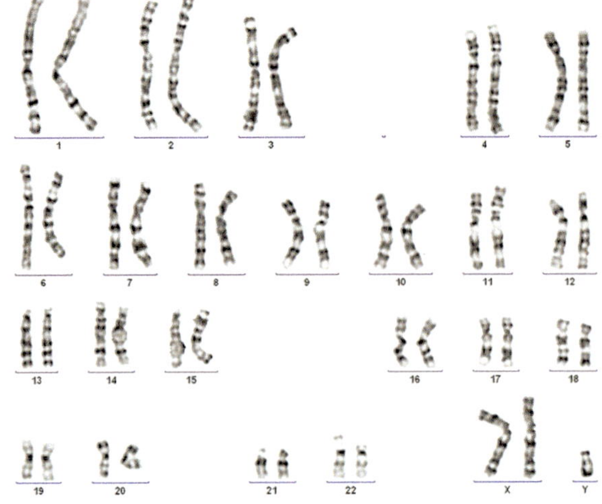

Fig. 4.7B: Karyotype of a patient with Klinefelter syndrome
Source: Courtesy of the Institute of Human Genetics, National Institute of Health, University of the Philippines-Manila

TURNER SYNDROME

The characteristic features of Turner syndrome are short stature, absence of secondary sexual characteristics and amenorrhea. This phenotype results from female gonadal failure and maldevelopment attributed to a faulty chromosomal distribution leading to an individual with a monosomy for the X chromosome. In the majority of cases, it is the paternal X chromosome that is missing. There is no increased maternal age risk factor for this aneuploidy and it is generally a sporadic event in families. The typical karyotype is 45X accounting for 65% of the cases (Fig. 4.7A); however, 20% have structural abnormalities of the X at another 20% present with a mosaic karyotype such as 45X or 46XY. At birth, patients with Turner syndrome has edema of the dorsum of the hands and feet and also present with webbed neck, low posterior hairline and broad chest with widely-spaced nipples. Cardiac defects are common including bicuspid aortic valve and coarctation of the aorta. The ovaries, which appear as streak gonads reflect a failure of ovarian maintenance. Patients with Turner syndrome have normal intelligence but may display visual-spatial organization deficits.

KLINEFELTER SYNDROME

Patients with Klinefelter syndrome present with lack of sexual maturation during adolescence, i.e. small testes and underdeveloped secondary sexual characteristics. They are also often identified through infertility clinics with failure of germ cell development causing the infertility. Characteristic physical features include tall, thin stature with relatively long legs. In half of the cases of Klinefelter syndrome, the sex chromosome aneuploidy results from errors in paternal meiosis I due to the failure of normal recombination in the pseudoautosomal regions of X and Y. Of those of maternal origin most are due to errors in maternal meiosis I, meiosis II or from postzygotic mitotic error leading to mosaicism. The most common mosaicism is a 46XY or 47XXY karyotype as shown in the Figure 4.7B. Variants of Klinefelter syndrome include 48XXXY, 48XXYY and 49XXXXY. The additional X chromosome is thought to produce a more abnormal phenotype, a greater degree of dysmorphism, more defective sexual development and mental impairment. Performance of XXY individuals varies but generally, learning difficulties and poor psychosocial adjustments are frequent.

BIBLIOGRAPHY

1. Evaluation of the Newborn with Developmental Anomalies of the External Genitalia. American Academy of Pediatrics. Committee on genetics. Pediatrics 2000;106:138-42.
2. Jones KL. Smith's Recognizable Patterns of Human Malformation, 6th edn. USA: Elsevier Saunders, 2006.
3. McGillivray B. Genetic aspects of ambiguous genitalia. Pediatric Clinics of North America 1992;39(2):307-17.
4. Moore K, Persaud T. The Developing Human: Clinically Oriented Embryology, 6th edn. Philadelphia: WB Saunders Company, 1998.
5. Nussbaum R, McInnes R, Willard H. Thompson & Thompson Genetics in Medicine, 6th edn. Philadelphia: WB Saunders Company, 2001.
6. Philippine Newborn Screening Program, 2008. (Unpublished data)
7. Pinsky L, Erickson R, Schimke RN. Genetic Disorders of Human Sexual Development. UK: Oxford University Press, 1999.
8. Simpson J, Elias S. Genetics in Obstetrics and Gynecology, 3rd edn. USA: Elsevier Science, 2003.

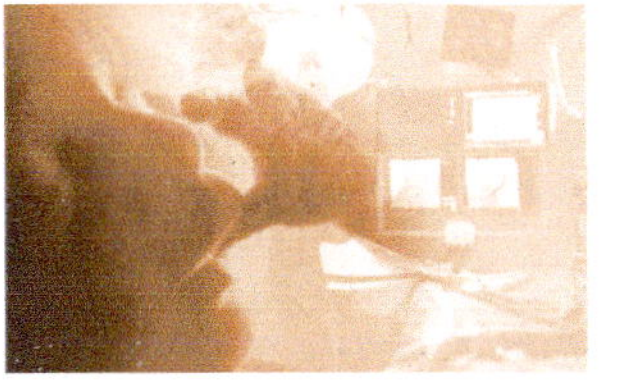

5 Vulvovaginal Disorders

Ma Socorro C Bernardino, Annebelle Dimatulac-Aherrera

Vulvovaginal disorders in children are different from that of adults. Many factors are to be considered in the diagnosis and treatment of these conditions. Among these factors the following are: anatomy and physiology of the reproductive tract; growth and development; and the hormonal milieu of the patient. Clinical features are age dependent. These may be categorized into neonatal, infancy, prepubertal and peripubertal age-group.

VULVOVAGINAL INFECTIONS IN CHILDREN

Ma Socorro C Bernardino

VULVOVAGINITIS

The most common gynecologic condition in children is vulvovaginitis. It is defined as inflammation of the vulva and vagina (Figs 5.1 and 5.2). The vulva or vagina may be involved alone or both at the same time. The symptoms may vary with each child. The parent or caregiver may notice a discharge on the child's diaper or underwear, an abnormal odor, or redness of the vulva.

Vaginal discharge in neonates may be physiologically secondary to the influence of maternal estrogens as shown in the Figures 5.3 and 5.4. The discharge is characterized to be whitish mucoid and without odor and gradually disappears by six weeks postnatally. The presence of vaginal discharge in prepubertal children is almost always considered to be abnormal. They are anatomically, physiologically and behaviorally at relative risk for vulvovaginitis.

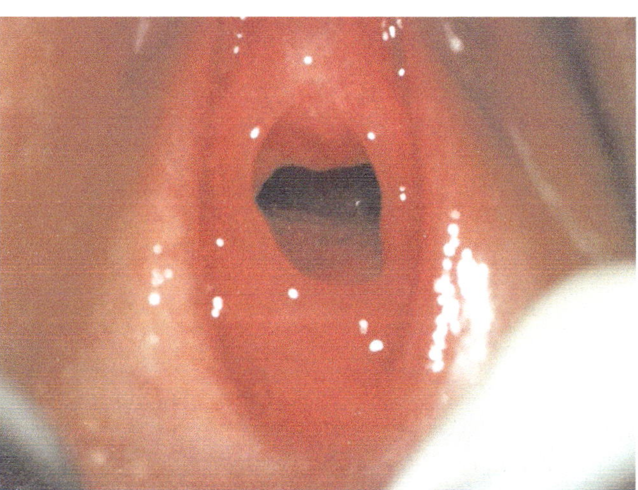

Fig. 5.1: Inflammation of the perihymenal and vaginal tissues

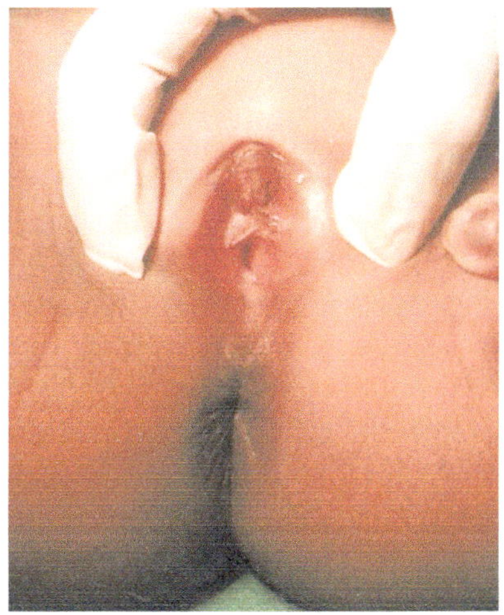

Fig. 5.2: A 2-year-old child patient presenting with vulvitis

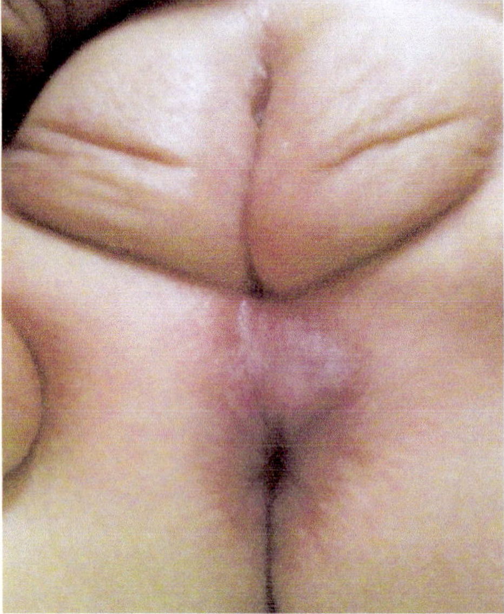

Fig. 5.3: Characteristics of a newborn vulva and vagina relate to high estrogen levels. Puffy labia majora, thickened labia minora, redundant hymenal folds and vaginal mucosa that is moist and pink with an acidic pH

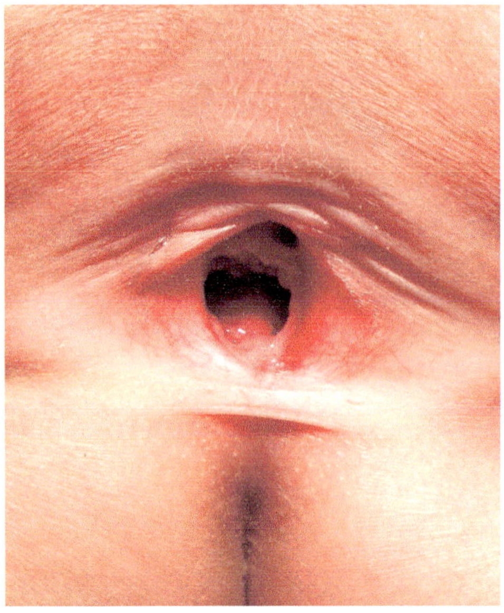

Fig. 5.4: Prepubertal vulva. Characteristics, relate to low estrogen levels. Labia majora losses its fullness, labia minora become thinner and flatter and do not cover the vestibule fully; perineum and perivaginal tissues are rigid and inelastic

Clinical Manifestation of Vulvovaginitis

Signs and symptoms of vulvovaginitis: the sign and symptoms of vulvovaginitis are as follows:

- Vaginal discharge is the most common presenting sign and symptoms in vulvovaginitis
- Vulval pain
- Abnormal odor
- Vulval and vaginal bleeding
- Pruritus

Risk Factors for the Susceptibility of Prepubertal Children to Vulvovaginitis

Behavioral factors: following are the behavioral factors responsible for vulvovaginitis:

- Inadequate front-to-back wiping
- Inattention to perineal hygiene (Fig. 5.5) at home or day program
- Over vigorous vulval cleansing
- Deodorant soaps or adult feminine washes
- Masturbation

Anatomic factors: the anatomic factors responsible for vulvovaginitis are as follows:

- Lack of protective fat pads
- Thin vulval skin
- Atrophic vaginal mucosa
- Neutral vaginal pH
- Proximity of the anus to the vaginal opening

Physiologic factors: following are the physiologic factors

- Respiratory or GI illness
- Diabetes mellitus or immunodeficiency state
- Limited antibodies in vaginal secretions
- An estrogenic vaginal epithelium
- Neutral pH
- Sexual abuse
- Dermatologic conditions

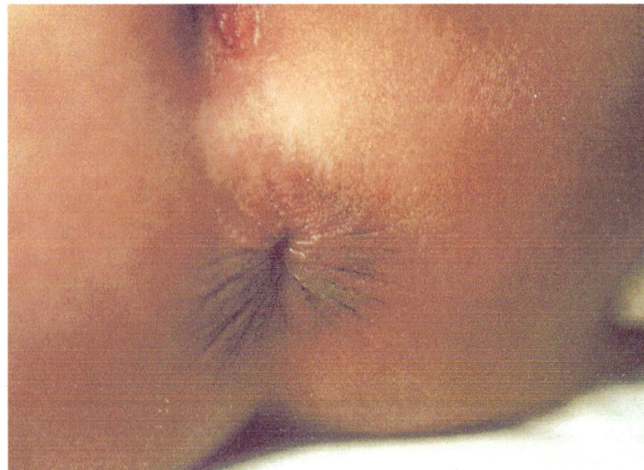

Fig. 5.5: Poor perineal and anal hygiene

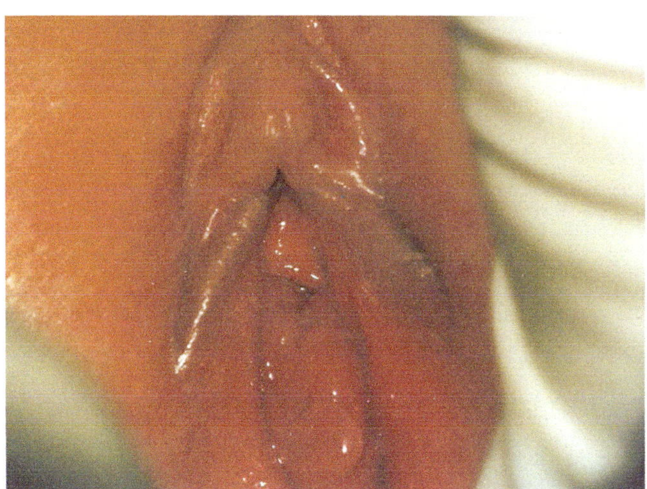

Fig. 5.6: A 5-year-old child patient with nonspecific vulvovaginitis

CAUSES OF VULVOVAGINITIS

At the Pediatric and Adolescent Gynecology Unit of the Philippine Children's Medical Center, a total of 125 prepubertal children were included in a study from April 2002 to April 2004 to determine the causative factors of vulvovaginitis. Age range was between 2 to 10 years with a mean age of 5.1 years. Isolated organisms in the vaginal culture were 62%, with the remaining attributed to noninfectious causes of vulvovaginitis. Among the isolated organisms, 70% were considered to be nonpathologic or part of the normal cervico-vaginal flora, hence, termed as nonspecific vulvovaginitis as shown in the Figures 5.6 and 5.7. Several studies provided information on the normal cervicovaginal flora of prepubertal girls (Table 5.1).

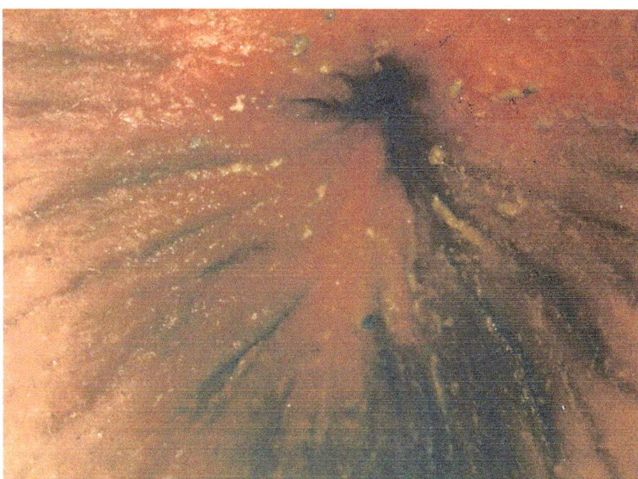

Fig. 5.7: Magnification of the anus in a 5-year-old child patient with nonspecific vaginitis

Table 5.1
Normal flora of the prepubertal vagina

Staphylococcus aureus	*Lactobacillus*	*Bacteroides species*
Staphylococcus epidermidis	Proteus	Peptococcus species
Alpha-hemolytic streptococci	Gardnerella vaginalis	Peptostreptococcus species
Escherichia coli	Non-hemolytic streptococci	Veilonella species
Klebsiella species	Enterococci	Diphtheroids

Noninfectious Causes of Vulvovaginitis

Most common noninfectious causes of vulvovaginitis still relate to poor perineal hygiene. Most common causes of vulvovaginitis are given below:

- Poor perineal hygiene
- Poor perineal aeration
- Chemical irritants
- Contact Dermatitis
- Parasites
- Anatomic Anomalies
- Neoplasms
- Systemic Illnesses

SPECIFIC VULVOVAGINITIS

Cultures of organisms that are not part of the normal flora are considered to cause specific vulvovaginitis. These may be categorized as either being respiratory, intestinal or sexually transmitted.

Candida Vulvovaginitis

Vaginal yeast infection in children is usually rare, however, certain risks factors may contribute to its occurrence. Among these are histories of recent antibiotic intake, diabetes mellitus, immunocompromised state and diaper use. The child usually presents with vulvar pruritus followed by vulvar pain because of inflammation as shown in Figure 5.8. At times, there may be presence of a whitish, curd like, nonfoul smelling vaginal discharge.

Group A Beta Hemolytic Streptococcal Infection

Patients with group A beta hemolytic streptococcal vulvovagintis (Fig. 5.9) often present with a distinctive fiery red inflammation of the vulva or perihymenal area. The discharge, which may be present, is usually blood tinged. This condition usually follows a history of sore throat or upper respiratory tract infection.

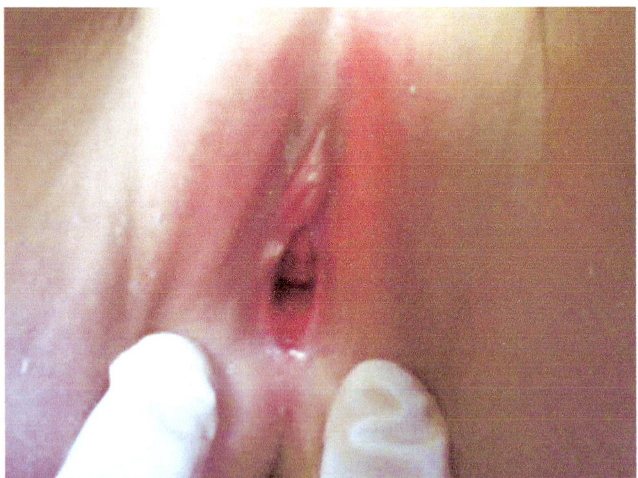

Fig. 5.8: A 4-year-old girl patient complaining of vulvar pruritus and pain. KOH smear of vaginal discharge shows hyphal elements

Shigella Infection

An enteric pathogen can spread to the genital region following a bout of diarrhea. Patients usually present with a malodorous, mucopurulent discharge that may be blood-tinged.

Sexually Transmitted Causes

The possibility of sexual abuse should always be considered when a child presents with genital symptoms. If confirmed, further investigation and reporting to child protective services is necessary. Once an STI-related organism is isolated, several factors should be considered such as the mode of transmission and anatomic characteristics in children that differ in the clinical manifestations as that of adults. It should be noted that the cervix of children is longer than the uterus and there are no endocervical glands in the ectocervix thereby protecting them from upper genital tract infection.

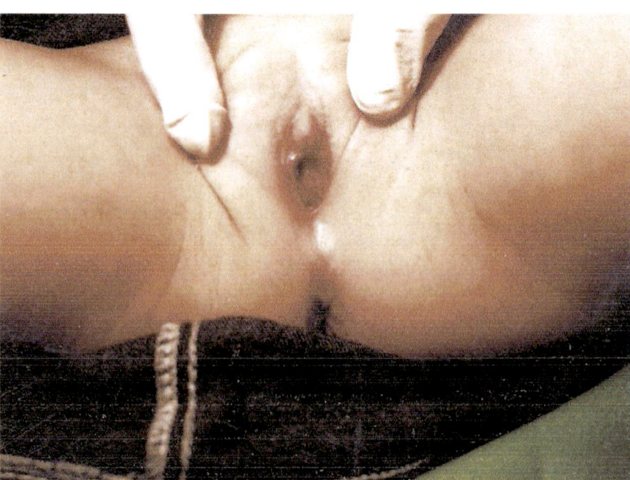

Fig. 5.9: Group A beta hemolytic streptococcal infection

Mode of Transmission

There are several modes of infection and is listed below.

- Sexual transmission
- Perinatal transmission (vertical)
- Possibility of fomite transmission
- Causal transmission.

Neisseria Gonorrhea

Gonococcal infection in children usually presents with yellowish to greenish mucopurulent discharge as shown in the Figure 5.10. It is rare for it to cause upper genital tract infection. Perinatally acquired infection may manifest in the first few weeks of life in a newborn. Transmission from one child to another has been reported secondary to genital exploratory behavior. Gold standard for the diagnosis is based on culture of the organism.

Trichomonas Vaginalis

Trichomonas infection outside of the newborn period rarely occurs because the organism prefers to thrive in an estrogenic environment. The vaginal discharge is usually profuse, whitish to yellowish, flocculent and has a distinctive fishy odor. Diagnosis is made by the presence of trichomonads in a saline wet smear of the vaginal discharge.

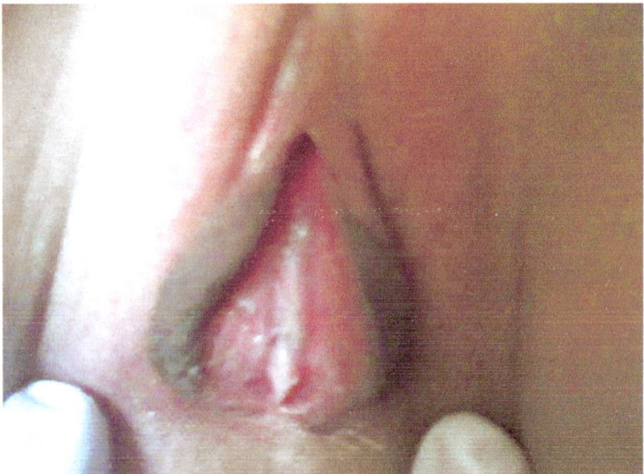

Fig. 5.10: A 10-year-old peripubertal child presented with persistent yellowish-green vaginal discharge. Gram stain results show the presence of gram negative intracellular diplococci. This is later confirmed with a positive culture of Neisseria gonorrhea

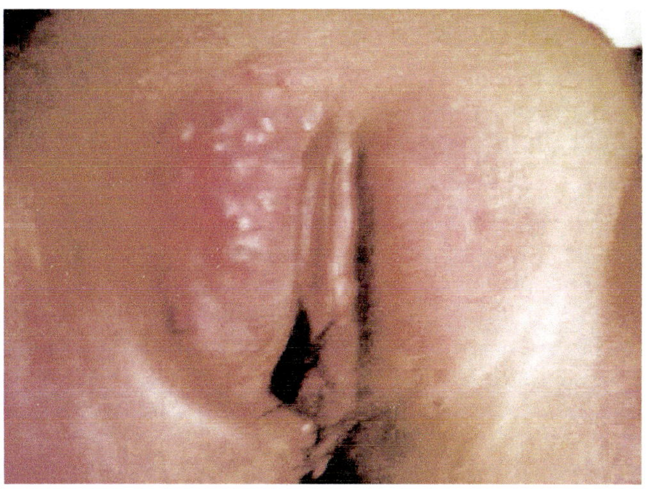

Fig. 5.11: A 9-year-old girl presented with HSV lesions with secondary bacterial infection. Patient had a history of gingivostomatitis a week before the occurrence of genital symptoms

Herpes Simplex Infection

The most common clinical manifestation of herpes simplex I infection is gingivostomatitis as shown in the Figure 5.11. However, both HSV 1 and 2 infections have been reported to occur in lesions in the genital area leading to the possibility of autoinoculation. Diagnosis is made by detection of ulcers and confirmed by culture.

Genital Warts

Condyloma acuminate (Figs 5.12 to 5.14A and B) are caused by the human papilloma virus and can occur in the genital area. They often present as fleshy verrucous growths in the mucosal membranes in the periurethral and perianal areas.

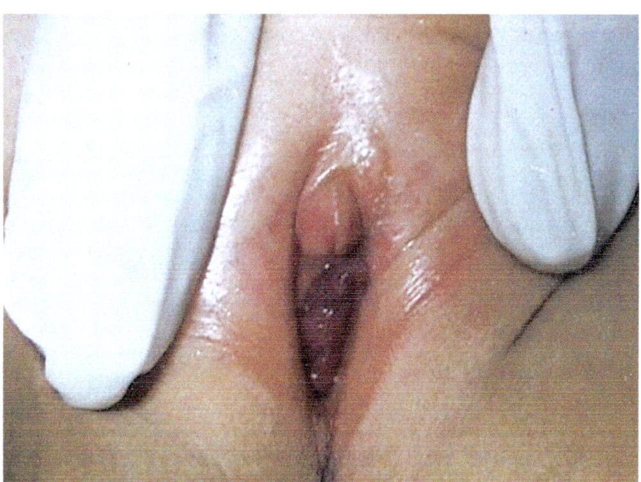

Fig. 5.12: A 4-year-old girl presented with a fleshy mass at the perihymenal area

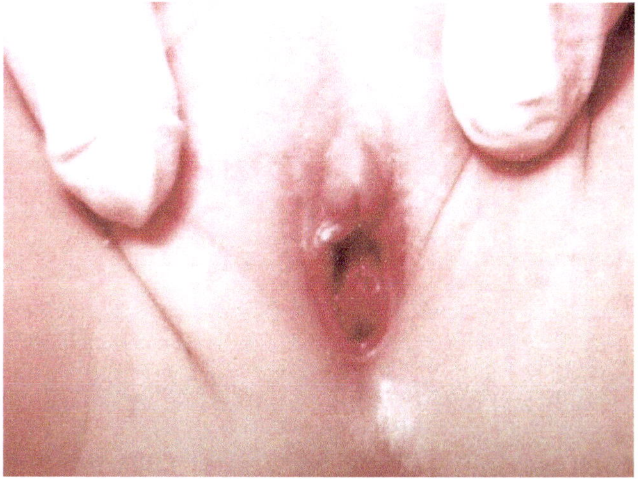

Fig. 5.13: Same patient S/P excision of the mass. Histopathologic findings revealed condyloma acuminata

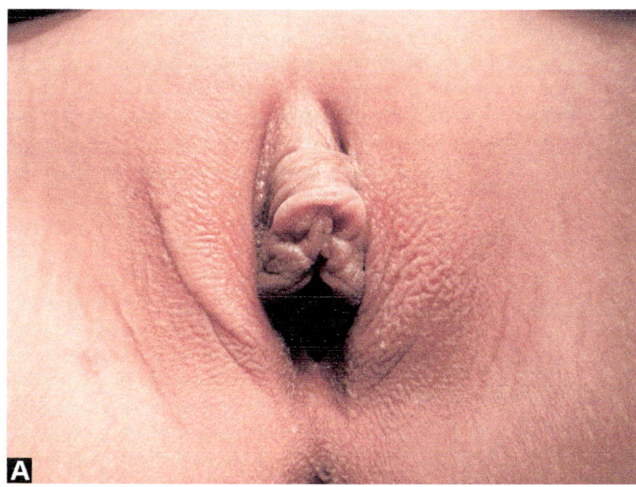

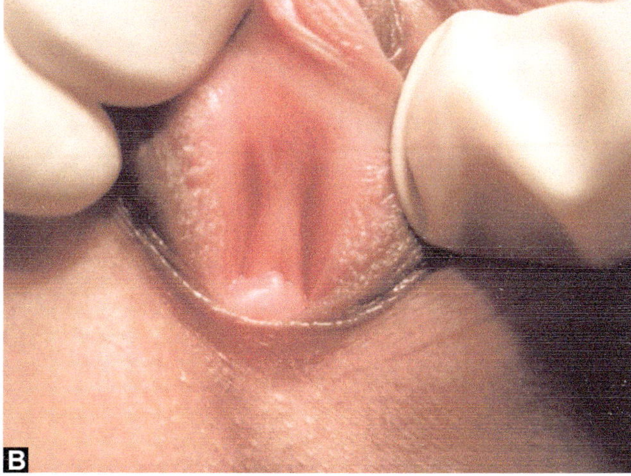

Figs 5.14A and B: A 4-year-old girl patient complains of persistent vulval pruritis. Cautery and excision is done revealing condyloma acuminata

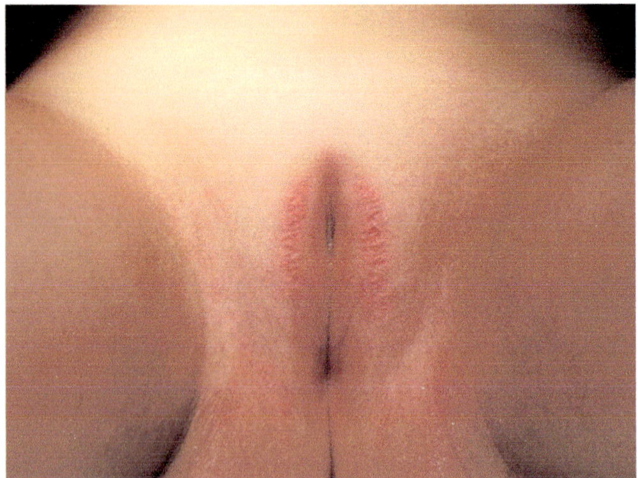

Fig. 5.15: Vulva of a 4-year-old girl presenting with persistent foul smelling vaginal discharge of 3 months duration

Foreign Body in The Vagina

Foreign bodies inside the vaginal canal (Figs 5.15 to 5.18) have been implicated in a majority of cases if the child reported with persistent or recurrent vaginal discharge and the passage of blood streaked foul smelling discharge (Figs 5.15 and 5.16). A number of foreign bodies have been documented through vaginoscopy (Fig. 5.17).

Commonly Seen Foreign Bodies

Types of foreign bodies extracted from vaginas of prepubertal girls with vaginal discharge:

- Tissue paper
- Pieces of cloth or paper
- Cotton fibers

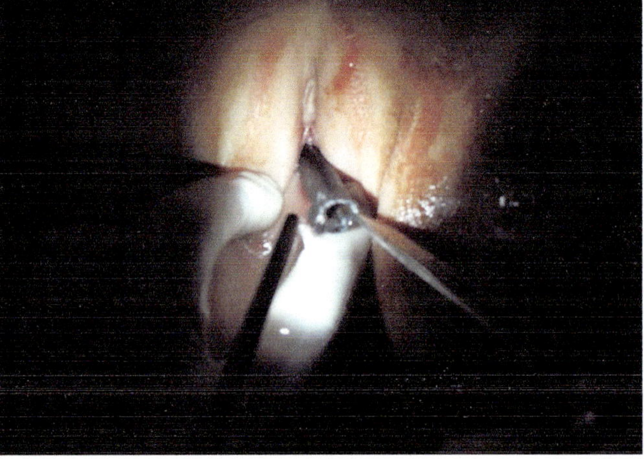

Fig. 5.17: Vaginoscopy done showing a black object embedded in the anterior vaginal wall. Retrieval of the object revealed a ball pen cap. Same patient shown in the Figure 5.15

- Small fragments of bed foam
- Eraser
- Cigarette butts
- Safety pin (closed)

DIAGNOSIS OF VULVOVAGINITIS

Microbiologic investigation should be carried out if there is visible discharge or the presence of inflammation. Vaginal discharge sampling may be done with the use of a small cotton tip moistened with sterile saline to minimize pain and trauma upon collection. A small feeding tube may likewise be used to retrieve washings located inside the vaginal canal.

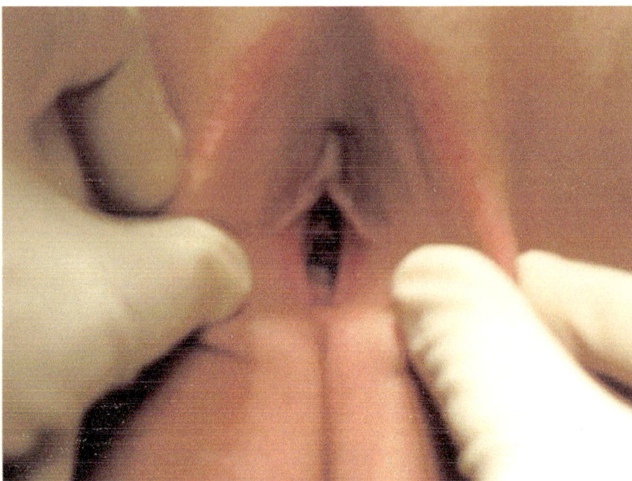

Fig. 5.16: Examination of the vestibule of the same patient has shown in the Figure 5.15

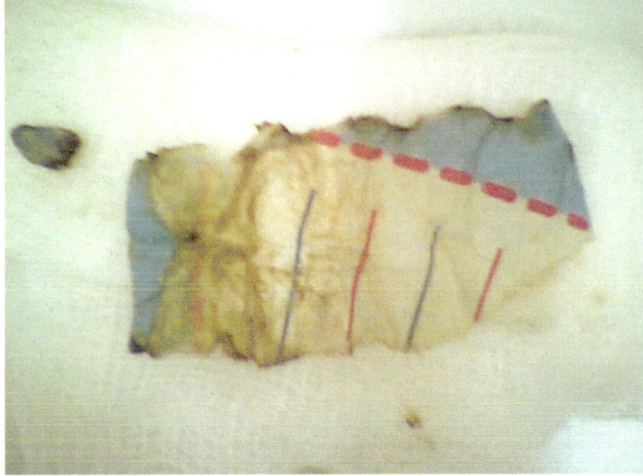

Fig. 5.18: Folded piece of cloth retrieved from a 6-year-old girl presenting with blood streaked foul smelling discharge. Sexual abuse is confirmed in this case

Diagnostics Tests for Vaginal Discharge Samples

Following diagnostic tests are used for vaginal discharge sample:

- Gram stain
- Culture and sensitivity
- KOH smear
- Direct saline wet preparation.

TREATMENT OF VULVOVAGINITIS

If no specific cause is found in prepubertal girls with vulvovaginal symptoms (nonspecific vulvovaginitis), then initial treatment should focus on improved perineal hygiene.

Initial Treatment for Nonspecific Vulvovaginitis

1. *Good perineal hygiene:* Wiping from front to back after bowel movement.
2. *Tub sitz bath with warm water:* Immerse buttocks for 10 to 15 minutes. If present with inflamed vulva, it is advisable to use warm water mixed with baking soda. If there is heavy purulent discharge then it is advisable to use water mixed with a small amount of povidone-iodine solution, however, minimize use because it can cause drying of the vulva.
3. Advise frequent changes of white cotton underwear to absorb discharge.
4. Daily perineal wash with mild unscented soap.
5. Loose fitting shorts, pants or skirts especially when sleeping.
6. Urination with legs spread apart and labia separated.

Treatment for Persistent Nonspecific Vulvovaginitis

- Antibiotic use is preferred if the relevant pathogen is identified
- Broad spectrum antibiotics may be used
- Antibacterial cream, if lesion is located outside the vulva, may be applied
- Estrogen cream preparations applied at night for a maximum of two weeks
- Petroleum cream can help alleviate vulvitis.

Other Infections of the Vulva

There are other infections like labial abscess, incision and drainage, and labial ulcer with secondary bacterial infection that are shown in the Figures 5.19 to 5.21.

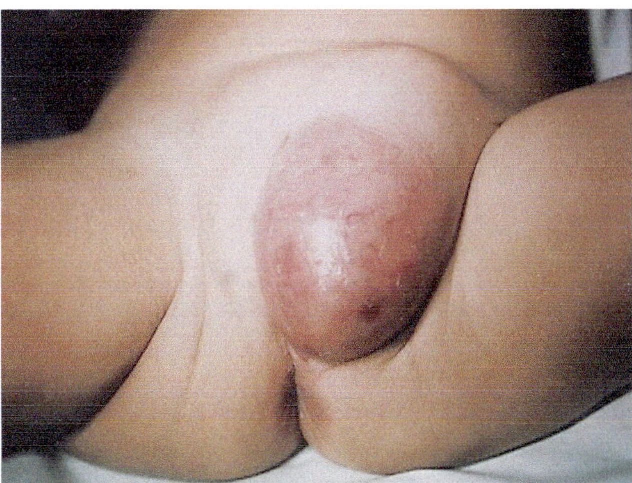

Fig. 5.19: Labial abscess in a 10-month-old female

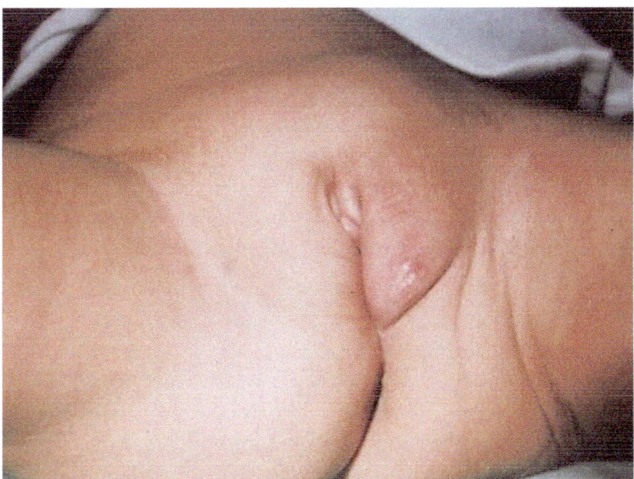

Fig. 5.20: S or P incision and drainage 1 week after

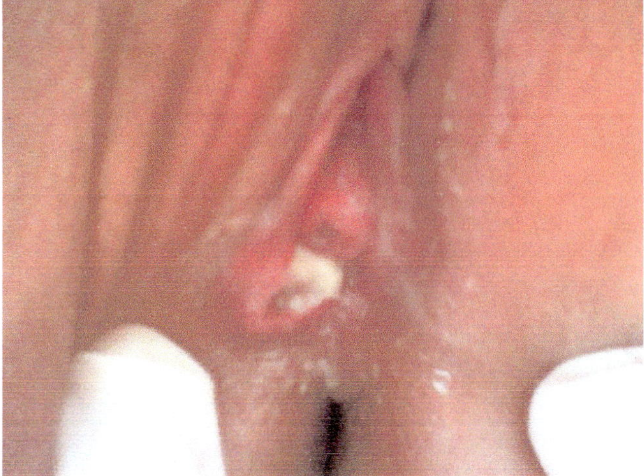

Fig. 5.21: Labial ulcer with secondary bacterial infection in 9-year-old prepubertal girl

DERMATOLOGIC PROBLEMS AND OTHER DISORDERS OF THE VULVA

Annebelle Dimatulac-Aherrera

LABIAL FUSION OR LABIAL ADHESION

A common benign pediatric gynecologic condition is adhesion or fused [inner vaginal lips, (Figs 5.22 and 5.23)] labia minora. It often gives the appearance that the opening of the vagina has closed off. The adhesion results in a formation of smooth membrane over the vulval opening with a thin, pale translucent streak usually found in the midline as shown in the Figure 5.24.

This surface membrane usually starts forming at the rear of the opening and "zippers" closed toward the front. Usually, a sufficient opening at the front remains to permit urine and vaginal secretions to exit. It may be noticed incidentally by a parent or by a physician during a medical examination, or the child may complain of irritation or difficulty in urinating.

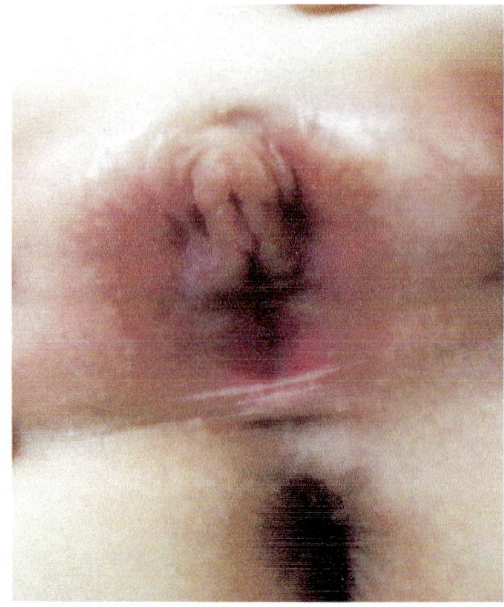

Fig. 5.23: Labial adhesion in a prepubertal child

Age Group

- Commonly found in young girls between the age of 3 months and 6 years old
- Uncommon in the newborns and after 6 years of age
- Peak incidence of 13 to 24 months of age.

Etiology

- Cause is unknown
- May result in the inflammation of the labia minora creating two raw surfaces at the edges of the lips, which eventually heal together in the middle, partly or fully covering the opening of the vagina
- Lack of estrogen (which is normal before puberty) probably plays a role in this process.

Other Factors

- Exposure to irritants like fabric softener residue, perfumed soaps, or bits of stool
- Prolonged exposure to damp (as in wet diapers) can cause irritation in the area
- Urine, stool, diaper rash, infections, irritants, or mechanical trauma commonly cause chronic inflammation of the labia.

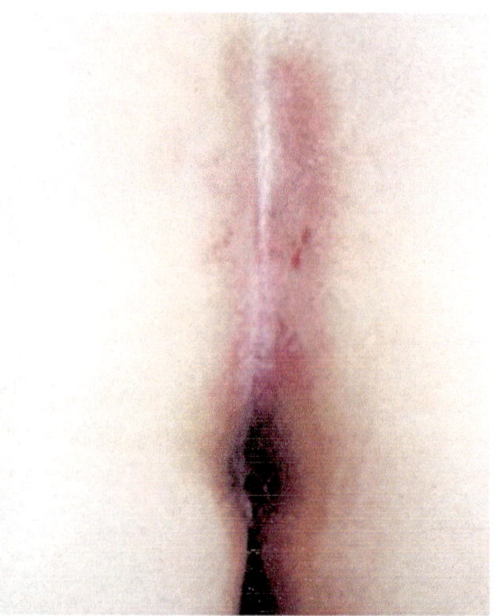

Fig. 5.22: Typical adhesion or fused labia minora (inner vaginal lips)

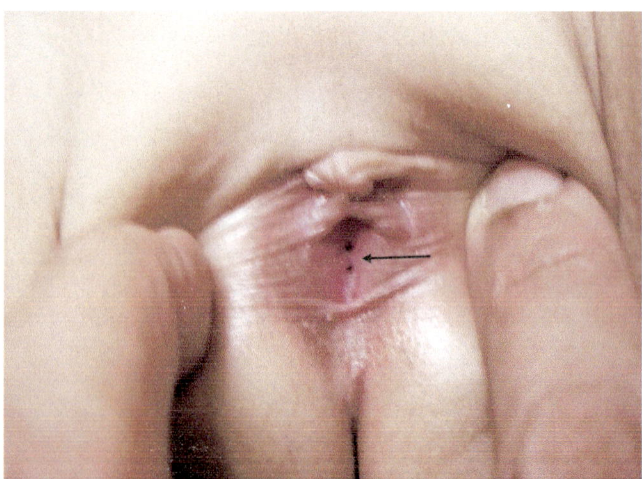

Fig. 5.24: Partially resolved labial fusion of the same child as in Figure 5.23. Note the thinning and small openings in the inter-labial line marked by an arrow

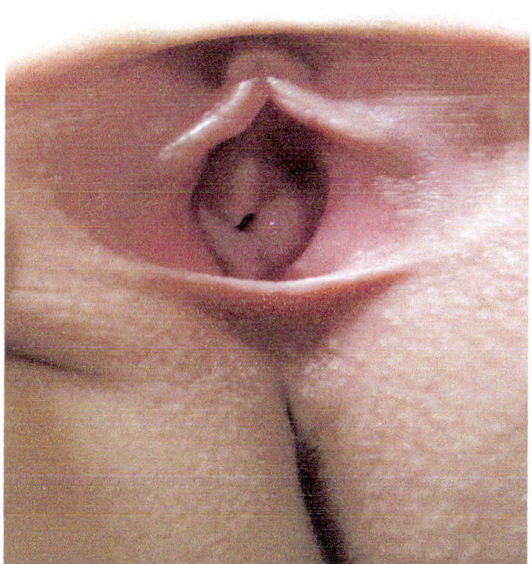

Fig. 5.25: The same child as shown in the Figure 5.23 after estrogen applications for 4 weeks

Management

- Therapy is not always required as spontaneous resolution can occur in 6 to 18 months
- If treatment is necessary, a topical estrogen cream may be used and often effective. Apply twice a day at the fused portion, labia get separated within 3 to 8 weeks as shown in the Figure 5.25
- Avoid irritants, those that cause inflammation. Include daily baths in plain water.

Associated Symptoms

Associated urinary tract infection (UTI) and a symptomatic bacteriuria.

CONTACT DERMATITIS

Contact dermatitis is a type of acute or chronic skin reaction in which sensitivity is manifested by reactivity to materials or substances coming in contact with the skin. It may involve allergic or nonallergic mechanisms.

Age Group

- Almost all children in diapers get some diaper rashes
- Peak age group is between 8 and 10 months old.

Diagnosis

- Clinical appearance is often eczematous and oozing
- It may involve congruent areas.

Symptoms

Skin wetness is the common denominator underlying the various causes of diaper rash.

1. *Friction:* The most common form of affecting almost all babies, mostly seen in areas where friction is most pronounced like the inner thighs or under the elastic of diapers (Figs 5.26A and B). Resolve spontaneously to frequent diaper changes airing out and protective barriers.
2. *Irritant:* This results from constant contact with irritants such as harsh soaps, baby wipes, detergents, stool, urine or topical medicines. Seen mostly on the exposed areas such as round part of the buttocks or

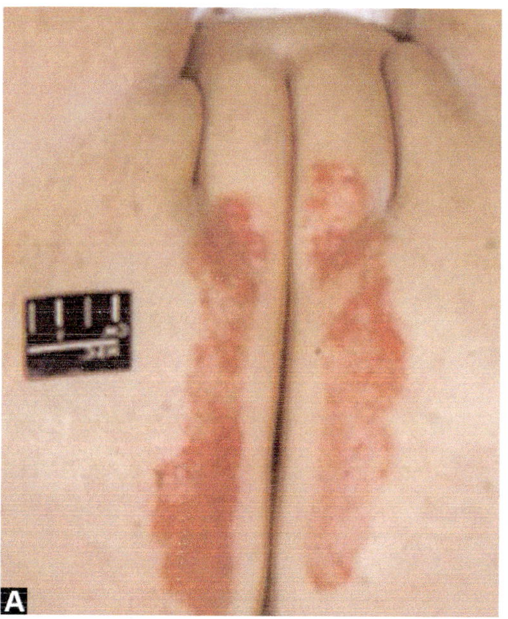

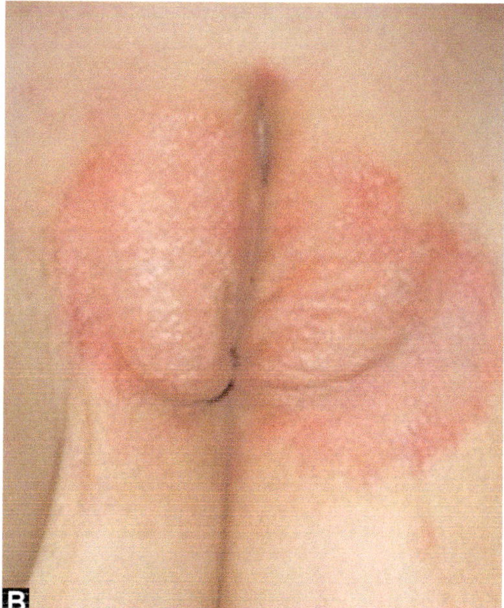

Figs 5.26A and B: Friction contact dermatitis from diapers seen in a 2-month-old infant

the front of vulval area sparing intertriginous folds and creases.

3. *Allergic:* Commonly seen in the exposed areas and occurs in combination with an irritant or by itself.
4. *Psoriasis:* This stubborn rash doesn't necessarily look distinctive. Other signs of psoriasis usually accompany the diaper rash like well-demarcated erythematous plaques with or without fine silvery scale, on the neck, face scalp and with pitting of the nails.

Therapy

- Cool compresses
- Mild cleanser (Cetaphil)
- Topical steroid (low to mid potency)
- Avoid allergens
- Frequent diaper changes, airing out
- Protective lotions or creams

VULVAL HEMANGIOMA

Hemangiomas are benign tumors of the vascular endothelium that occur in infants (Figs 5.27 and 5.28). They enlarge by active proliferation of endothelial cells due to still unknown factors.

Symptoms

Following are the presenting symptoms of vulval hemangioma:

- Most genital hemangiomas involve the labia majora, but the labia minora, the perineal area and the perianal area may also be involved to varying degrees

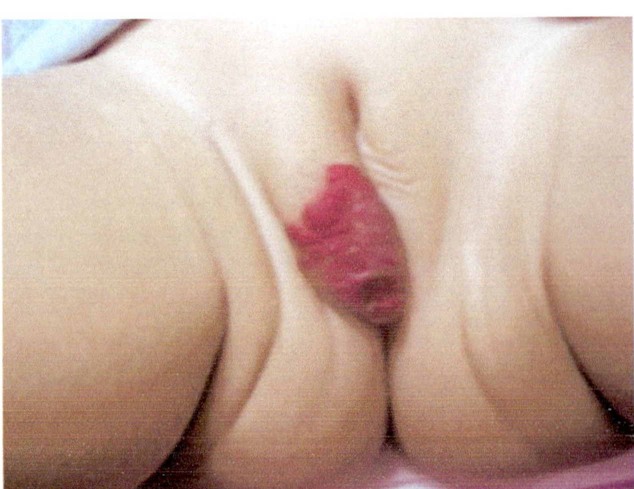

Fig. 5.27: A large labial hemangioma with ulceration in a 1-year-old child patient. Lesion has been present since birth

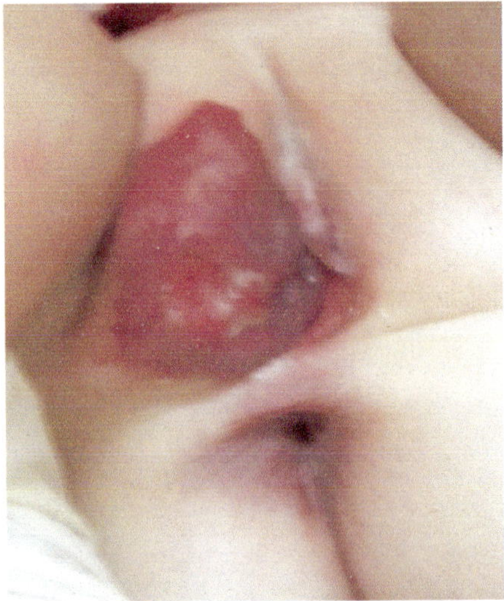

Fig. 5.28: Ulcerated hemangioma of the right labia majora in a prepubertal child

- Appear as red macules that rapidly progress to well-circumscribed, raised, red, and soft lesions of variable size
- Lesions may regress over time with involution and fibrosis
- Possible complications include ulceration, bleeding, urethral obstruction, and Kasabach-Merritt syndrome (a consumptive coagulopathy mainly described in association with large hemangiomas).

Diagnosis

- Diagnosis is clinical
- Biopsy of lesions is discouraged due to propensity for bleeding.

Management

- No therapeutic measures are required
- Close monitoring toward spontaneous regression is done
- No therapeutic measures are required unless complications occur. Corticosteroids and interferon, both systemic and intralesional have been used in severe cases.

GRANULOMA GLUTEALE INFANTUM

Granuloma gluteale infantum is an uncommon skin disorder characterized by oval, reddish purple granulomatous nodules on the gluteal surfaces and the groin areas of infants. A history of a previous or preceding inflammatory skin conditions (dermatitis—contact, irritant) that have been treated with some steroid-like agents is a causative factor.

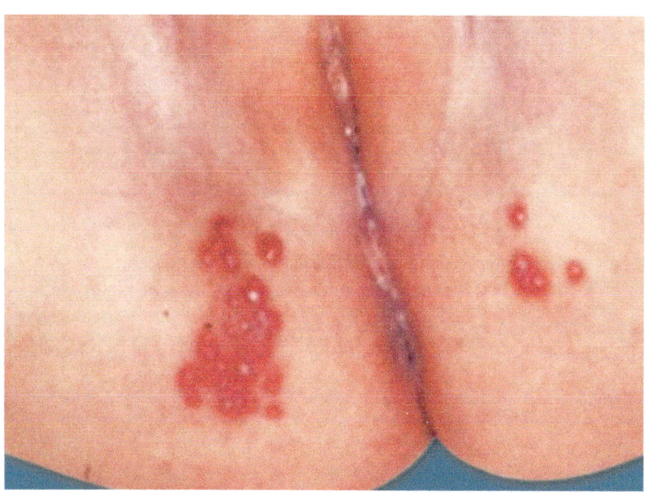

Fig. 5.29: Granuloma gluteale infantum. Erythematous nodules on the gluteal area with a smooth surface of a 5-month-old infant

Physical Appearance

Physical appearance of granuloma gluteale infantum is shown in the Figure 5.29.

- Usually 1–30 lesions are seen in the affected area
- They appear red-purple to red-brown with oval, firm to hard discrete nodules with smooth or lichenified surface measuring about 5–40 mm diameter
- The lesions are aligned with the long axis parallel to the skin folds; located on the gluteal surfaces, with no involvement of the inguinal folds and the gluteal cleft (absence of diaper contact).

Causes

The etiology of granuloma gluteale infantum is unclear. It is believed to be a cutaneous response to local inflammation, maceration and secondary infection.

Diapering-related items (e.g, diapers, plastic pants, paper napkins, laundry detergents, starch and powder), halogenated corticosteroids, candidal infection and urine and feces are possible etiologies.

Sparing of deep body folds suggests that contact occlusion is predisposing.

Age

The condition develops in the diaper area of infants aged between 4 and 9 months.

Treatment

Lesions spontaneously resolve generally not requiring treatment.

Treatment of any initiating inflammatory process, with its associated maceration and secondary infection, is beneficial.

Protectants

Use of zinc oxide (desitin cream) 15% ointment or 25% paste.

GENITAL ULCERS

The differential diagnosis for genital ulcers in children includes not only sexually transmitted diseases, but also other nonsexually related infections and autoimmune disorders [such as Behcet's disease, (Fig. 5.30)].

There has been a recently-reported condition called "vulval aphthosis" which is nonspecific and not associated with sexually transmitted infections. A viral etiology is implicated like Epstein Barr virus, Cytomegalovirus and Influenza A. These patients would present with a previous history of fever or upper respiratory tract infection and would go to the gynecologist's clinic with a painful erythematous ulcer of the labia (Fig. 5.31). Further investigation would yield a negative history of sexual contact. Treatment consist of addressing the pain and swelling with NSAIDs. The role of antibiotics and antivirals for these cases is controversial.

APHTHOUS LESION IN BEHCET'S DISEASE

Behcet's disease is a chronic multisystemic inflammatory disorder classically characterized by a triad of symptoms that include recurring crops of mouth ulcers (aphthous

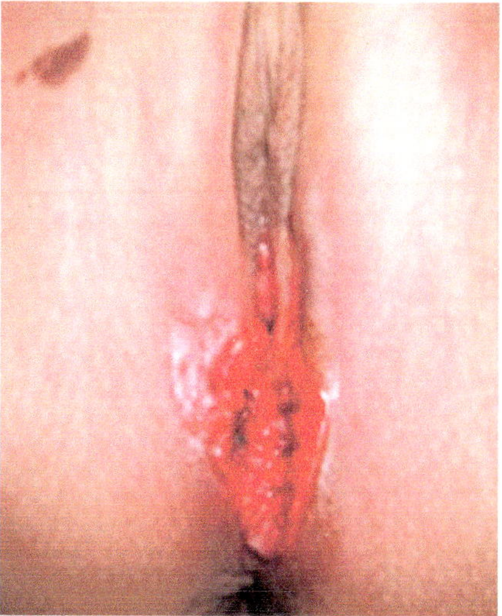

Fig. 5.30: Huge genital ulcer in a patient with Behcet's disease, postdebridement

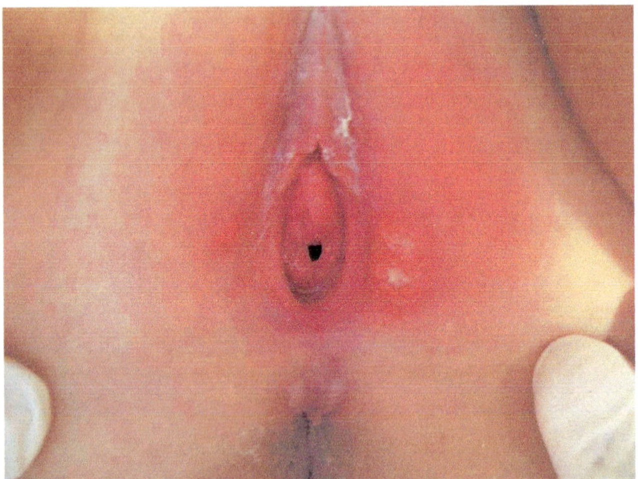

Fig. 5.31: Genital ulcer in a child with a history of upper respiratory tract infection

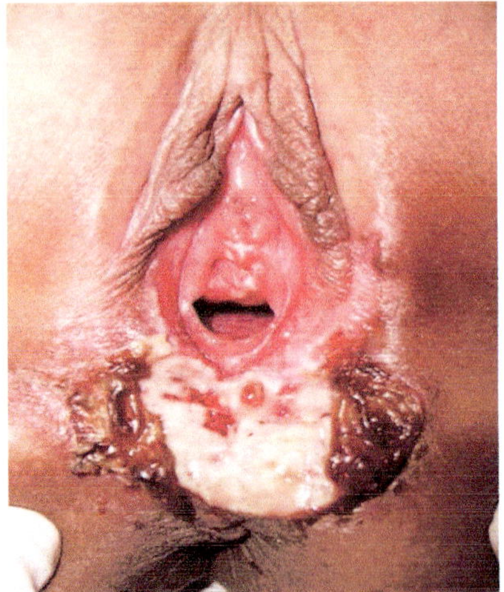

Fig. 5.33: Genital ulcer in an adolescent with the Behcet's disease. Ulcers may be necrotic with purulent material

ulcers), genital ulcers and inflammation of a specialized area around the pupil of the eye (the uvea).

Etiology

- Cause is unknown
- There is probable altered immunity in genetically predisposed patients
- Racial predilection for individuals of Asian or Middle Eastern descent
- Disease is not contagious

Symptoms

- Ulcers in the mouth (gums, tongue and inner lining of the mouth) are usually multiple and recurrent and may be extensive showing a pseudomembranous coating as shown in the Figure 5.32.

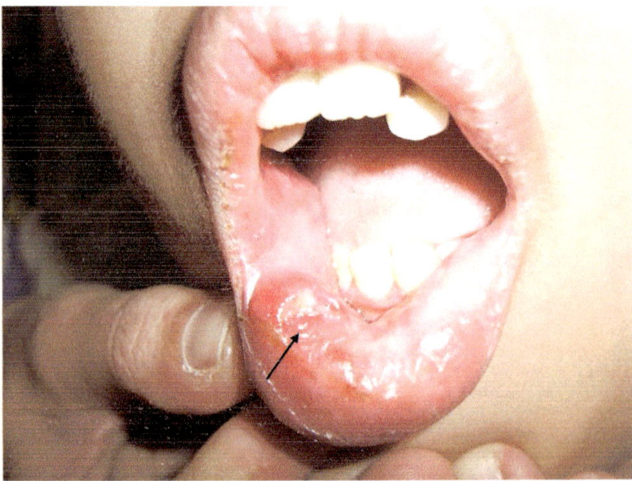

Fig. 5.32: Oral ulcer in a patient with Behçet's disease marked by an arrow

- Genital areas (scrotum and penis of males and vulva in females) are painful and generally recur in crops that are well-defined and very tender with fibrinous bases ranging in size from a few millimeters to 30 mm in diameter. Fistulae with partial or complete destruction of the labia may develop as shown in the Figure 5.33.
- To complete the triad, inflammation of the eye involving the front of the eye (uveitis) or back of the eye (retinitis) can lead to blindness
- Associated symptoms like fever, malaise, acneiform lesions or cutaneous nodules on the skin, arthritis, synovitis, and thrombophlebitis. Associated erythema nodosum and erythema multiforme have been reported.
- Other areas of the body that can be affected by the inflammation of Behcet's syndrome include the retina, brain, joints, skin and bowels.

Diagnosis

Behcet's disease is diagnosed based on the finding of recurrent mouth ulcerations combined with any two of the following: eye inflammation, genital ulcerations, or skin abnormalities.

Management

Treatment is based on the severity and location of lesions in an individual patient.

1. For local symptoms, topical superpotent steroids applied twice a day.
2. For mouth and genital ulcers, steroid (cortisone) gels, pastes and creams can be helpful. Extremely painful ulcers may be treated with an injection of intralesional triamcinolone.

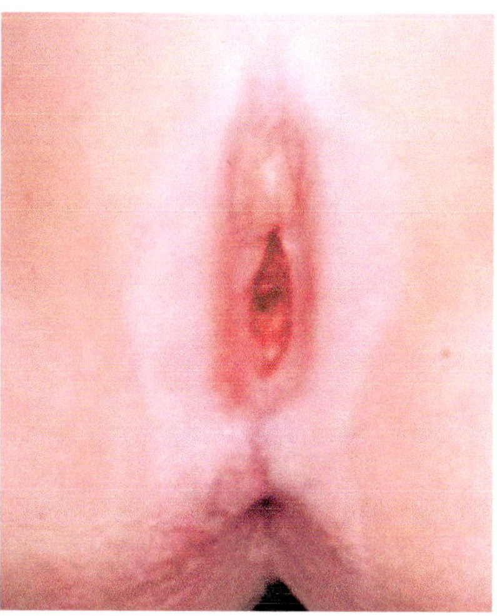

Fig. 5.34: Labial atrophy from chronic steroid use

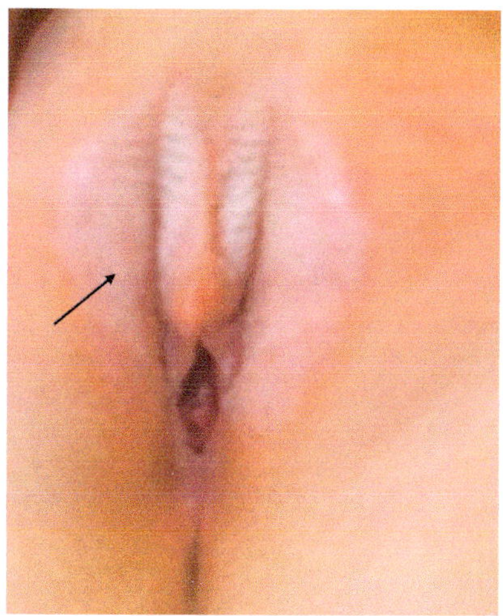

Fig. 5.35: "Keyhole" pattern of involvement from the skin of the vulva to the skin around the anus shown by arrow

3. For joint inflammation, nonsteroidal anti-inflammatory (NSAID) drugs or oral steroids are useful.
4. For eye inflammation, exhaustive and consistent monitoring by an ophthalmologist is warranted.
5. In systemic cases where arteries, eyes and brain may be difficult to treat, use of immunosuppressive agents is helpful. These include Chorambucil (Leukeran), Azathioprine (Imuran), Cyclophosphamide (Cytoxan), methotrexate and colchicines.

LICHEN SCLEROSUS

Lichen sclerosus is an uncommon condition that creates patchy, white wrinkly [atrophic, (Fig. 5.34)] skin that's thinner than normal. Lichen sclerosus may affect skin on any part of a body, but most often involves skin of the vulva, skin around the anus and keyhole or hourglass pattern as shown in the Figure 5.35.

Symptoms

- Itching (pruritus), may result in erosions, petechiae, fissures and small purpura
- Discomfort, on or around the genital or anal areas
- Tenderness of the affected areas on skin
- Easy bruising or tearing
- In severe cases, bleeding, blistering or ulcerated lesions.

Appearance

Early in the disease, small white spots appear on the skin. The spots are usually shiny and smooth. Later, the spots grow into bigger patches. The skin on the patches becomes thin and crinkled. Then, the skin tears easily and bright red or purple bruises are common. Sometimes, the skin becomes scarred. If the disease is a mild case, there may be no symptoms.

Etiology

The exact cause of lichen sclerosus is not known. However, the condition may be related to a lack of sex hormones in the affected skin or to an overactive immune system. Previous skin damage at a particular site on your skin may increase the likelihood of lichen sclerosus at that location. Lichen sclerosus is not contagious (it can't be caught from another person).

Diagnostic

- Cutaneous appearance
- Biopsy

Management

- Topical steroid (high potency clobetasol propionate 0.05% ointment) BID for six weeks; then taper, monitor for topical steroid side effects (i.e. labial atrophy)
- Proper hygiene; emollients
- Consider immune modulating medications such as tacrolimus (Protopic) and pimecrolimus (Elidel).

BIBLIOGRAPHY

1. Bernardino MS. Clinical features and microbiology of vulvovaginitis in Filipino prepubertal children. (Unpublished).
2. Emans SJH, Laufer M, Goldstein G. Pediatric and Adolescent Gynecology, 4th edn. Philadelphia: Lippincot Williams & Wilkins, 2005.
3. San Filipo J, Muram D. Clinical Pediatric and Adolescent Gynecology. New York: Informa Healthcare, 2009.

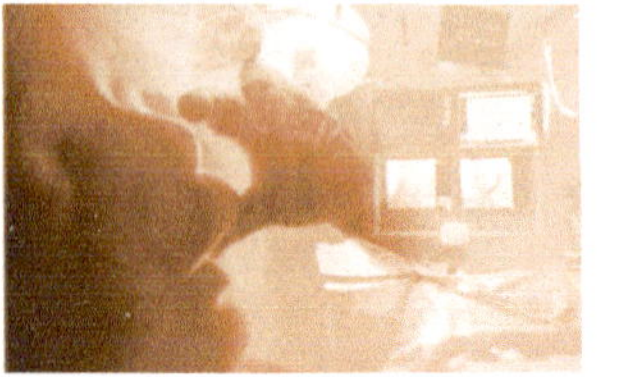

6 Normal and Precocious Puberty

Blanca C De Guia

Puberty is the transition between childhood and adulthood and the attainment of the ability to reproduce. The start of puberty was pegged by Marshall and Tanner to be 8–13 years in girls and 9 6/12 to 13 6/12 years in boys. Among females, the first sign of puberty is breast budding or thelarche. This is followed by the development of pubic hair, a period of growth spurt and the onset of menstruation (menarche).

Normal puberty starts with the awakening of complex neuroendocrine mechanisms, which depends on the activation of the hypothalamic-pituitary-gonadal axis as shown in Figure 6.1. Changes in the frequency and the amplitude of pulsatile gonadotropin releasing hormone (GnRH) secretion affect the release of pituitary follicle stimulating hormone (FSH) and luteinizing hormone (LH). Signals from the environment such as nutrition, light, stressors and endocrine disrupters might impinge on the hypothalamic signaling network directly or through peripheral signals.

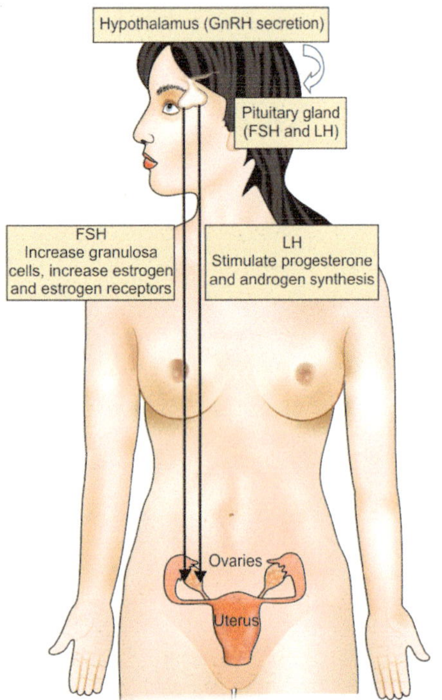

Fig. 6.1: The hypothalamic-pituitary axis

Thelarche, which is the first appearance of breast development, marks the onset of puberty in girls. This is followed by the appearance of pubic hair (pubarche), which is dependent on adrenal androgens. This increase in androgen production is also referred as adrenarche and may occur independently of the pituitary-gonadal maturation or gonadarche. The next phase is manifested by acceleration in growth velocity. This may difficult to ascertain because it requires several accurate measurements of height. The onset of menstruation is the last phase in the puberty process. In the Pediatric and Adolescent Gynecology Unit, review of records of all pubertal patients seen from 2002 to 2008 showed that the average age of menarche in this group is 11.96 years.

Tanner staging assessment by professionals provides reliable information regarding puberty stages; although this may be limited by interobserver variation as shown in the Figures 6.2 to 6.5.

PRECOCIOUS PUBERTY

Precocious puberty (Fig. 6.6) has been defined as the onset of breast or pubic hair development before the age of eight years.

Traditionally, classification as to etiology differentiates between central and peripheral precocious puberty. Several variants of precocious puberty have also been identified, which include isolated premature thelarche, premature adrenarche or premature menarche. Tables 6.1 and 6.2 show the different etiologies of precocious puberty.

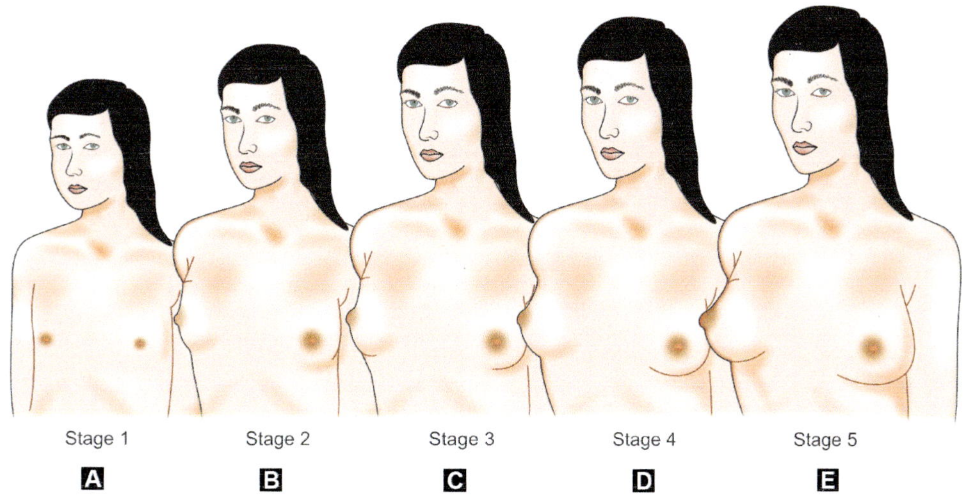

Figs 6.2A to E: Breast Tanner stages: (A) Stage-1 preadolescent; (B) Stage-2 breast and papilla elevated as small mound; areolar diameter increased; (C) Stage-3 breast, areola enlarged, no contour separation; (D) Stage-4 areola and papilla form secondary mound; (E) Stage-5 mature nipple projects, areola part of general breast contour

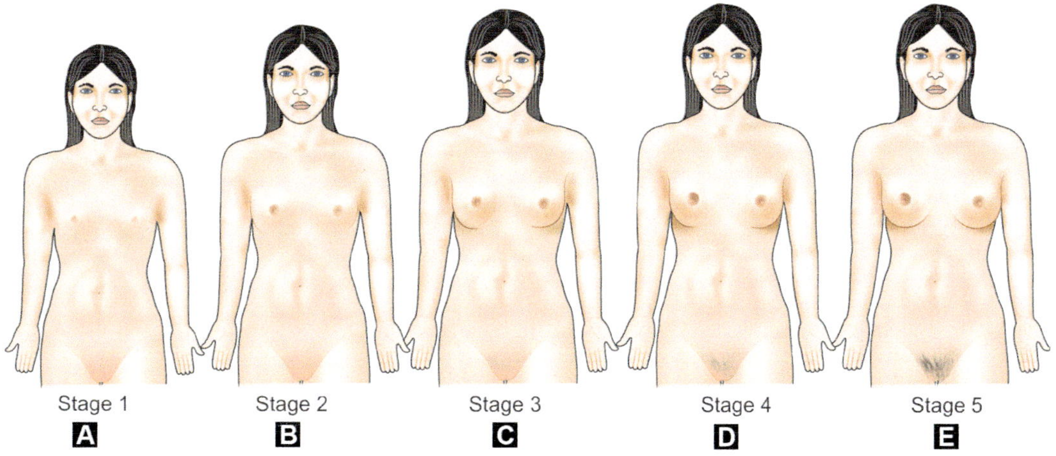

Figs 6.3A to E: Pubic hair Tanner stages: (A) Stage-1 preadolescent; (B) Stage-2 sparse, lightly pigmented, straight medial border of labia; (C) Stage-3 darker, beginning to curl, increase in amount; (D) Stage-4 coarse, curly, abundant; (E) Stage 5 adult feminine triangle, medial surface of the thigh

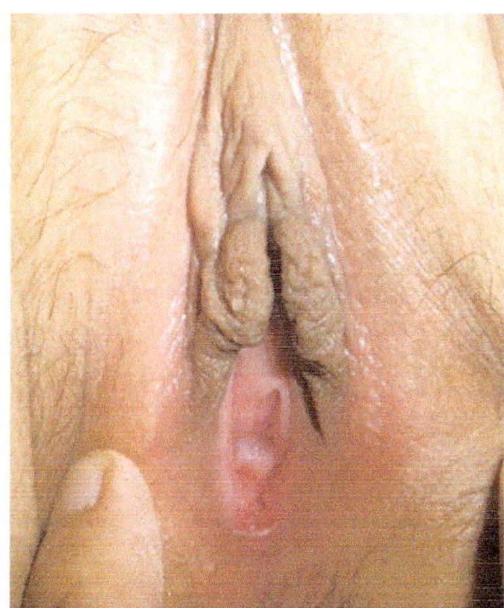

Fig. 6.4: Tanner stage 2 pubic hair. Sparse growth of long, downy, slightly pigmented pubic hair, straight or slightly curved, appearing chiefly along the labia

Fig. 6.5: Tanner stage 1 breast, prepubertal. There is only elevation of the papilla

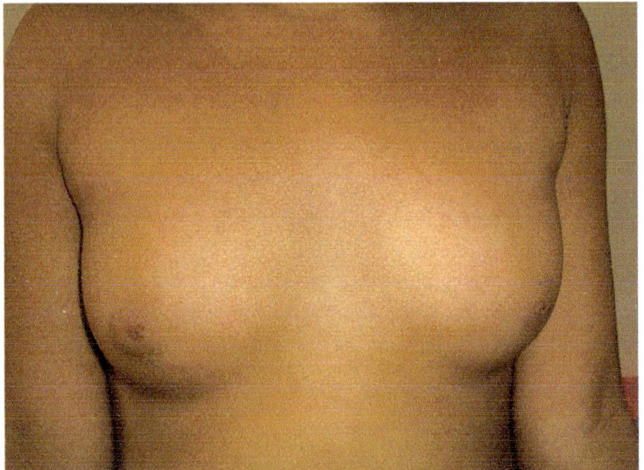

Fig. 6.6: Precocious puberty in a 3-year-old girl with Tanner stage 3 breasts

Case of Precocious Puberty

A 3-year-old girl patient consulted for vaginal bleeding. At one year of age, she was noted to have bilateral breast budding. When she was two years old, she had an episode of vaginal bleeding, which was scanty (around 3 panty changes) and lasted for four days. She was not brought for medical evaluation during that time. Four days prior to consult, there was recurrence of the vaginal bleeding, moderate in amount. Review of systems was unremarkable. The patient had no history of genital trauma or sexual abuse.

The patient weighed 23 kg (> 95 percentile for age) and had a height of 106.5 cm (> 95 percentile for age). Basal metabolic index (BMI) was normal at 20.28. She had no skin lesions. There was no enlargement of the thyroid gland. Breasts were enlarged and had a Tanner stage of 3. The abdomen was flat, soft, with no masses noted as shown in the Figures 6.7 and 6.8.

The patient had no pubic hair (Tanner stage 1). On examination of the genitalia, the hymen was found intact with an annular shape. The vaginal mucosa was pink. There was no note of vaginal discharge. There were multiple white-colored papules at the inferior aspect of both labia majora as shown in the Figures 6.9A and B.

Ultrasound of the pelvis (Figs 6.10 to 6.12) revealed a uterus, which measured 3.37–4.37 x 1.75–1.88 x 1.57 cm. Endometrial thickness was 0.51 cm. No adnexal masses were noted.

Final Diagnosis

Central precocious puberty (No CNS lesion).

Follicular Cyst Causing Precocious Puberty

A 2-year and 11-month-old girl patient was having breast enlargement and vaginal bleeding. On initial examination, she had Tanner stage 3 breasts and estrogenized vulval and vaginal mucosa (Figs 6.13 and 6.14). Her serum FSH, LH and estradiol were normal. Subsequent follow-ups showed

Table 6.1:
Central causes of precocious puberty

Central causes (Gonadotropin dependent, may be progressive)	*Distinguishing history and physical examination*	*Important diagnostic workups*
1. Central nervous system pathology		
A. Injury—pregnancy related, trauma, radiation, infection	History of injury signs of pituitary deficits	On magnetic resonance imaging (MRI), there is either evidence of injury of normal findings
B. Hypothalamic hamartroma	Seizure	On MRI, there is mass involving hypothalamus and/or optic chiasm
C. Hypothalamic mass, such as glioma, germ cell tumor and other cerebral lesions affecting hypothalamus	Neurologic symptoms, such as headache, altered sensorium, visual impairment, etc.	On MRI, there is no lesion
2. Non central nervous system (CNS) pathology	History of adoption (probably chemical exposure). History of familial precocity (i.e. possible chromosome 14 changes)	On MRI, there is no lesion
3. Sex steroid exposure	History of central precocity and treatment	On MRI, there is no finding

Table 6.2:
Peripheral causes of precocious puberty

Peripheral causes (gonadotropin-independent)	*Distinguishing history and physical examination*	*Important diagnostic workups*
1. Ovarian pathology		
A. Granulosa cell tumor	Sudden breast enlargement, abdominal tumor with or without pain	Pelvic ultrasound showing tumor
B. Ovarian edema	Breast and pubic hair development	Pelvic ultrasound showing enlargement
2. Adrenal disorders		
A. Adrenal tumors	Virilization, rarely estrogen producing	CT scan of adrenal mass Elevated dehydroepiandrosterone (DHEAS) and other adrenal steroid precursors
B. Congenital adrenal hyperplasia	Virilization	Activated adrenal steroid precursors especially 17-OH progesterone (basal or after corticotrophin stimulation test)
3. Iatrogenic		
A. Exogenous sex steroid (usually topical)	History of exposure sometimes with visualization	Not reliable sex steroid levels
B. Estrogenic endocrine disrupting chemicals (modulated timing of HPO activation)	History of exposure on adopted children. Early pubertal changes	None
4. Primary hypothyroidism	Clinically hypothyroid	Elevated TSH, low thyroxine. Normal bone aging
5. Autoimmune activation of the gonads (somatic mutation of GNAS gene)		
A. Recurrent autonomous ovarian cysts	Sudden breast enlargement and early vaginal bleeding. May be isolated pubertal changes	Pelvic ultrasound showing ovarian cysts which may be large
B. McCune-Albright syndrome	Above plus café-au-lait skin lesions or bone pain due to polyostotic fibrous dysplasia	Above bone lesions or fibrous dysplasia

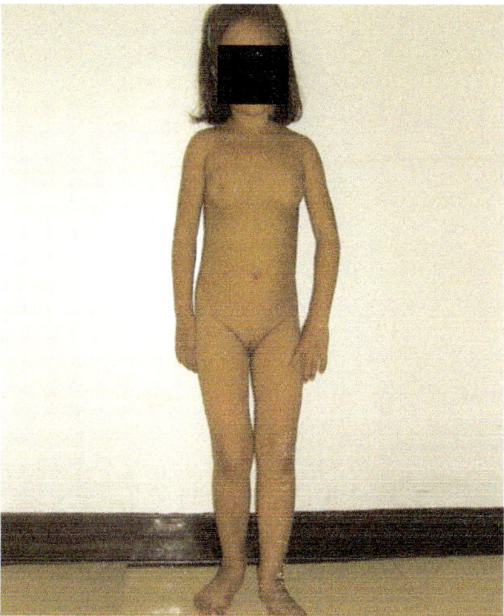

Fig. 6.7: The patient at 3 year of age with normal BMI, but with breast budding

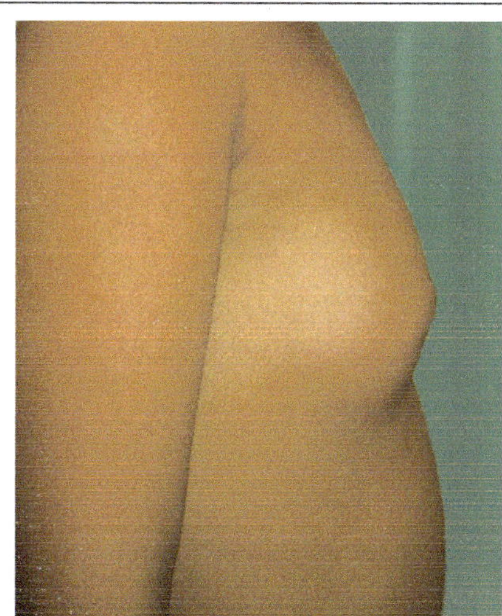

Fig. 6.8: Tanner stage 3 breasts are noted

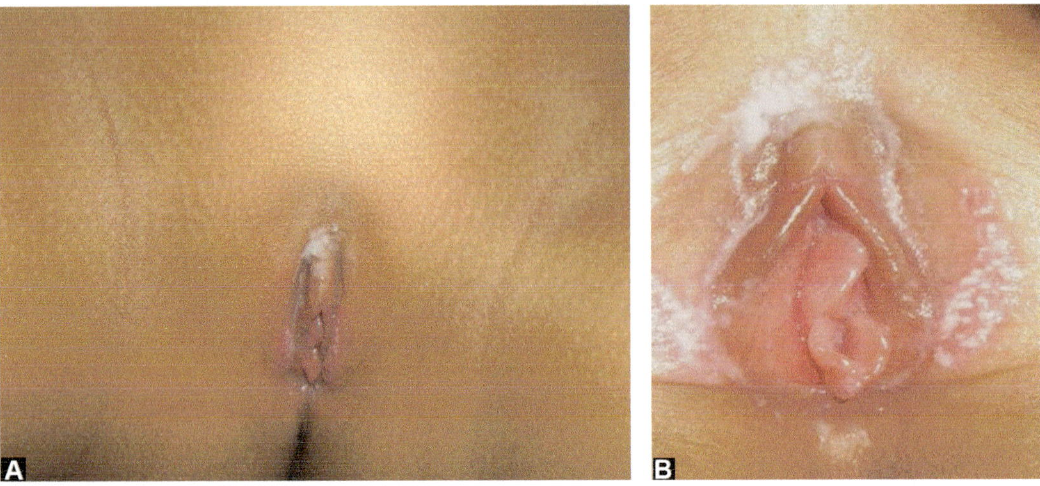

Figs 6.9A and B: Presence of multiple white colors at the inferior aspect of both the labia majora

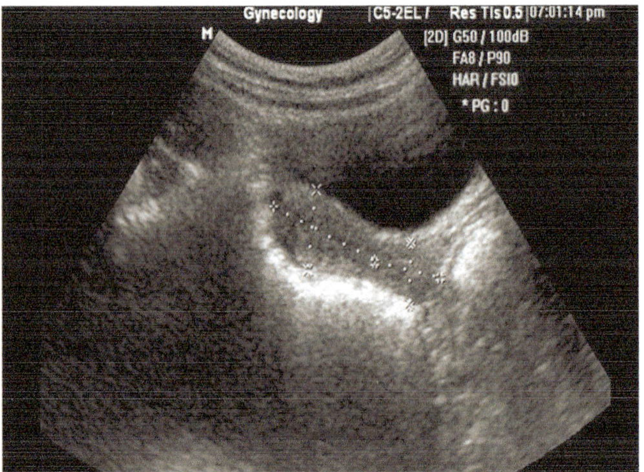

Fig. 6.10: Uterus

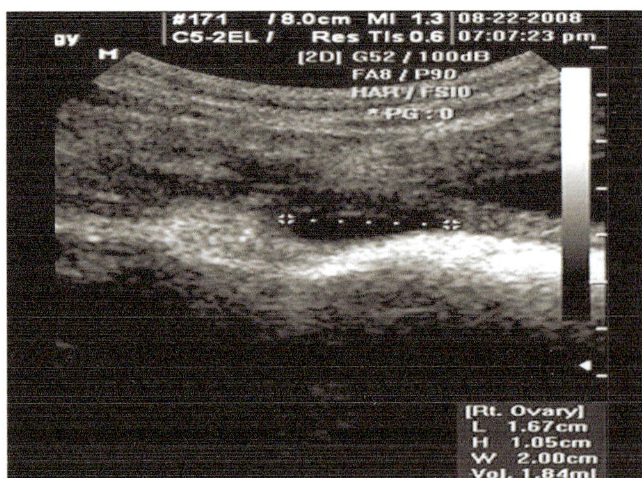

Fig. 6.12: Right ovary

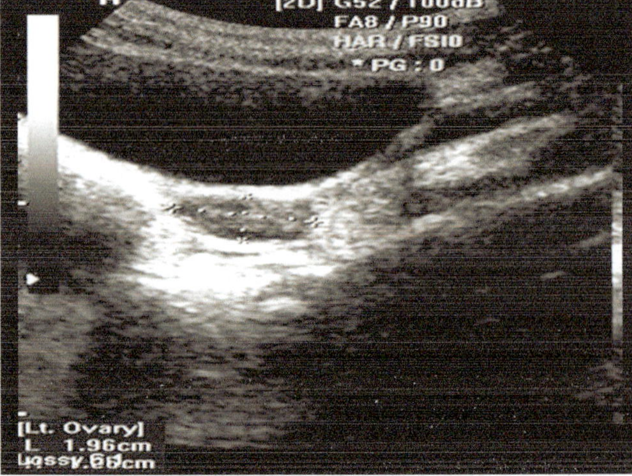

Fig. 6.11: Left ovary

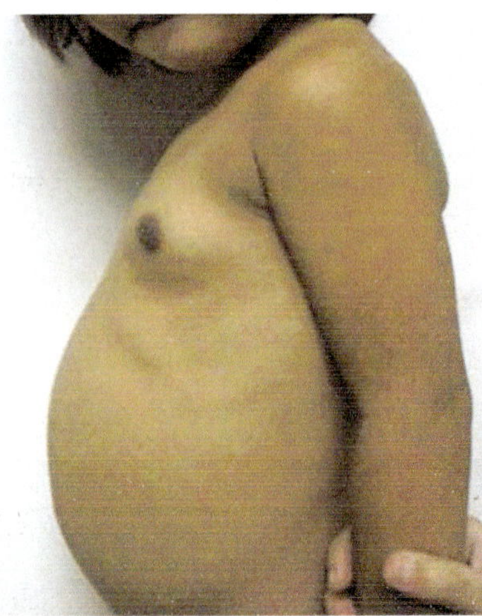

Fig. 6.13: Tanner stage 3 breasts in a 2-year and 11-month-old girl

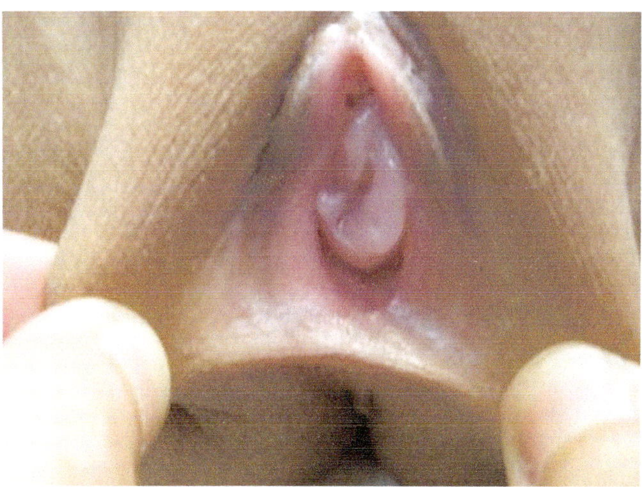

Fig. 6.14: Genital examination showed an estrogenized looking vulval and vaginal mucosa

an increasing trend on the serum estradiol with decreased serum FSH.

One year after the onset of breast enlargement, a 5 x 4 cm cystic left ovarian mass was noted on pelvic ultrasound. The cyst was initially observed but there was no change in its size even after four months. The bone age of the patient was also advancing.

On exploratory laparotomy, there was note of a 5 x 4 cm cystic mass (Fig. 6.15), thin-walled with serous fluid. Histopathologic examination of the mass revealed the presence of follicular cyst as shown the Figure 6.16.

Postoperatively, there was no recurrence of vaginal bleeding. There was also note of decrease in the breast size as shown in the Figures 6.17 and 6.18.

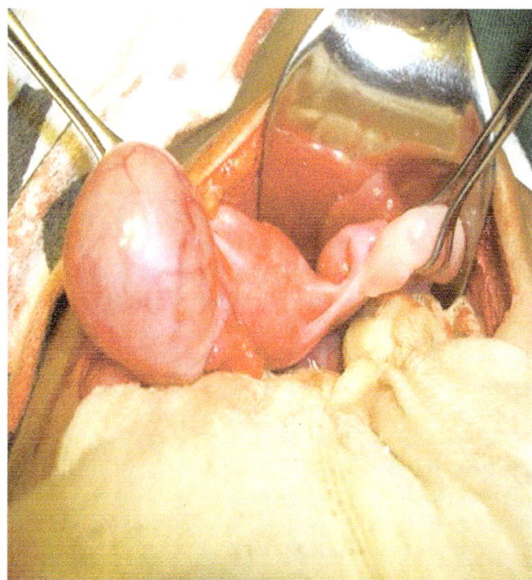

Fig. 6.15: A 5 x 4 cm thin-walled cystic mass is noted on operation

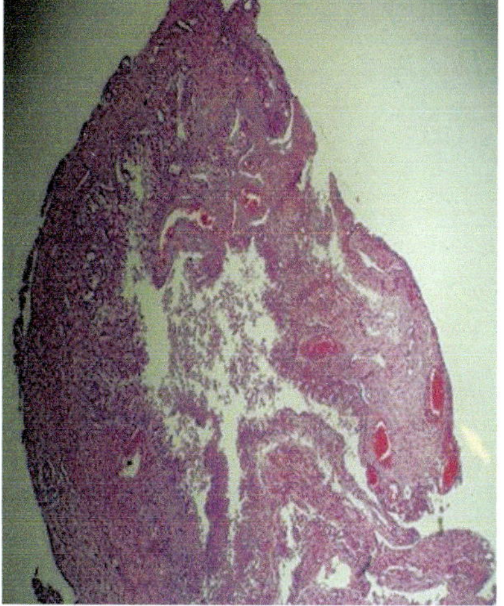

Fig. 6.16: Histopathology shows follicular cyst

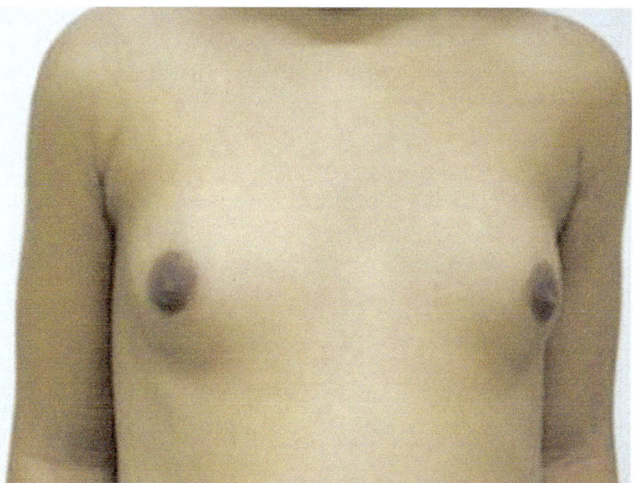

Fig. 6.17: Breasts (preoperative)

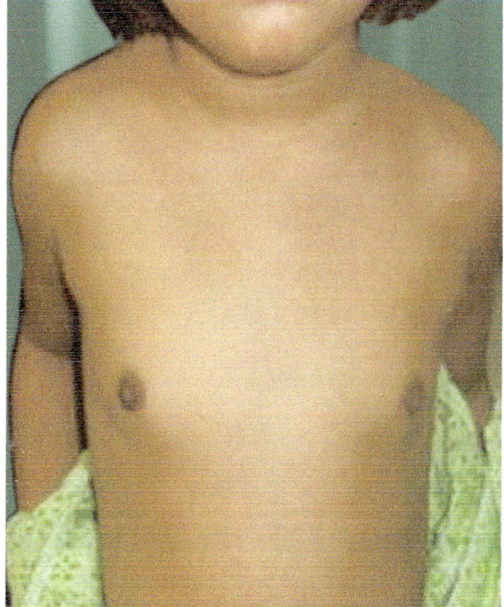

Fig. 6.18: Breasts (postoperative)

Table 6.3:
Benign variants of precocious puberty

Variants (usually isolated secondary sexual characteristics)	Distinguishing history and physical examination	Important diagnostic workups
1. Precocious thelarche	Unilateral or bilateral breast enlargement	Observe
2. Precocious pubarche	Pubic hair growth with or without axillary hair	Normal adrenal steroid precursors such as cortisol, 17-OH progesterone, dehydroepiandrosterone (DHEAS)
3. Precocious menarche	No breast or pubic hair growth	Normal bone aging
4. Nonprogressive precocity	If one or more pubertal changes occurred, there is note of regression	Normal bone aging Regular follow-up is important

Benign Variants of Precocious Puberty

Benign variants of precocious puberty are listed in the Table 6.3.

Isolated premature menarche in a 7-month-old girl patient shown in the Figure 6.19. This girl presented with irregular vaginal bleeding. The breasts are at Tanner stage 1 and show no enlargement (Fig. 6.20). The uterus is pre-pubertal on ultrasound examination, and there is no note of ovarian cysts as shown in the Figure 6.21. The hormone examination is all prepubertal levels; bone aging is at par with age and no vaginal lesion is seen on vaginoscopy.

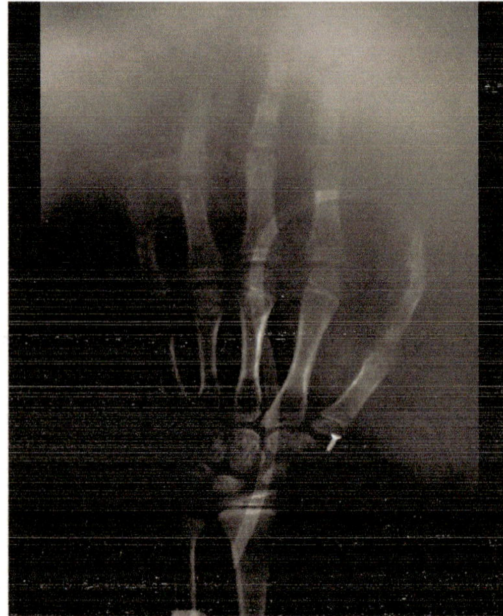

Fig. 6.19: Bone aging X-ray of the wrist of a 7-year-old girl with isolated premature menarche. Based on the Greulich and Pyle method, the bone age is consistent with chronologic age

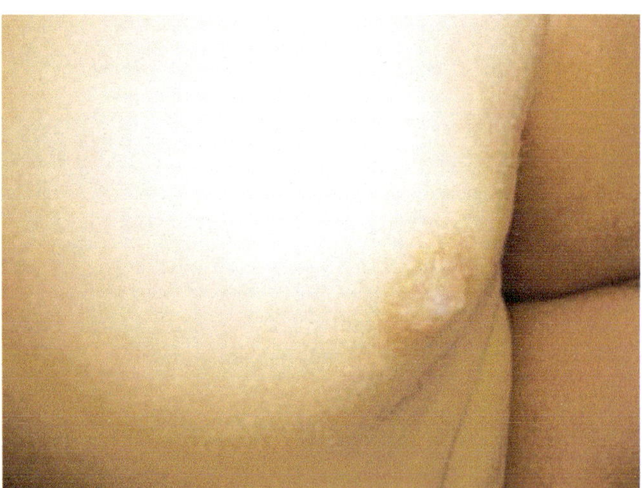

Fig. 6.20: The breast at Tanner stage 1 shows no enlargement

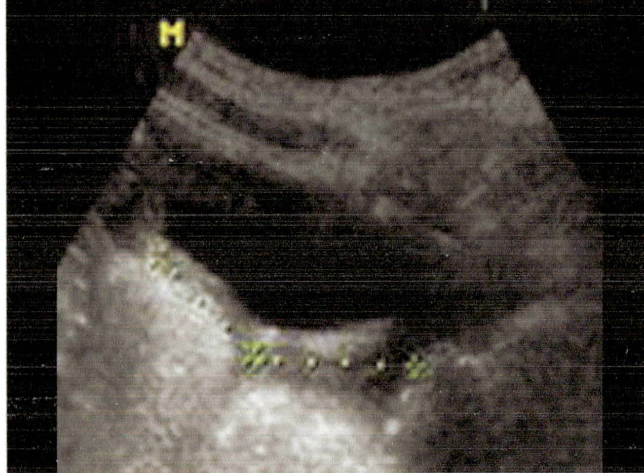

Fig. 6.21: Uterus is prepubertal on ultrasound examination with no note of ovarian cysts

Table 6.4:
Approach in the diagnosis of the precocious puberty

Pertinent findings on history
• Age of onset and timing of pubertal changes
• Check the child's growth rate based on standard growth charts (usually WHO growth chart is used)
• Exposure to hormones
• Central nervous system abnormalities, neurologic symptoms
• Past medical/family/social/psychological history
• Pubertal history, height and growth rates of family members
General physical examination
• Height, weight, body proportions, body mass index
• Neurologic deficit such as visual impairments
• Thyroid gland enlargement
• Café-au-lait spots
• Galactorrhea
Hormonal evaluation
• Gonadotropins
• LH:FSH ratios
• If < 1 prepubertal
• If >1 pubertal
• GnRH or GnRHa stimulation
• LH at 20, 30 or 40 minutes > 7
• Sex steroids
• Estradiol > 5 pg/ml suggestive of puberty
Bone aging
• If bone X-ray is advanced with > 2 standard deviations (SD), this is suggestive of early puberty
Pelvic sonography
• Check for uterine size and endometrial stripe
• Check for ovarian size and presence of cyst
Other relevant tests
• Cranial MRI or CT scan
• Thyroid function tests
• Serum prolactin
• DHEAS, 17-OH progesterone

Approach in the Diagnosis of the Precocious Puberty

Approach in the diagnosis of the precocious puberty is listed in the Table 6.4.

BIBLIOGRAPHY

1. Annual Reports 2002-2008. Pediatric and Adolescent Gynecology Unit. Philippine Children's Medical Center.
2. Brito VN, Latronico AC, Arnhold IJ, et al. Update on the etiology, diagnosis and therapeutic management

of sexual precocity. Arq Bras Endocrinol Metabol 2008;52:15-31.

3. Carel JC, Leger J. Precocious puberty. N Eng J of Med 2008;358:2366-77.
4. De Sousa G, Wunsch R, Andler W, et al. Precocious pseudopuberty due to autonomous ovarian cysts: a report of ten cases and long-term follow-up. Hormones 2008;7: 170-4.
5. Diamantopoulos S, Bao Y. Gynecomastia and premature thelarche: a guide for practitioners. Pediatrics in Review 2007;28(9):57-68.
6. Kaplowitz P. Clinical characteristics of 104 children referred for evaluation of precocious puberty. The Journal of Clinical Endocrinology and Metabolism 2004;89(6):3644-50.
7. Lee PA, Hook CP. Precocious puberty. In: Altchek A, Deligdisch L (Eds). Pediatric, Adolescent and Young Adult Gynecology. West Sussex, UK: Blackwell Publishing; 2009 pp. 159-70.
8. Merke DP, Cutler GB. Evaluation and management of precocious puberty. Archives of Disease in Childhood 1996; 75:269-71.
9. Midyett LK, Moore WV, Jacobson JD, et al. Are pubertal changes in girls before age 8 benign? Pediatrics 2003;111:47-51.
10. Natarajan A, Wales JK, Marven SS, et al. Precocious puberty secondary to massive ovarian oedema in a 6 month old girl. Eur J Endocrinol 2004;150:119-23.
11. New MI. Nonclassical 21-hydroxylase deficiency. The Journal of Clinical Endocrinology and Metabolism 2006; 9:4205-14.
12. Parent AS, Teilmann G, Juul A, et al. The timing of normal puberty and the age limits of sexual precocity: variations around the world, secular trends, and changes after migration. Endocrine Rev 2003;24:668-93.
13. Smith S, McClanahan K, Omar H. Adolescent pubertal development. In: San Filipo, et al. (Eds). Clinical Pediatric and Adolescent Gynecology. New York: Informa Healthcare 2009; pp. 20-39.

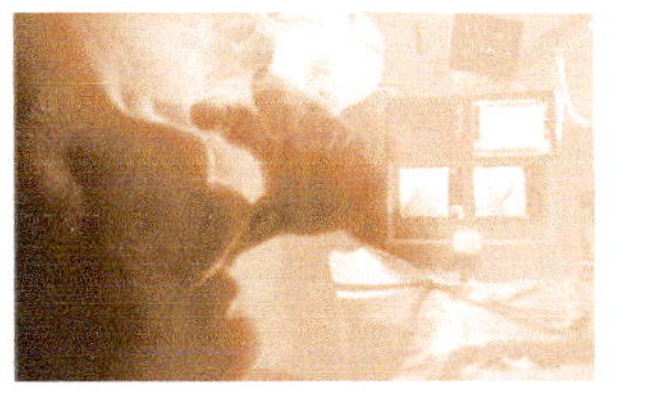

7 Delayed Puberty

Lorna F Ramos-Abad

DEFINITION

- Lack of the initial signs of sexual maturation by an age that is more than 2–2.5 SD above the mean for the population (~13 years in girls and 14 years in boys)
- Failure to reach Tanner stage 5 in 4 years from onset is also considered as delayed puberty

It is important to know the normal pattern of pubertal development (Fig. 7.1) to be able to pick up aberrant patterns when examining adolescent girls.

CAUSES OF DELAYED PUBERTY

Factors which determine pubertal onset includes genetic, sex, environment and metabolic.

- Delay in puberty is usually due to a state of hypogonadism which necessitates thorough investigation
- The first step is to determine whether the patient is hypergonadotropic or hypogonadotropic as shown in the Flow chart 7.1 and Figure 7.2.

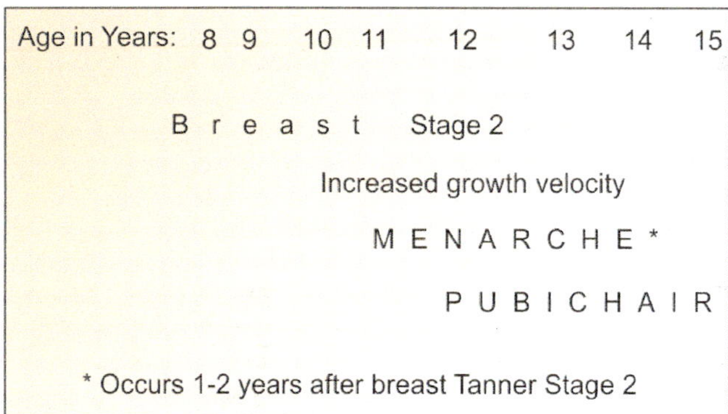

Fig. 7.1: Normal pubertal events

Flow chart 7.1: Approach to delayed puberty

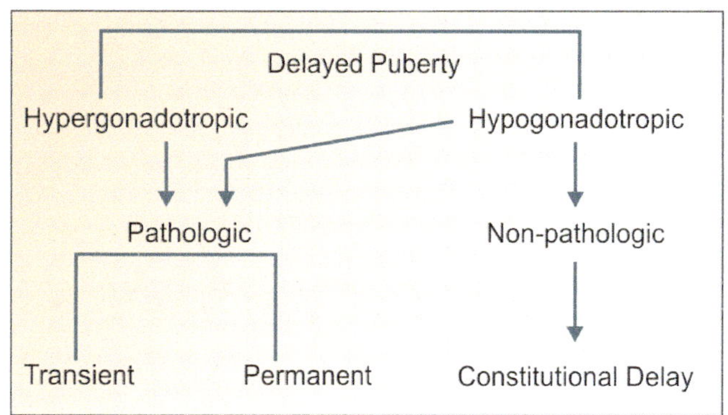

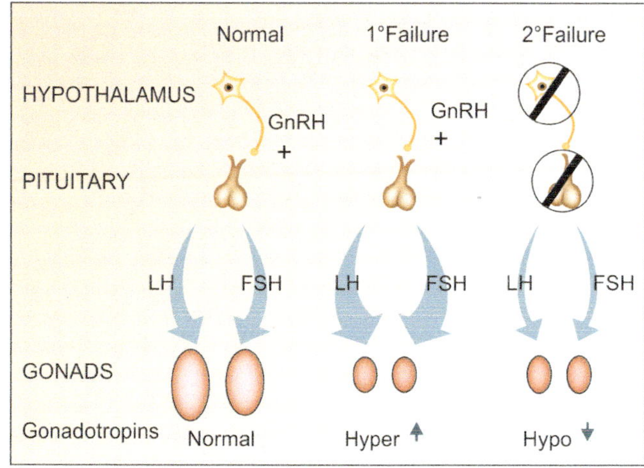

Fig. 7.2: Illustration of the hypothalamic-pituitary-gonadal axis. Both forms of hypogonadism result in smaller than normal gonads leading to pubertal delay

Constitutional Delay

Constitutional delay (CD) is the most common cause of delay and is usually associated with delayed growth. When the adolescent has no underlying illness or endocrinopathy and their growth rate is consistent with delayed growth curves on the longitudinal growth charts, then this assessment is made, which virtually is a diagnosis by exclusion. Growth velocity is normal at least 5 cm per year for children above 3 years old. There is a family history of constitutional delay in growth and puberty (CDGP) and predicted height is within mid-parental height.

Hypogonadotropic Hypogonadism

Hypogonadotropic hypogonadism (Table 7.1) is a secondary form of delayed puberty due to failure of the pituitary and hypothalamus to produce luteinizing hormone (LH) or follicle stimulating hormone (FSH) and gonadotropin releasing hormone (GnRH) respectively.

SAMPLE CASE 1

Systemic Illness Causing Pubertal Delay

This is the case of an 18-year-old girl patient (Fig. 7.3) with primary amenorrhea. Her height is below the 50th percentile for her age. She has juvenile rheumatoid arthritis. At her age, no secondary sexual characteristics are developed. Breasts and pubic hair remained at Tanner stage 1 (Figs 7.4A to C). Ultrasound evaluation showed prepubertal uterus and ovaries as shown in the Figures 7.5 and 7.6.

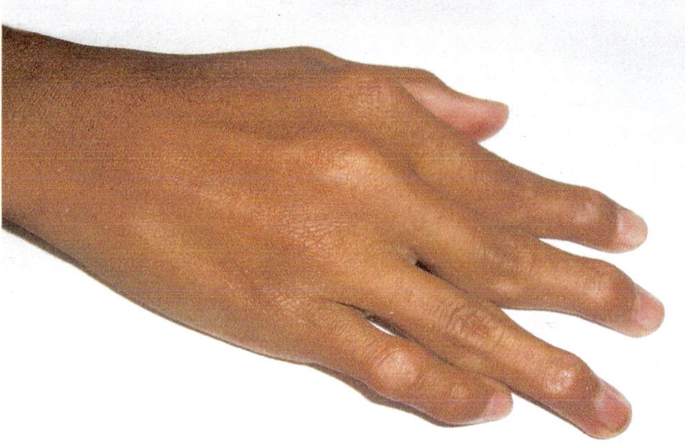

Fig. 7.3: Fingers show swan neck deformity which is typical feature of rheumatoid arthritis. She is also small for her age

Table 7.1: Causes of hypogonadotropic hypogonadism

Temporary causes with potential for normal function	*Permanent causes*
Constitutional delay of growth and puberty	Kallman syndrome Idiopathic HH
Chronic systemic illness, drug abuse	DAX-1 gene mutation GPR 54 gene mutation
Excessive energy or exercise expenditure	Multiple pituitary hormone deficiencies
Exogenous obesity	
Endocrinopathies (growth-hormone deficiency)	
Hypercortisolism	
Hypothyroidism	
Hyperprolactinemia	
Uncontrolled DM	
Malnutrition or malabsorption	
Psychiatric illness	

Hypergonadotropic Hypogonadism

This is due to the failure of the ovaries to develop normally and is associated with chromosomal, genetic and syndromic causes, usually congenital in origin.

Causes Include

The causes include Turner's syndrome (Figs 7.7 to 7.9), congenital adrenal hyperplasia, androgen receptor (AR) mutations, androgen insensitivity syndrome (AIS), autoimmune, chemotherapy, galactosemia, infectious, infiltration, irradiation and surgical.

SAMPLE CASE 2

Turner's Syndrome

The patient is a 17-year-old girl with primary amenorrhea and lack of secondary sexual characteristics.

EVALUATION OF DELAYED PUBERTY

History

- Assess general health and growth
- Exposure to irradiation or chemotherapy
- Physical activity
- Family history of pubertal timing and menarche.

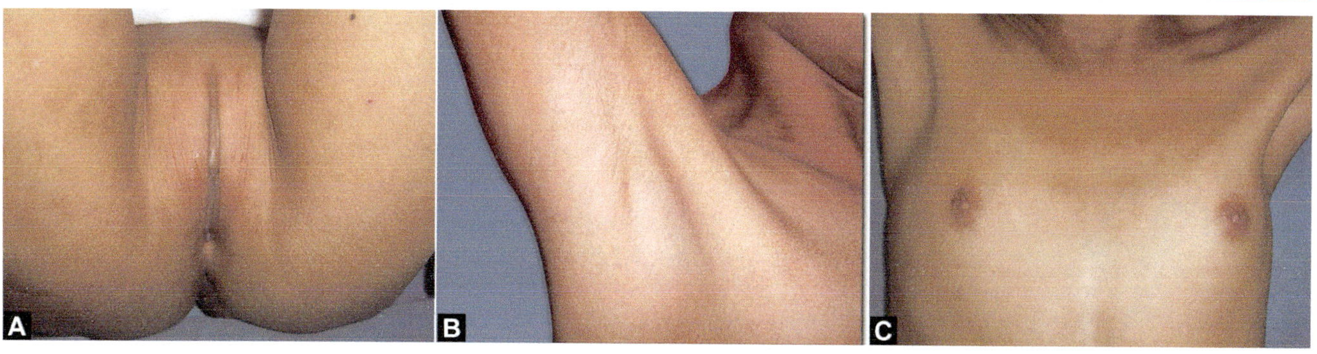

Figs 7.4A to C: (A) Lack of pubic hair; (B) Lack of axillary hair; (C) Breasts are under-developed

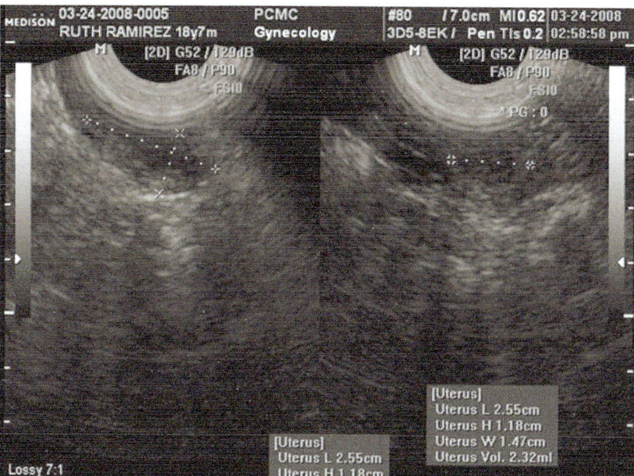

Fig. 7.5: Prepubertal uterus

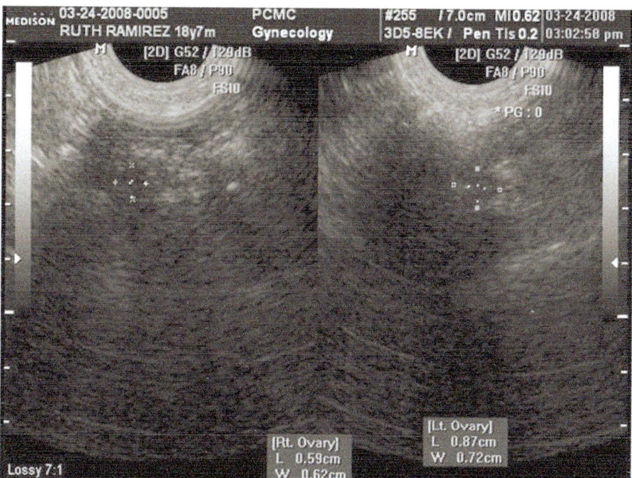

Fig. 7.6: Prepubertal ovaries

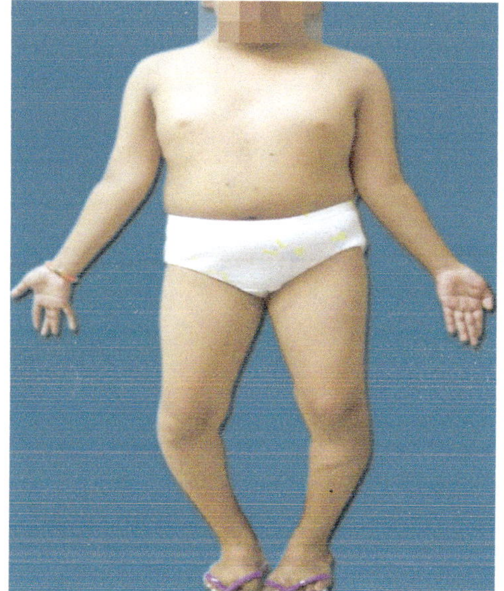

Fig. 7.7: Increased carrying angle of the arm, short stature

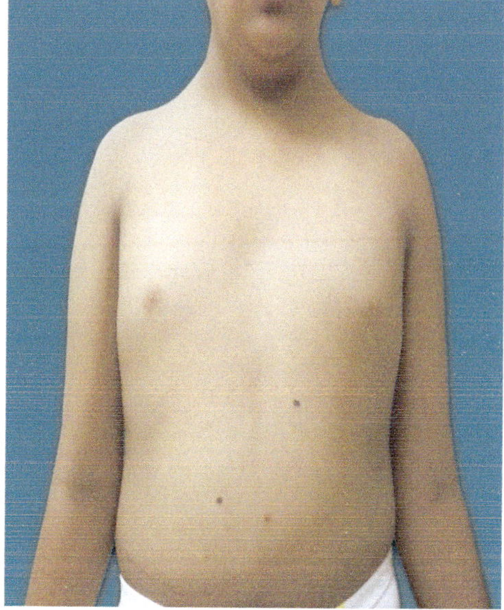

Fig. 7.8: No breast budding, shield-like chest

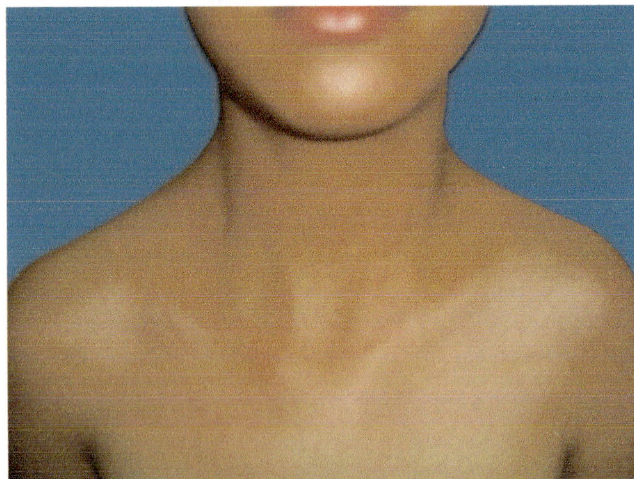

Fig. 7.9: Another patient with webbed neck

Physical Examination

- Measure height, weight and indices of nutrition
- Determine upper segment to lower segment ratio (US/LS ratio)
- Pubertal staging
- Testing of sense of smell.

Laboratory Tests

- Initial tests include LH, FSH which, if elevated, denote gonadal failure; if low, a GnRH stimulation test should be done
- To assess skeletal age, an X-ray of the left hand should be done
- CBC, electrolytes, liver function tests, ESR, prolactin and cortisol
- Insulin like growth factor-1 (IGF-1)
- TSH, free T4
- Sex steroids
- Cranial magnetic resonance imaging (MRI)
- BHCG stimulation testing
- Chromosomal analysis should be done in all girls with severe short stature (more than 2.5 SD from normal).

Management

- Depends on the cause

Induction of Puberty 10–12 years

- Estrogen: 0.3 mg conjugated E2 OD
- Ethinyl Estradiol: 5 µg daily
- Transdermal E2: (0.025 mg) 2x/week
- Increase dose q 6–12 months until full replacement dose is reached (0.625 E2; 20 µg EE).

BIBLIOGRAPHY

1. Rosenfeld RL, Cooke DW, Radovick S. Puberty and its disorders. In: Sperling M (Ed). Pediatric Endocrinology, 3rd edn. Pennsylvania: Saunders Elsevier, 2008.
2. www.endotext.org/male5.htmCJ [Accessed September 1, 2009].

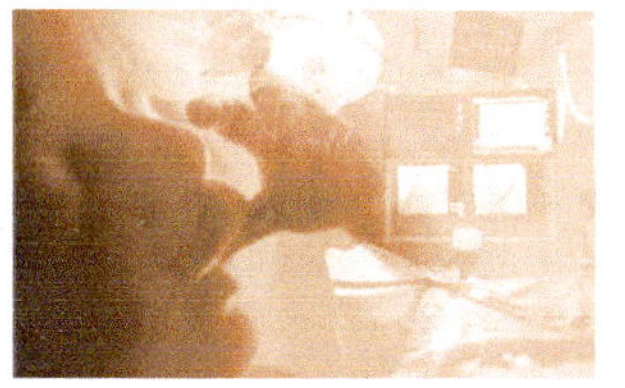

8

Hyperandrogenism in the Adolescent

Lorna F Ramos-Abad

Hyperandrogenism is the most common cause of menstrual disturbances in an adolescent in the face of normal estrogen (Table 8.1). Most cases arise from either an ovarian or adrenal dysfunction or a few from an abnormal peripheral formation of androgens. The manifestations include menstrual irregularity, hirsutism, acne, alopecia, deepening voice and clitoromegaly, central obesity.

Table 8.1
Causes of hyperandrogenism

Functional gonadal hyperandrogenism
Primary (dysregulation) functional ovarian hyperandrogenism
Secondary polycystic ovarian syndrome
• Poorly controlled classic congenital adrenal hyperplasia
• Ovarian steroidogenic blocks
• Syndromes of severe insulin resistance
• Portohepatic shunting
• Epilepsy or valproic acid therapy
Adrenal rests
Ovotesticular disorder
Chorionic gonadotropin related
Functional adrenal hyperandrogenism
Primary (dysregulation) functional adrenal hyperandrogenism
Congenital adrenal hyperplasia (Fig. 8.1)
Prolactin or growth hormone excess
Cushing syndrome
Peripheral androgen overproduction
Obesity
Idiopathic hyperandrogenism
Polycystic ovarian syndrome (PCOS)
Common form of PCOS
Uncommon form of PCOS

EVALUATION OF HYPERANDROGENISM

History

- *Menstrual history:* age at menarche, length of time between periods, quantity of menstrual flow, presence of dysmenorrhea
- *Onset:* onset at menarche suggests PCOS, idiopathic hirsutism or 21-hydroxylase deficiency. Onset distinct from menarche suggests tumor
- *Progression:* rapid progression of hirsutism or other symptoms suggests tumor
- History of development of secondary sexual characteristics
- Onset of hyperandrogenic manifestations
- Growth history
- Family history of diabetes and PCOS
- Social history, dietary intake or habits, exercise patterns, alcohol intake.

Physical Examination

- Measurement of height, weight, BMI and plotting on corresponding charts
- Obtain blood pressure
- If obese, get waist-to-hip ratio (value > 0.72 indicates central obesity)
- Look for hirsutism, acne, alopecia, acanthosis nigricans [suggestive of PCOS or idiopathic hirsutism (Fig. 8.2)]
- Look for virilization (degree of virilization could be assessed using Ferriman-Gallwey score; clue for ovarian or adrenal tumor, hyperthecosis).

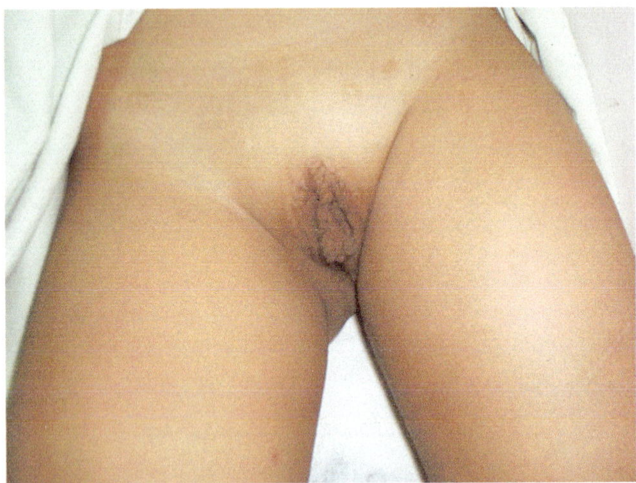

Fig. 8.1: A 13-year-old female with virilization (growth of beard and enlarged clitoris) due to simple virilizing congenital adrenal hyperplasia secondary to 21-hydroxylase enzyme deficiency

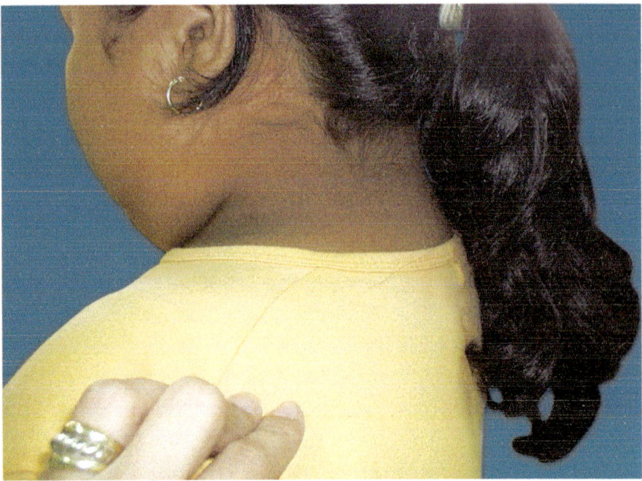

Fig. 8.2: Obese adolescent with acanthosis nigricans and hyperinsulinism

Laboratory Tests

- Total and free testosterone, dehydroepiandrosterone-sulfate (DHEA-S) and androstenedione tests to confirm hyperandrogenism
- 17-hydroxyprogesterone test to rule out mild 21-hydroxylase deficiency
- Prolactin
- Thyroid stimulating hormone test in all patients with oligo-amenorrhea or dysfunctional bleeding
- Fasting blood glucose and serum insulin
- Serum cortisol diurnal pattern test for suspicion of cushing syndrome
- Pregnancy test.

Imaging

- Transvaginal ultrasound: confirm polycystic ovaries, rule out ovarian tumor
- Computed tomography of adrenal glands: if ovarian ultrasound is normal and tumor is suspected.

Management

- Individualized according to etiology, symptoms and patient's goals
- For hirsutism: cosmetic measures such as bleaching, shaving, depilatory agents, waxing, LASER therapy
- Dermatological and menstrual abnormalities
  - Combination oral contraceptives (OCPs): Suppress plasma androgens, free testosterone particularly, by inhibiting ovarian function
  - Progestin monotherapy: Alternative to OCP to control menstrual irregularities
  - Micronized progesterone 100–200 mg daily at bedtime for 7 to 10 days induces withdrawal of bleeding in most patients
  - Antiandrogen: Improves hirsutism
  - Spironolactone 100 mg BID
  - Cyproterone acetate: Used with estrogen at 50 to 100 mg OD on days 1 to 10 when estrogen is given on days 1 to 21
  - Topical minoxidil for alopecia

BIBLIOGRAPHY

1. Buggs C, Rosenfeld RL. Polycystic ovary syndrome in adolescence. Endoc Metab Clin North Am 2005;34:677-705.
2. Rosenfeld RL, Cooke DW, Radovick S. Puberty and its disorders. Sperling Med, Pediatric Endocrinology, 3rd edn. Pennsylvania: Saunders Elsevier, 2008.

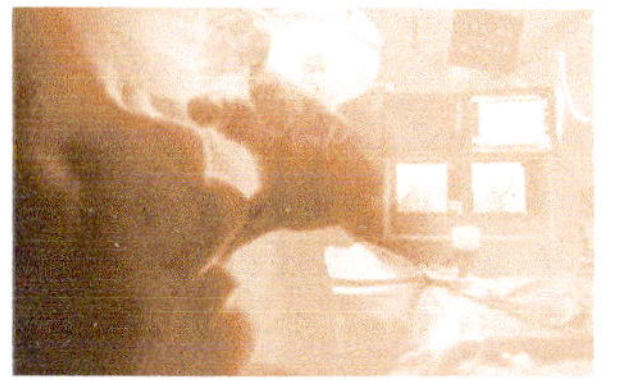

9 Polycystic Ovary Syndrome in Adolescents

Angela Sison-Aguilar

DIAGNOSIS

Polycystic ovary syndrome (PCOS) among adolescents with menstrual irregularity can be diagnosed using the same Rotterdam criteria as in adults.

Revised 2003 criteria (two out of three):

1. Oligo-ovulation and/or anovulation
2. Clinical and/or biochemical signs of hyperandrogenism
3. Polycystic ovaries (Fig. 9.1) and exclusion of other etiologies (congenital adrenal hyperplasia, androgen-secreting tumors and Cushing's syndrome).

CLINICAL PRESENTATION AND NATURAL COURSE

Amenorrhea may be the presenting symptom of PCOS in adolescence, but menstrual disorders, such as oligomenorrhea, and sometimes heavy menstrual bleeding occurs. Marked increased weight gain during puberty may be a manifestation of adolescent PCOS as shown in the Figure 9.2.

A more profound alternation in hypothalamic-pituitary-ovarian hormones exists among non-obese adolescent patients with PCOS compared with their obese counterparts. Their hormonal, lipid and metabolic profiles are similar to adult women. Among those who are obese, insulin resistance is more pronounced in the adolescent patient with PCOS compared to the non-obese counterpart.

LONG-TERM IMPLICATIONS

While adolescents and eventually adult women with PCOS are at increased risk for developing diabetes mellitus type II, especially those with the obese phenotype, it is uncertain whether modifying this risk factor during adolescence will reduce the incidence of DM type II in adulthood. Also, the link between PCOS and cardiovascular risk is uncertain as of present time.

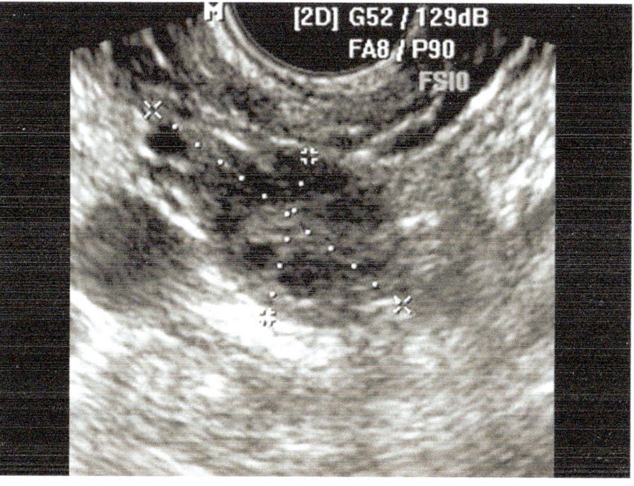

Fig. 9.1: Ultrasound of ovaries

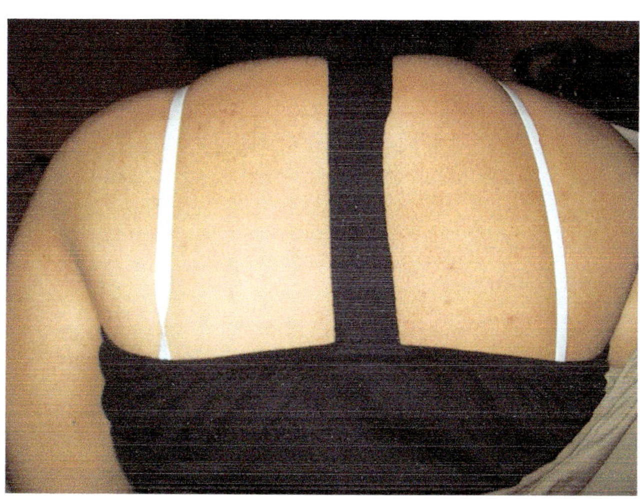

Fig. 9.2: Obesity

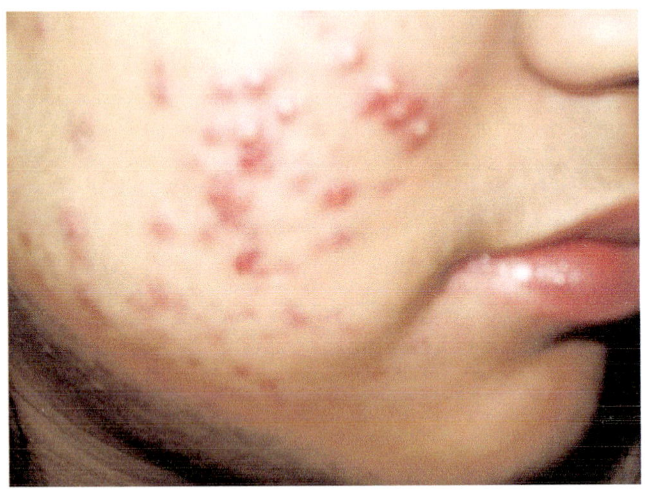

Fig. 9.3: Acne

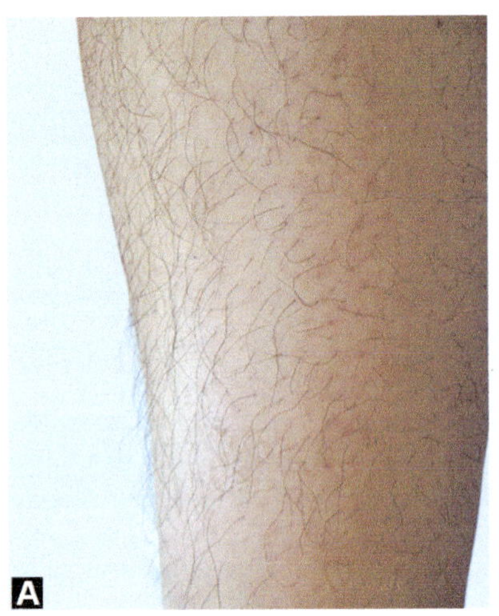

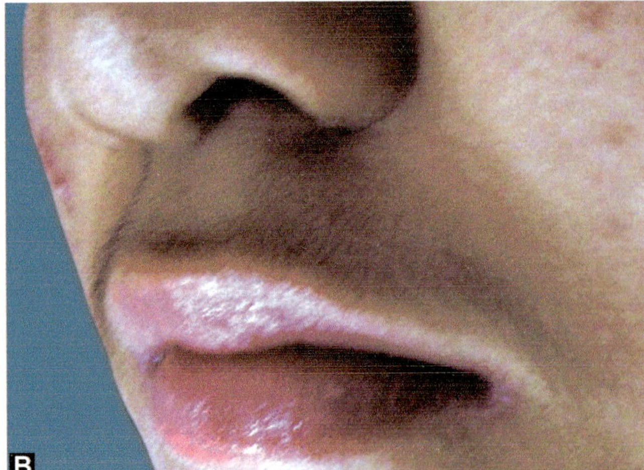

Figs 9.4A and B: Hirsutism

MANAGEMENT

Amenorrhea and Oligomenorrhea

Progesterone withdrawal bleeding is recommended for amenorrheic or oligomenorrheic adolescents. Mere weight loss may result in regular menstrual periods among obese girls with PCOS. Cyclical progestogen treatment for 10 days, every 4 to 6 weeks generally lead to withdrawal bleeding and prevent hyperplasia.

Weight Gain

Lifestyle changes are a first-line intervention in obese adolescents with PCOS. Glucose intolerance can be managed by diet and exercise, and appropriate weight control.

Acne and Hirsutism

Cyproterone-containing contraceptive pills are cost effective methods of managing adolescent PCOS patients with acne (Fig. 9.3) and hirsutism (Figs 9.4A and B). Drug treatments may take 6 to 9 months to show tangible results hence adjunctive measures, such as waxing, bleaching, depilation by electrolysis or LASER, may be resorted too. For adolescents who may additionally require contraception, oral contraceptive pills containing drospirenone, which is a derivative of spironolactone, may be prescribed.

Role of Insulin Sensitizers

Metformin given to adolescents showed decrease in testosterone levels, increase in HDL levels and improvement in menstrual cycles in small scale studies. No significant effect on insulin sensitivity has yet been demonstrated.

BIBLIOGRAPHY

1. Hickey M, Balen A. Menstrual disorders in adolescence: investigation and management. Human Reproduction Update 2003;9(5):493-504.
2. Legro R. Polycystic ovary syndrome and cardiovascular disease: a premature association? Endocrine Reviews 2003;24:302-12.
3. Mastorakos G, Koliopoulos C, Deligeoroglou E, et al. Effects of two forms of combined oral contraceptives on carbohydrate metabolism in adolescents with polycystic ovary syndrome. Fertility Sterility 2006;85:420-6.
4. Mathur R, Levin O, Azziz R. Use of ethinylestradiol/ drospirenone combination in patients with the polycystic ovary syndrome. Ther Clin Risk Manag 2008;4(2):487-92.
5. Norman RJ, Davies MJ, Lord J, et al. The role of lifestyle modification in polycystic ovary syndrome. Trends in Endocrinol Metab 2002;13:251-7.
6. Rittmaster R. Antiandrogen treatment of polycystic ovary syndrome. Endocrinology and Metabolism Clin North Am 1999;28:409-21.
7. Silfen M, Denburg R, Manibo A, et al. Early endocrine, metabolic and sonographic characteristics of polycystic ovary syndrome (PCOS): comparison between non-obese and obese adolescents. J Clin Endocrinol and Metab 2003;88:4682-8.
8. The Rotterdam ESHRE/ASRM-sponsored PCOS consensus workshop group. Revised 2003 consensus on diagnostic criteria and long-term health risks related to polycystic ovary syndrome (PCOS). Hum Reprod 2004;19(1):41-7.

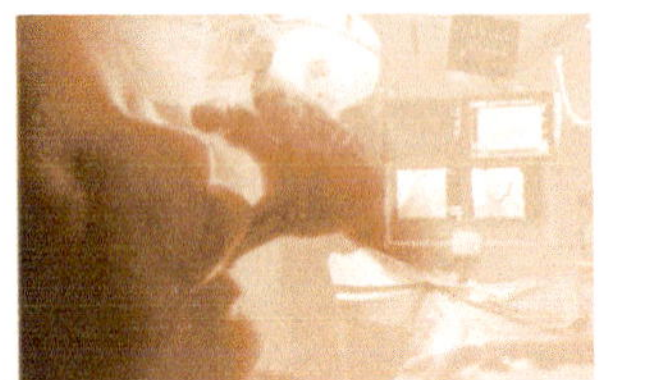

10

Menstrual Dysfunction in Adolescents

Corazon Yabes-Almirante

The menstrual cycle is a result of an interaction of hormones occurring simultaneously in inter-related events in the hypothalamic-pituitary-ovarian (HPO) axis (Fig. 10.1). The nucleus arcuatus in the medial basal hypothalamus generates signals, which results in the pulsatile secretion of gonadotropin releasing hormone (GnRH) in the neurons. In the adenohypophysis, release of follicle stimulating hormone (FSH) and luteinizing hormone (LH) is induced by GnRH, which regulates the production of estrogen and progesterone in the ovary. The cause of the mechanism of the activation of nucleus arcuatus oscillator accelerator is unknown.

The preovulatory peak of gonadotropins induces ovulation. The dominant follicle (mechanism still unknown) produces estrogen to a peak, which exerts positive feedback on LH causing LH surge. Luteinizing hormone surge: (1) induces release of proteolytic enzymes; (2) degrades cells at follicular surface; (3) stimulates angiogenesis in follicular wall; (4) induces secretion of prostaglandin causing follicle to swell and rupture and (5) converts granulosa and theca cells into progesterone-synthesizing cells. High levels of progesterone cause atresia of corpus luteum by negative feedback on GnRH inhibiting follicle growth. Estrogen enhances stimulating action of progesterone creating high levels of endogenous opiates (beta endorphin during luteal phase). Luteolysis interrupts progesterone blockade and cycle continues with menstruation. Inhibin and follistatin secreted by granulosa cells in response to FSH directly suppress the pituitary FSH secretion. Activin, originating from both granulosa cell and pituitary, increases the FSH secretion.

The length of the menstrual cycle is determined by the rate and quality of follicular growth and development. The approximate length of the menstrual cycle is 29 days plus 3 days. Blood loss should not exceed 1 ml/kg of body weight (1%) of total amount of circulating blood equivalent to not more than 80 cc as shown in the Figure 10.2.

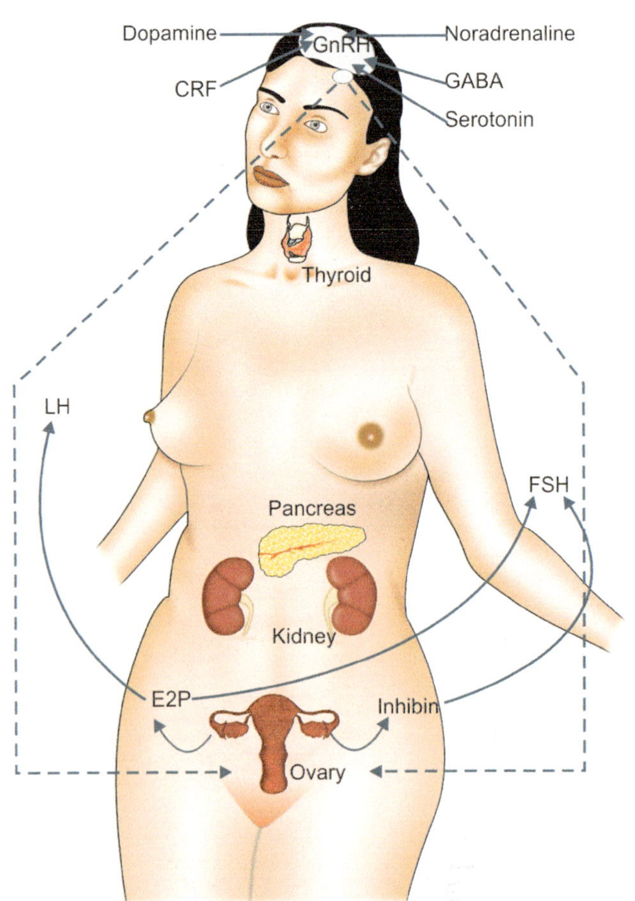

Fig. 10.1: Schematic representation of the HPO Axis. Pulsatile GnRH discharge determines pulsatile release of FSH and LH from pituitary. Ovary secretes estradiol (E2), progesterone and inhibin

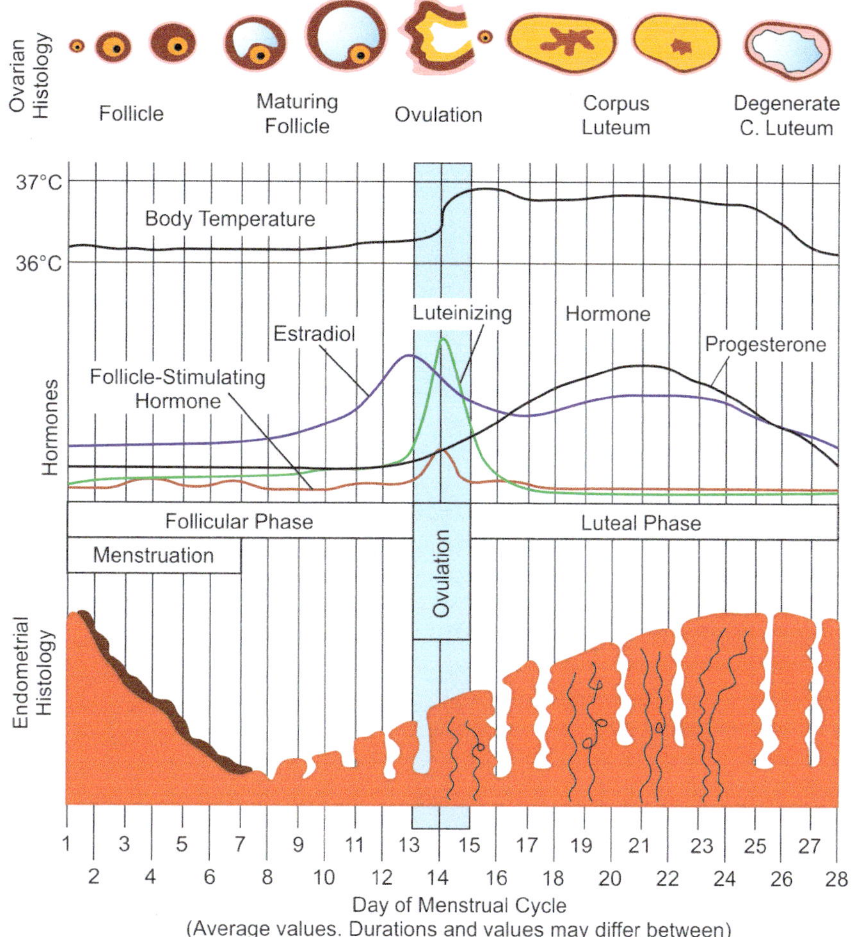

Fig. 10.2: The normal menstrual cycle

MENARCHE

The onset of menses follows a period of 4.5 years (1.5-6 years) from the start of growth spurt, breast development and adrenarche. The age at menarche in 1948 was 16.2 years, in 1982 was 13.3 years. The reduction of 2.5 years of onset of menarche was attributed to early sexual activity and improvement in food technology in the Philippines. The latest survey (2003) showed a mean average of 13.3 years influenced by the woman's general health and nutritional status. Younger women had the menarche earlier than the older women thus, in the 15-19 years old age group, mean menarche was 12.8 years while, in the 45-49 years old age group, it was 13.6 years. In the rural areas in the Philippines like the continuing study of Linda Adair 1 out of 997 girls in 14-15 years of age from the cohort followed up since birth from 1983 to 1984, in a community in Cebu, Philippines; age at menarche was found 12.4-13.9 years with a median age of 13.1 years. Menarche occurred earlier in girls living in urban area and higher socio-economic status. Girls who were relatively long and thin at birth (> 49 cm; < 3 kg) had menarche 6 months earlier than girls who were short and light (< 49 cm; < 3 kg); another evidence of the intrauterine fetal programming of later health outcomes.

A review of the menarche of 244 patients seen in a government hospital shows that those born after 1989, menarche is at 11.89 years, while those born before 1988, the menarche occurred at 13.58 years. Among patients seen in a private facility, totaling to 472, those born before 1969 had a menarche of 12.7 years while those born after 1969 had an onset of menses at 11.9 years.

DISORDERS OF THE MENSTRUAL CYCLE

It takes 5 to 7 years from menarche for the menses to become regular like that of the mature woman. The disorders of the menstrual cycle are listed in the Table 10.1.

Table 10.1

Disorders of the menstrual cycle

Disorders	Definations
Polymennorrhea (shorter cycles)	Less than 21 days interval
Oligomenorrhea (longer cycles)	More than 35 days interval
Hypermenorrhea	Excessive blood flow and prolonged more than 8 days
Hypomenorrhea	Scanty flow and short duration
Metrorrhagia	Irregular interval, prolonged and profuse bleeding
Menorrhagia	Irregular interval, prolonged and profuse bleeding

Platelets and fibrin are important in the hemostasis of the bleeding menstrual endometrium. Deficiencies cause increased blood loss, as in von Willebrand's disease and thrombocytopenia.

Anovulatory bleeding is related to high sustained levels of estrogen as in polycystic ovaries, obesity and immaturity of the HPO axis as in postpubertal teenagers. The bleeding could be excessive because without progesterone and periodic desquamation, the endometrium attains a height without structural support and lead to irregular shedding thus the prolonged and profuse menses.

Other pathologic causes of abnormal bleeding should be ruled out, such as abortion, medications that have an effect on the endometrium, such as ginseng, which has been associated with estrogen activity, and other herbal medicines such as evening primrose. Cancers of the cervix and endometrium, although rare in young women, should be ruled out, as are submucous myomas and endometrial polyps.

Abnormal menstrual cycles could also be the first sign of hypothyroidism or hyperthyroidism or blood dyscrasia (20%) especially in adolescents, although anovulatory bleeding is the most common. Irregular serious bleeding can occur in severe organ disease such as renal and liver failure. Genital injury and foreign body should also be ruled out.

Curettage is not the first mode of treatment in these cases, but the last, unless there is pathology. Use of appropriate hormones or prostaglandin synthetase inhibitors to reduce bleeding should be the first options.

AMENORRHEA

At age of 14 without growth of secondary sex characteristics, at age of 16 even with growth and development of secondary sex characteristics and in women previously menstruating, but no period for 6 months, work-up for amenorrhea should be done. Turner's syndrome is obvious, as there is absence of vagina or Müllerian anomalies. Progesterone challenge, TSH and prolactin level should be performed first. Combination of estrogen and progesterone challenge; if still no bleeding, FSH and LH assay. If FSH and LH are normal or low consider hypothalamic amenorrhea; or if high, ovarian problem. Karyotype can rule out ovarian agenesis or dysgenesis. Premature ovarian failure (early exhaustion of ovarian follicles) can occur in 1% of women. The cause is unknown. A genetic disorder can be the possible cause with an increased rate of follicle disappearance. This could be caused by autoimmune process or by destruction of follicles by infection such as mumps oophoritis or irradiation or chemotherapy.

Hypothalamic Amenorrhea—GnRH Deficiency

It is the failure of withdrawal bleeding, low or normal gonadotrophin, normal prolactin. If associated with psychological stress or weight loss, spontaneous recovery after 6 years in 72% of women can occur. Metabolic disorder—chronic renal disease with steroid therapy—causes growth of pubic hair and enlargement of the clitoris. Another case with hepatosplenomegaly and early cirrhosis, FSH and estrogen levels are low at 15 years, no menses, absent sexual development, bone age lower than chronologic age and primary amenorrhea.

Assessment of girls with amenorrhea entails a thorough history of maternal menarche, as well as that of siblings and other relatives. Past histories of endocrinopathies, autoimmune disorders and surgeries should be elicited. Headaches, weight changes, medications, acne, hirsutism, eating disorders and intense athletic activities should be ruled out.

A thorough physical examination that includes nipple discharge, Tanner staging of breasts and pubic hair, thyroid, weight and height and abnormalities of the external genitalia should be done. If physical examination shows a patent external genitalia and presence of uterus, an ultrasound examination may have to be done to rule out abnormalities of the vagina and ovaries. If ultrasound is normal, Flow chart 10.1 shows algorithm of the work-up of a girl with amenorrhea.

DYSFUNCTIONAL UTERINE BLEEDING OR ANOVULATORY UTERINE BLEEDING

Dysfunctional uterine bleeding is a diagnosis made by excluding all organic causes. The most common cause of anovulation is immaturity of the HPO axis. Hypothalamic dysfunction can also occur following stress, strenuous exercise, weight loss and systemic disease such as liver

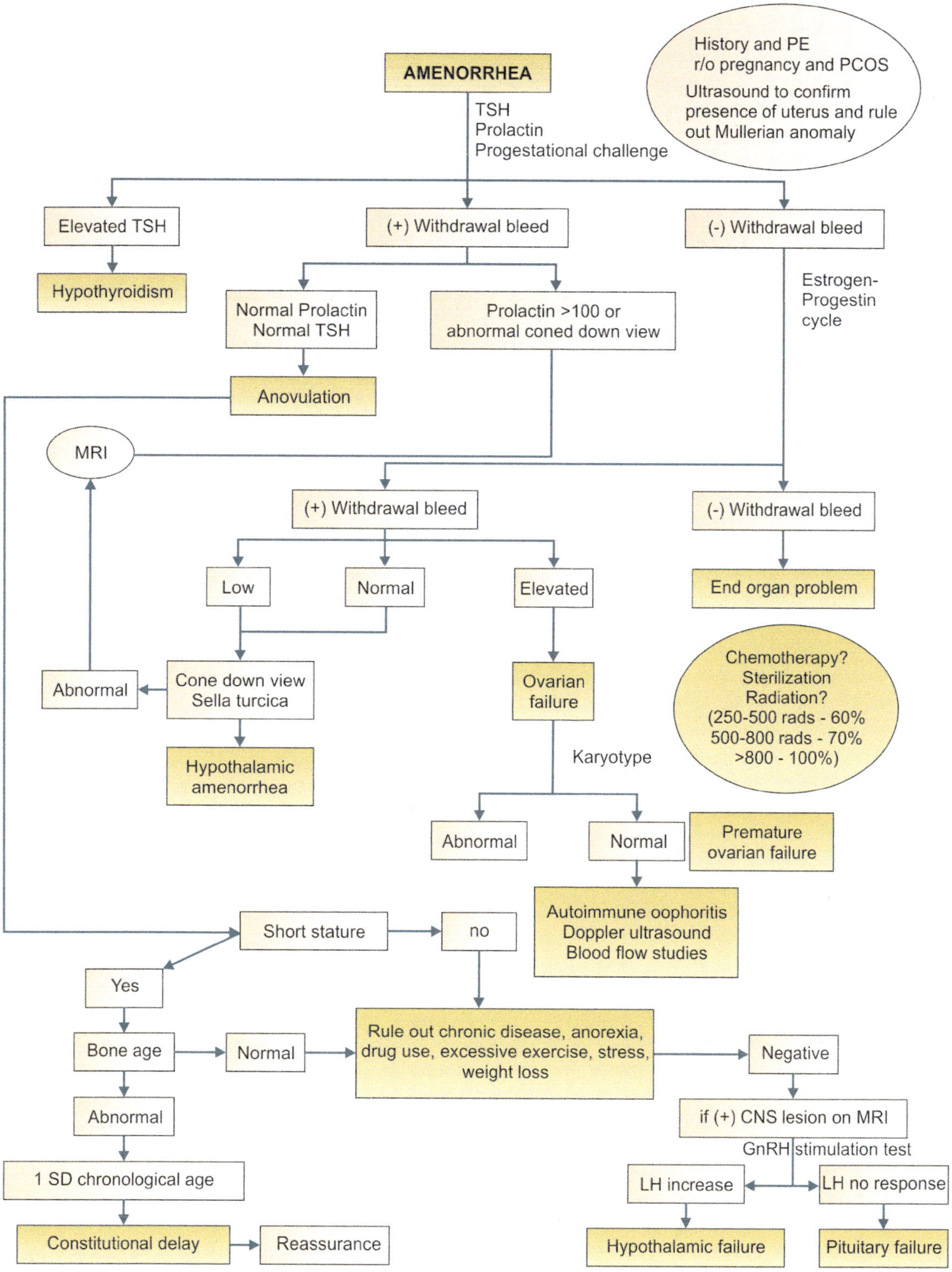

Flow chart 10.1: Algorithm for work-up of patients with amenorrhea

and kidney failure, adrenal and thyroid insufficiency. In the review of 244 patients in a government hospital, there were 42 or 17.2% cases of dysfunctional uterine bleeding.

Differential Diagnosis

1. *Abortion*: Every 5% of pregnant adolescent had at least one abortion experience in the Philippines. Among 244 patients in a government hospital, there were only 2 or 0.8%.
2. *Other pathologies*: Idiopathic thrombocytopenic purpura (3 or 1.2%), other blood dyscrasias (4 or 1.6%), steroid therapy (1 or 0.4%), myoma (1 or 0.4%) and ovarian cyst (2 or 0.8%).

BIBLIOGRAPHY

1. Adair LS. Size at birth predicts age at menarche. Pediatrics 2001;107(4):E59.
2. Annual Reports 2002 to 2008. Pediatric and Adolescent Gynecology Unit. Philippine Children's Medical Center.
3. Emans SJ, Laufer MR, Goldstein GP. Pediatric and Adolescent Gynecology. Philadelphia: Lippincott Williams and Williams, 2005.
4. Goldfarb AF, Creatsas G, Mastorakos G, et al. (Eds). The Future of Pediatric and Adolescent Gynecology. Annals of the New York Academy of Sciences 1997;816:1-3.
5. National Demographic Health Survey, 2003. National Statistics Office.
6. Sexual and reproductive health of adolescents and youths in the Philippines: a review of literature and projects 1995-2003. World Health Organization. Western Pacific Region.
7. Speroff L, Glass RH, Kase NG. Clinical Gynecologic Endocrinology and Infertility. Baltomore: W Williams and Wilkins, 1994.
8. Wikipedia. [http://commons.wikimedia.org/wiki/file:menstrual cycle.pNg].

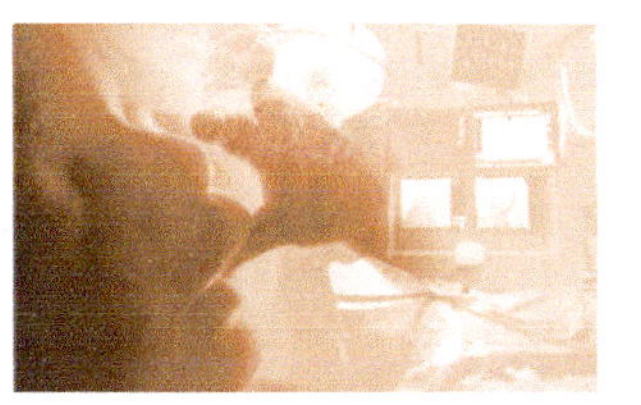

11 Urologic Causes of Pelvic Pain in Young and Adolescent Girls

David T Bolong

URINARY TRACT INFECTIONS

Urinary tract infection (UTI) remains to be the most common cause of dysuria in children and adolescents. As shown in Graph 11.1, 4.5% of females from 5 to 15 years of age have UTI and 18–25 of them have recurrent infections. After this age group they have increased propensity to infection reaching to 40% by the time they are 50 years of age. This susceptibility to infection is due to the unique anatomy of the female. The urethra is short and sits right above the vagina whose bacterial flora is extremely susceptible to changes. Sexual intercourse remains to be a very common cause in the adolescent. In the first year of life, infection rate in girls is at 0.5%, but suddenly shoots up to 4.5% from the age of 3 years onward.

This is the time when girls begin to control wetness; same reason why voiding dysfunction should be entertained as primary cause of recurrent UTI (RUTI) for older female children. Children become dry by progressively increasing their bladder capacity by holding on to their sphincter. Almost all evolve to have full coordination of the bladder and sphincter relaxes perfectly to allow full emptying of the bladder. A few of these children do not develop this full co-ordination as bladders remain to have low capacity, sphincter coordination is not achieved, holding of sphincter becomes a habit, etc. This disordered voiding seems to occur more often in girls, setting the reason for the higher incidence of UTI. Young girls and adolescents who have recurrent infections, therefore, need evaluation to identify congenital and acquired problems that may need to be corrected to avoid recurrent or persistent UTIs. In a setting of recurrent febrile UTIs, an ultrasound of the bladder and kidneys, and urodynamics must be done. Radionuclide scans to assess renal involvement and/or voiding cystourethrography to appraise presence of vesicoureteral reflux may also be needed to evaluate the full extent of the problem.

Graph 11.1: Comparison of the incidence of urinary tract infection in males and females (all age groups)

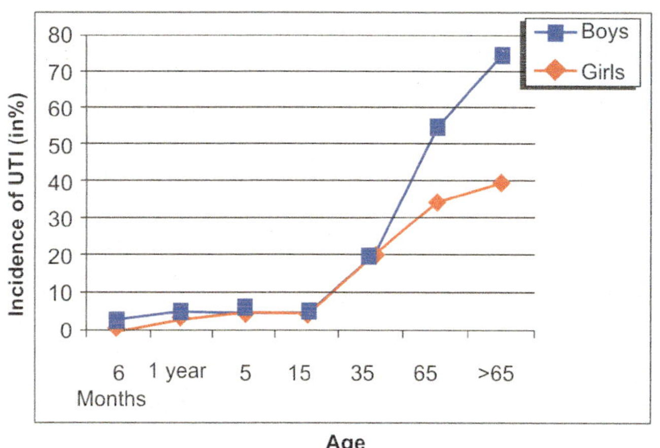

Most UTIs present with the typical dysuria, frequency and urgency symptoms in older female children. Neonates, infants and very young children do not present with the typical signs and symptoms; most present with just fever and other systemic symptoms like failure to thrive, jaundice and others.

Hemorrhagic Cystitis

Hemorrhagic cystitis manifests with alarming amount of blood in the urine and irritability of afflicted children. Most of the time urine cultures do not grow any bacteria as many of them are caused by virus. They present with a typical sudden onset of dysuria, frequency and bloody urine. Diagnostic workup alarms the uninitiated that a mass is found in the bladder (Figs 11.1 to 11.3). But with conservative management, use of analgesics, fluid intake and rest in 1 to 2 weeks, the patient becomes asymptomatic and the bladder mass disappears as suddenly as it came.

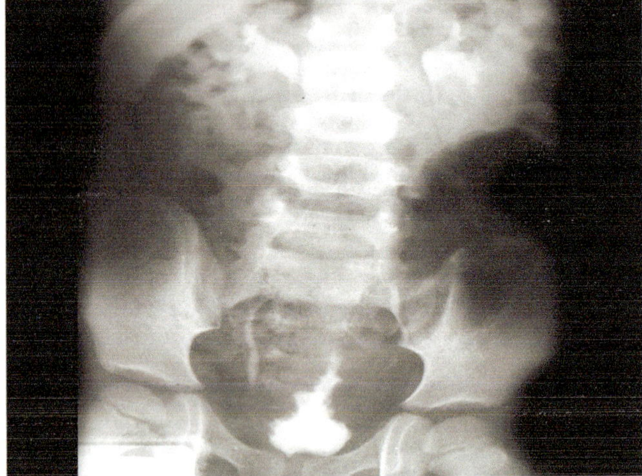

Fig. 11.1: Child presenting with severe hematuria. Intravenous urography shows a mass in the bladder

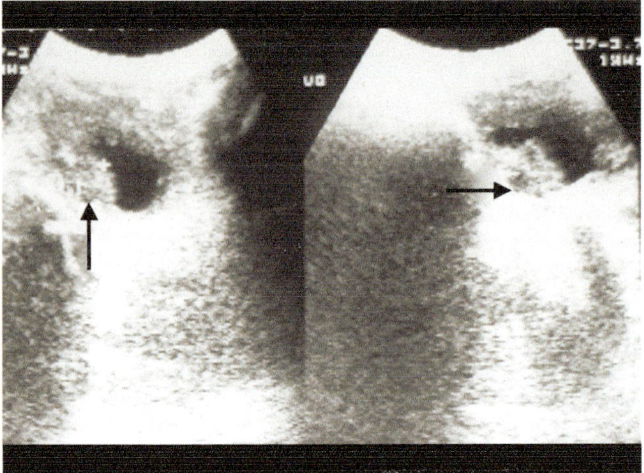

Fig. 11.2: Ultrasound of the bladder confirms the mass (arrows)

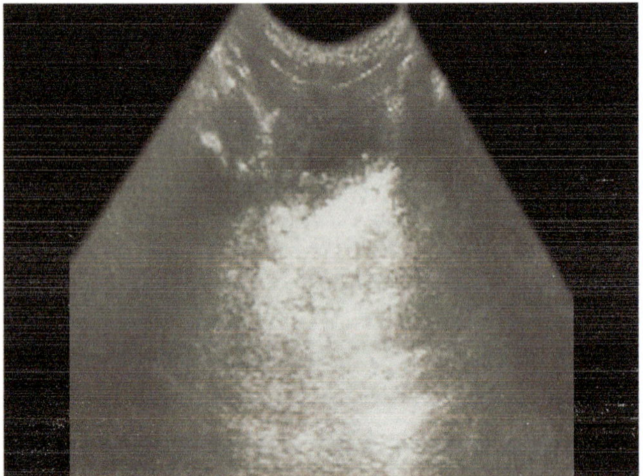

Fig. 11.3: Bladder mass completely disappears

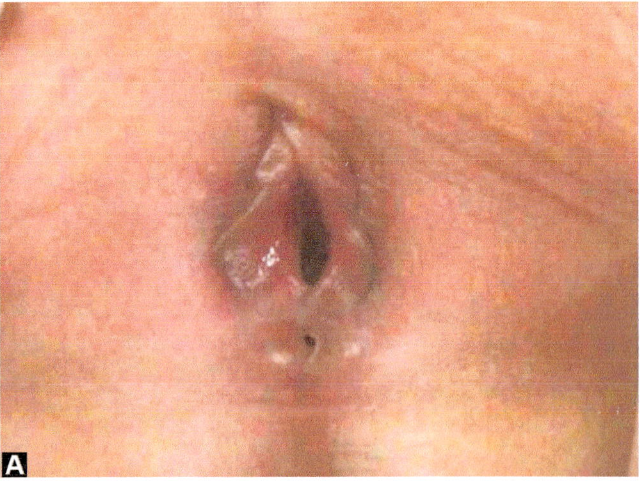

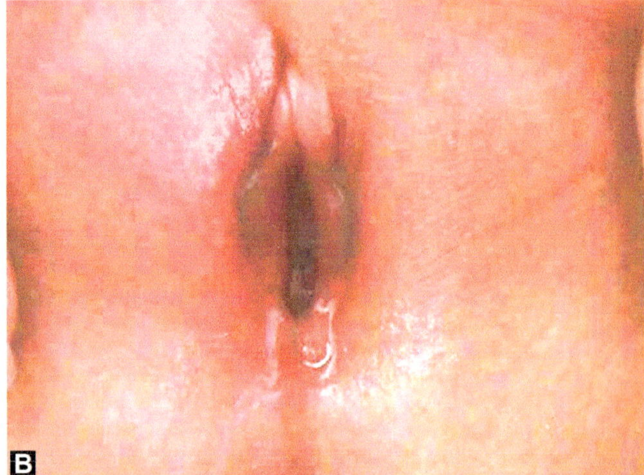

Figs 11.4A and B: Case of a 3-month-old with diagnosed RUTI. Estrogen trial failed and a cut-back is done to correct it

A common cause of RUTI (Figs 11.4A and B) in infants is vulvar synechiae. The synechiae should be cut or severed as it pools urine in the vagina and encourages infection.

CONGENITAL ANOMALIES

Introital masses are disturbing cysts or masses often causing discomfort and pain to the child. Differential diagnoses range from paraurethral cysts, remnants of the mesonephric duct (such as Gartner's duct cysts), a covered ectopic ureter, urethral prolapse or rhabdomyosarcoma of the genital or lower urinary tract. Physical examination and ultrasound of the pelvis, urinary bladder and kidneys confirm the diagnosis.

Paraurethral Cysts

Paraurethral cysts displace the urethral meatus to one side. The urethral meatus has to be identified as completely separate from the cysts. Urinary stream usually deviates to one side. In the very young, these cysts are self-limiting and often rupture on their own. The size can be disturbing or may get infected, necessitating excision especially in the adolescent.

Gartner's Duct Cysts

Gartner's duct cysts represent cystic remnants of the Wolffian duct system and can be found along the anteromedial wall of the vagina. At times the cyst is the termination of an ectopic urete. Diagnosis can be established by ultrasound. The ectopic ureter may come from a single small hydronephrotic kidney or more often is the ureter of the upper pole moiety of a double collecting system. This latter deformity can easily be diagnosed by the hydronephrotic upper pole of the ureter and a normal lower pole. Definite diagnosis is established with a CT urography or MR urography. Excision of the cyst is at times necessary. Those with communication to an ectopic ureter should be treated together with upper urinary tract abnormalities.

Ectopic Ureterocele and Ureters in Double Collecting System

An ectopic ureterocele is a cystic dilatation of the terminal portion of the ureter and in approximately 90%, that of the upper pole of a double collecting system. The cyst can at times be so large that they prolapse through the urethral meatus. Patients at times present with urinary retention, but more often patients complain of pain or incessant crying of small babies caused by the exposed ureterocele, which may vary from pink to purple and dusky. Ultrasound again helps in defining the anatomy of the double collecting system. Treatment is correction of the double collecting system either by removal of the usually poorly functioning upper pole and removing the ureter down to the bladder or excision of the ureterocele through the bladder and reimplantation of the ureter into the bladder (Figs 11.5 to 11.7).

Urethral Prolapse

Urethral prolapse is encountered predominantly in girls between 1 and 9 years of age (Figs 11.8 and 11.9). The most common signs are bloody spotting on the underwear or diaper, although dysuria or perineal discomfort may also occur. An inexperienced examiner may mistake the finding for sexual abuse. The usual therapy consists of application of estrogen cream two to three times daily for 3 to 4 weeks and sitz baths. Surgical excision and reapproximation of the mucosal edges is curative.

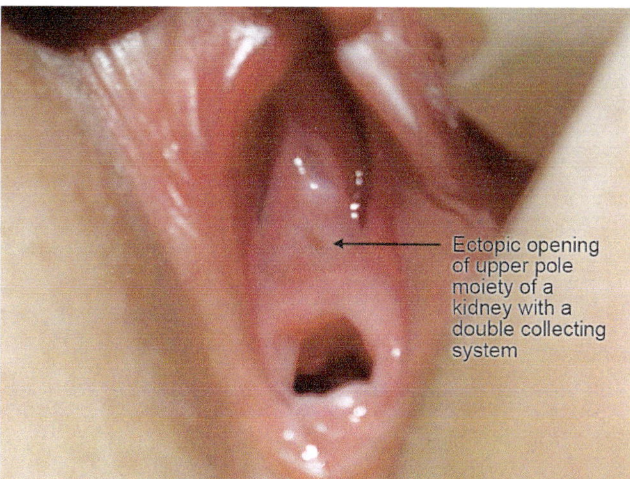

Fig. 11.5: The prolapsing ureterocele and ectopic ureter are part of one and the same anomaly of a kidney with a double collecting system (arrow) except that the ureter ends in a sac in the ureterocele

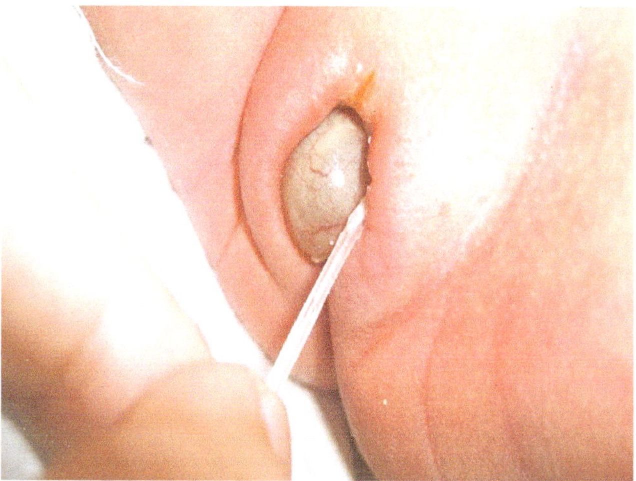

Fig. 11.6: Neonate presenting with UTI and the typical bulging ureterocele per vagina

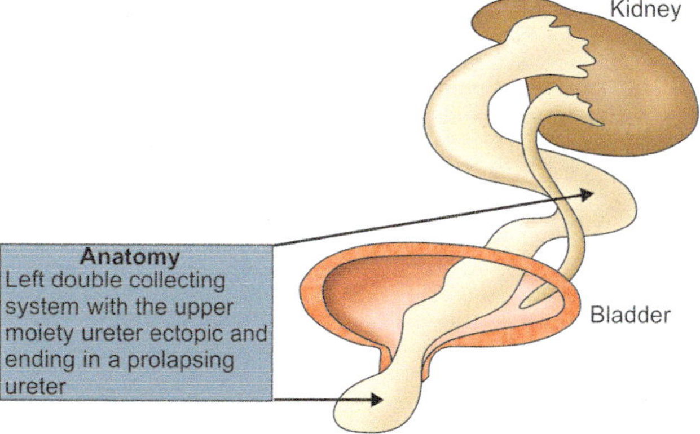

Fig. 11.7: Anatomic picture of a left double collecting system. The ureter of the upper pole moiety is usually ectopic and can end in a sac called an ureterocele

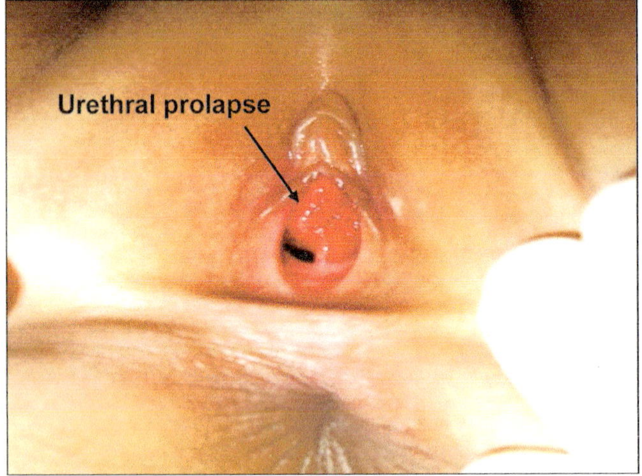

Fig. 11.8: Urethral prolapsed shown by arrow

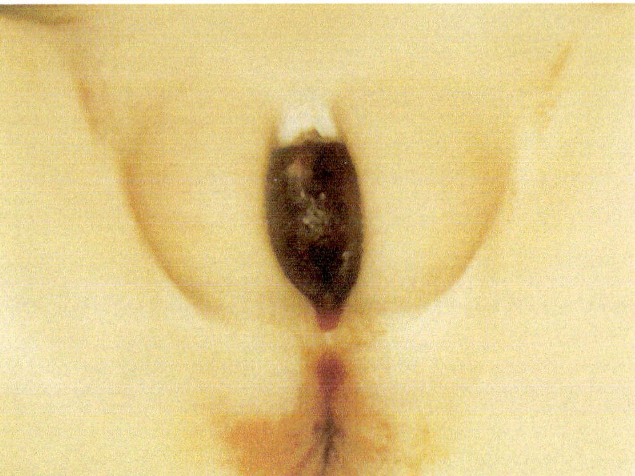

Fig. 11.9: Neglected prolapsed urethra causing necrosis

Urethral Polyp

Urethral Polyp is the pediatric equivalent of a urethral caruncle. It is a rare lesion that can manifest as an intralabial mass. The etiology of true lesions has not been completely elucidated, but in a young child they probably represent either hamartomatous growth or a response to inflammation.

Rhabdomyosarcoma

Rhabdomyosarcoma of the vagina, urethra and bladder appears as grapelike cluster of soft tissue emanating from the vagina or urethra. Physical examination must include a digital rectal examination and an abdominal bimanual palpation as this will give the extent of the mass. Most of the time children present with urinary retention. Placing a catheter will relieve these children. Tissue biopsy should be done. Proper staging with abdominal and pelvic CT scans, chest radiography and bone marrow biopsy are important (Figs 11.10A and B). A multispecialty involvement is a must if doctors are to ensure survival. After chemotherapy, local resection may be required.

Paraurethral Cysts

Paraurethral cysts come from either the Skene's gland which are tubular glands arising from the urethra (are considered counterparts of the male prostate) or from the Bartholin gland (which are vestibular glands arising from the urogenital sinus and open into either side of the hymen). Confronted with interlabial masses, gynecologic conditions have to be entertained (such as imperforate hymen, transverse septum). Please refer to chapter number three of this book.

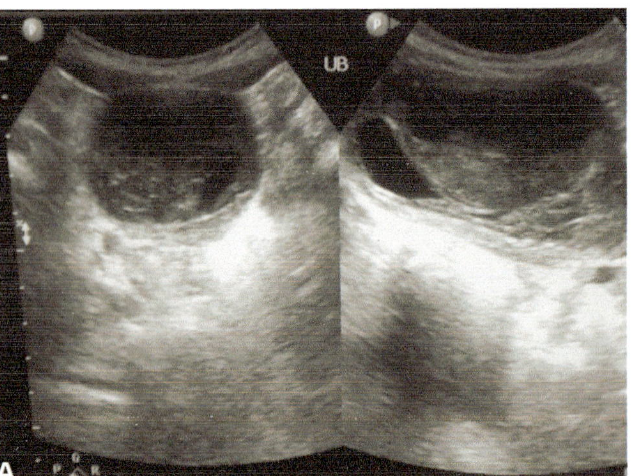

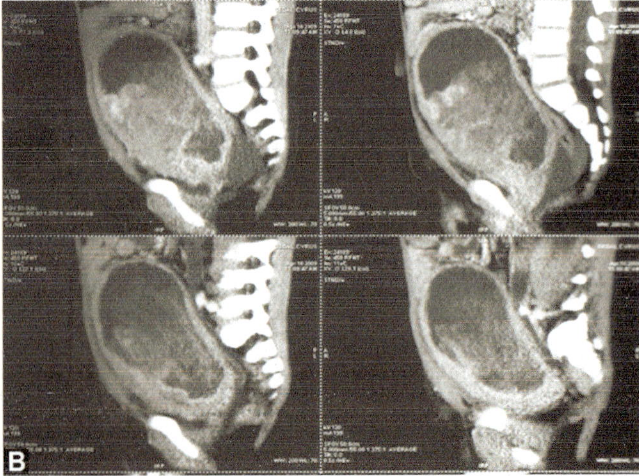

Figs 11.10A and B: Bladder rhabdomyosarcoma by ultrasound and CT scan. This causes gross hematuria, inability to urinate and severe dysuria

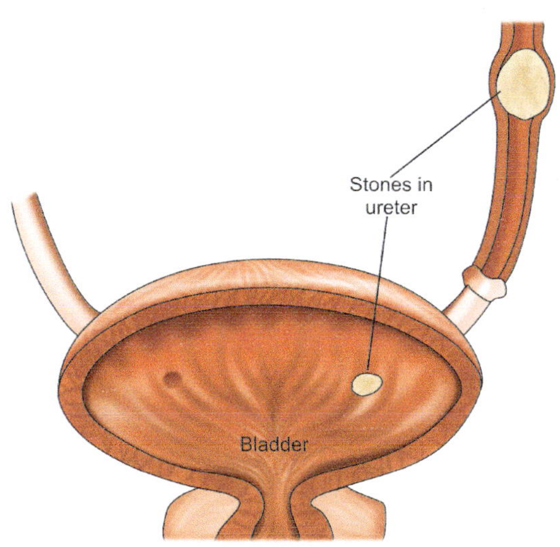

Fig. 11.11: A CT sonograph confirms the diagnosis

STONES AND URINARY OBSTRUCTION

Urolithiasis in the bladder and the distal ureter can manifest as dysuria, frequency, urgency; the same signs and symptoms as UTIs. Initial history of unilateral severe colicky flank pains manifested by older children can give away the diagnosis, but symptoms can be deceiving. A CT stonogram confirm the diagnosis as shown in the Figure 11.11.

INTERSTITIAL CYSTITIS/URETHRAL SYNDROMES/IRRITABLE BLADDER SYNDROMES

Lower urinary tract symptoms of frequency, urgency and urgency incontinence are common in the preadolescent and the adolescent age group. Many of these symptoms may or may not be preceded by urinary tract symptoms. Once the diagnosis of UTI is ruled out, a bladder diary (Fig. 11.12) make the distinction of a probable bladder problem. Differential diagnoses include functional polydipsia, diabetes insipidus, overactive bladder, dysfunctional voiders and/or dysfunctional elimination syndrome and extraordinary urinary frequency syndrome in children.

48 HOUR BLADDER CHART

Name				
Date of Start	Feb 5, 2000 (Sat)		Feb 6, 2000 (Sun)	
	in	out	in	out
07.00-08.00AM	30+150			
08.00-09.00		50		120+260
09.00-10.00			120	30
10.00-11.00	90+90	....	120+60	
11.00-12.00Noon		50		30
12.00-01.00PM	60+150+ 60 soup		120+60	
01.00-02.00		60	90	90
02.00-03.00		60		90
03.00-04.00				
04.00-05.00	90	60		
05.00-06.00	60+	30	50	30
06.00-07.00	60		100	
07.00-08.00			20+150	
08.00-09.00	150+30	30		
09.00-10.00	30		120	30
10.00-11.00	50	40		
11.00-12.00Mid night				
12.00-01.00AM				
01.00-02.00				
02.00-03.00				
03.00-04.00				
04.00-05.00				
05.00-06.00				
06.00-07.00				

Fig. 11.12: A 48 hour bladder chart of an 8-year-old girl with RUTI and urgency incontinence. This diary shows her small bladder capacity bladder with episodes of incontinence. A child at this age group could easily accommodate a capacity of 270 cc (age x 30 + cc = cc). The history of urgency and urgency incontinence is pathognomonic of overactive bladder

Functional Polydipsia

Functional polydipsia is diagnosed by frequent intake of fluids and has to be differentiated from diabetes insipidus by a trial of restriction of fluid and the persistence of increased urine output.

Overactive Bladders

The overactive bladders are easily identified by history. They frequently manifest with strong desire to void and at times wet themselves before they reach the bathroom. Children with this problem have developed tricks to squeeze their urethra to prevent leakage without socially being obvious. As they grow older they develop more subtle ways of squeezing, they have identified the malls where they go, as well as where the bathrooms are. They have limited social circle. The bladder chart shows small bladder capacities and episodes of slight wetting. Treatment involves use of anticholinergics and pelvic floor exercises. Pelvic floor exercises (Kegel's) develop a feedback to the bladder and in turn accommodate more urine.

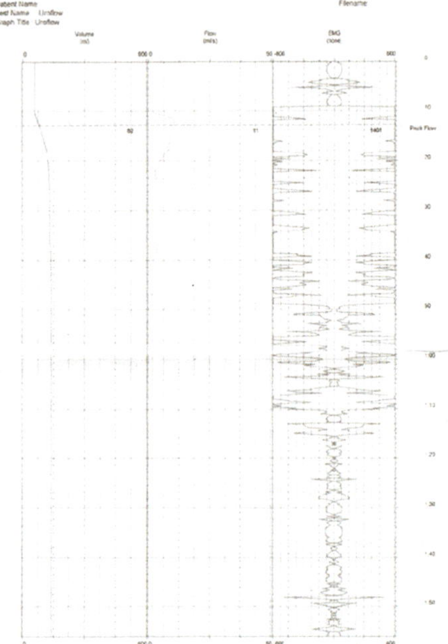

Fig. 11.13: This is the uroflow-electromyography (EMG) of a 7-year-old female with RUTI and frequency of urination. Normal children would urinate with a bell-shaped uroflow and the relaxation of the sphincter EMG. She voids in fractions accompanied by active contractions of the sphincter as shown by the EMG-acting as a functional obstruction to flow. She is diagnosed to have dysfunctional voiding. This child needs to learn how to urinate properly by means of biofeedback, fluid therapy and coaching

Dysfunctional Voiders

The dysfunctional voiders void with the sphincter closed (Fig. 11.13). This creates a turbulent flow and encourages inflammation and infections. Most likely, this problem is part of a spectrum with the overactive bladder on one end. Eventhough the overactive bladder has resolved, children and adolescents can carry this voiding pattern over. Urotherapy is the treatment. Urotherapy includes teaching these children to urinate by relaxing their sphincters; this includes pelvic floor exercises and biofeedbacks.

Dysfunctional Elimination Syndrome

Dysfunctional elimination syndrome is characterized by dysfunctional voiding (Fig. 11.14) and severe constipation. They usually manifest with frequent UTIs, voiding disorders such as hesitancy, frequency and severe constipation. Treating the constipation resolves the problem. Constipation, however, persists in most cases.

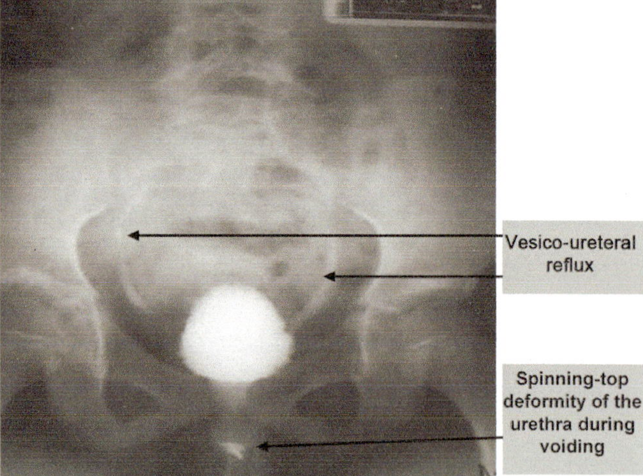

Fig. 11.14: This is the voiding cystourethrography (VCUG) of a 6-year-old female with dysfunctional voiding, RUTI and constipation. Typical spinning-top deformity of the urethra during voiding and the grade 2 bilateral reflux. Diagnosis is dysfunctional elimination syndrome

Extraordinary Urinary Frequency Syndrome

Extraordinary urinary frequency syndrome is an extreme frequency of voiding in children. Parents often describe that their children need to go sometimes every 5–10 minutes with so little urine evacuated. The frequent urination at daytime, however, stops immediately once they go to bed, and most sleep soundly and continuously until morning. Any deviation from this should be evaluated to rule out overactive bladder, dysfunctional voiding and dysfunctional elimination syndrome. Extraordinary frequency syndrome is a self-limiting syndrome and all it needs is assurance to the parents that this will disappear on their own.

BIBLIOGRAPHY

1. Bogen D, Gehris R, Bellinger M. Picture of the month. Archives of Pediatrics and Adolescent Medicine 2000;154(9):959-60.
2. Pradhan S, Tobon H. Vaginal cysts: a clinicopathological study of 41 cases. International Journal of Gynecological Pathology 1986;5(1):35-46.
3. Wein A, Kavoussi L, et al. Structural Anomalies of the Female Internal Genitalia. Campbell-Walsh Urology, 9th edn. USA: WB Saunders Company, 2007.

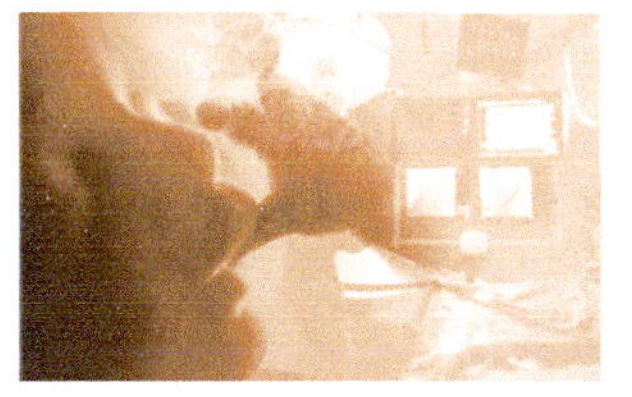

12 Gynecologic and Other Causes of Pelvic Pain

Dianalyn G Sazon-Carlos

Pelvic pain can be characterized as acute, chronic or recurrent. Acute pelvic pain is defined as pain lasting for less than 3 months, while chronic pelvic pain generally lasts longer than 3 to 6 months. This timeline is arbitrary, and patients with cyclic episodic pain may be best classified as having recurrent pelvic pain rather than acute or chronic pain.

GYNECOLOGIC CAUSES OF PELVIC PAIN

Acute Pelvic Pain

Possible source of pelvic pain in female is illustrated in the Figure 12.1.

Pelvic Inflammatory Disease

Pelvic inflammatory disease (PID) refers to infection and inflammation of the upper genital tract which is predominantly caused by Neisseria gonorrhea and/ or Chlamydia trachomatis, although other aerobic and anaerobic organisms may be involved. Pelvic examination findings include lower abdominal tenderness, adnexal tenderness and cervical motion tenderness. Patient is febrile and may complain of purulent vaginal discharge. Ultrasound evaluation may be helpful in evaluating for tubo-ovarian abscess, which may require surgery.

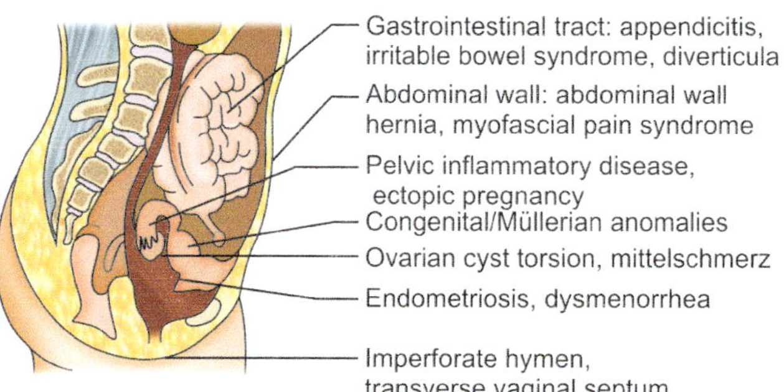

Fig. 12.1: The possible sources of pelvic pain in females

Ectopic Pregnancy

Ectopic pregnancy should be considered in sexually active female individuals presenting with the classic triad of pelvic pain, vaginal bleeding and an adnexal mass. Pregnancy test, serum beta-human chorionic gonadotropin and transvaginal ultrasound are indicated in order to confirm an extrauterine pregnancy. Medical or surgical management may be done as shown in the Figures 12.2A and B.

Ovarian Cysts and Torsion

Ovarian cysts and torsion adnexal masses are common in this age group, and physiologic cysts are frequent findings. Functional or physiologic cysts include follicular cysts, corpus luteum cysts and theca lutein cysts. Often, they go away on their own within a day or two after ovulation. However, some may persist and present as a dull ache or heaviness. Severe sharp and constant pain results when a large cyst twists. Adnexal torsion can lead to ovarian edema, ischemia, infarction and necrosis. The pain is acute in onset and unilateral in location. Large cysts and those that persist need to be removed by surgery (Figs 12.3A and B).

Chronic Pelvic Pain

Recurrent pelvic pain can be classified as chronic cyclic pain because of its intermittent nature. History is the key to making a diagnosis and patients should be asked about previous episodes of recurrent pelvic pain.

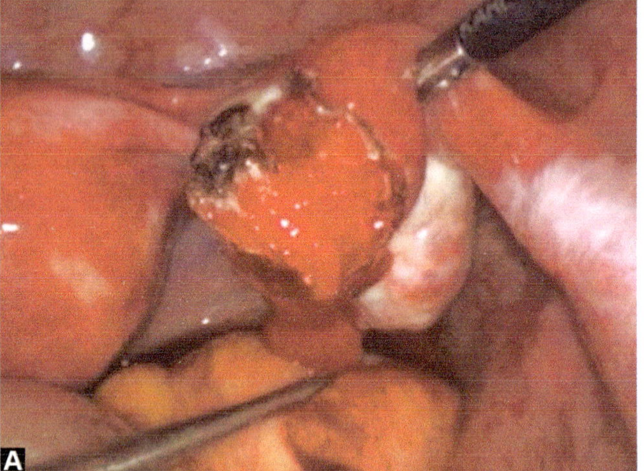

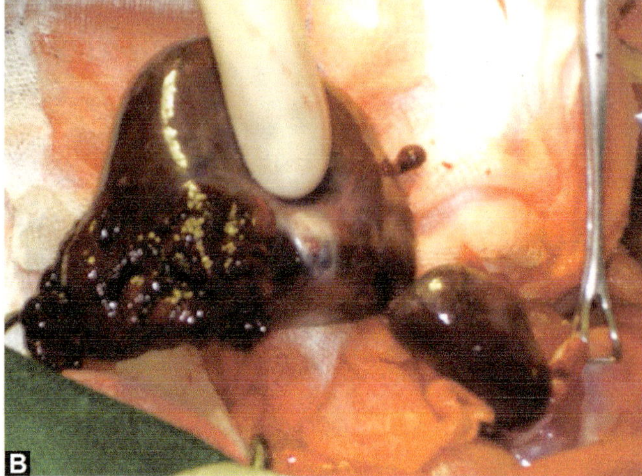

Figs 12.2A and B: Intraoperative pictures of ruptured ectopic (tubal) pregnancy

Dysmenorrhea

Dysmenorrhea is defined as painful menses causing severe sharp pain during a woman's menstrual period. Primary dysmenorrhea or functional dysmenorrhea is painful menstruation with no detectable organic disease and is common among adolescents. It may be caused by prostaglandins made by the lining of the uterus causing spasm and cramping of the uterus. Medical treatment may be given for symptomatic relief of pain.

Mittelschmerz

Mittelschmerz (German for "middle pain") is pain with ovulation; is usually a diagnosis of exclusion. It occurs midcycle and is characterized by unilateral lower abdominal or pelvic pain that is sharp in nature and lasts less than 24 hours. It probably results from a brief peritoneal irritation due to a ruptured follicular cyst.

Endometriosis

Endometriosis is defined as the presence of endometrial gland tissue in locations outside the uterus. Although various theories have been postulated to explain its etiology, none of them adequately explains its potential to occur in many diverse regions of the body. The pain generally increases during the menstrual period and declines after menstruation. The clinical diagnosis is presumptive and laparoscopy is necessary for establishing a definitive diagnosis (Figs 12.4 and 12.5). Treatment options include analgesics, oral contraceptives, progestin agents, danazol, GnRH agonists and, finally, surgery.

Congenital Anomalies

Congenital anomalies are the most obstructive genital tract anomalies to be diagnosed within a few months to years of the onset of menses.

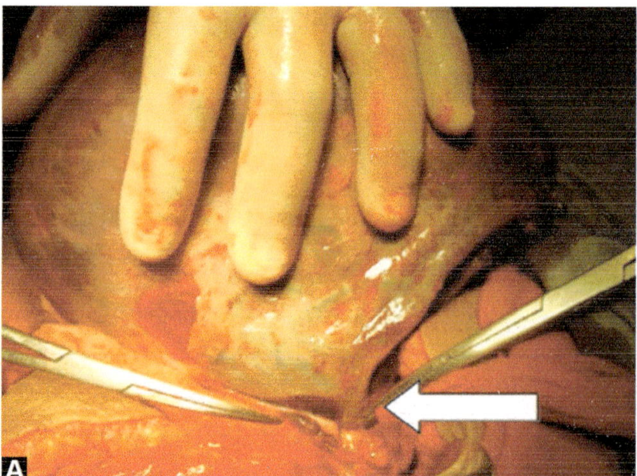

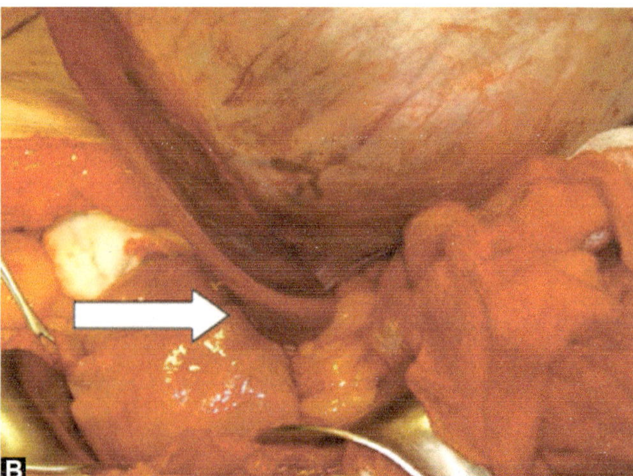

Figs 12.3A and B: Intraoperative pictures of ovarian cyst torsion (arrows)

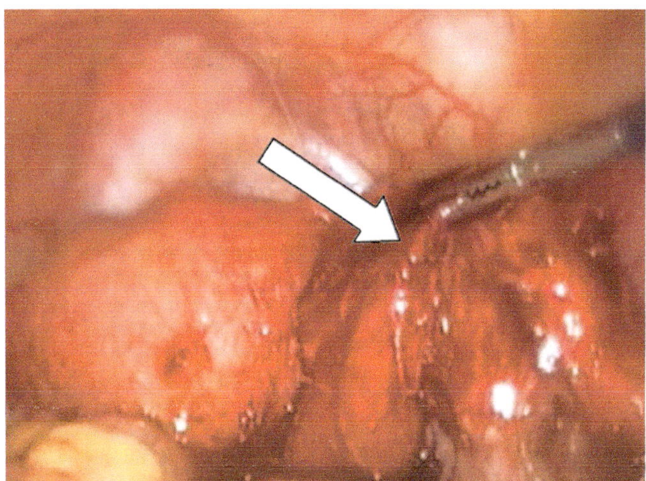

Fig. 12.4: Endometrial cyst of the ovary (collapsed), as seen laparoscopically

Imperforate Hymen and Transverse Vaginal Septum

In imperforate hymen and transverse vaginal septum pubertal development is present, but no menarche, with accompanying intermittent lower abdominal pain and/or suprapubic mass. With gentle pressure on the lower abdominal mass, while viewing the perineum, the hymen will be seen to bulge, if this is an imperforate hymen. Surgical intervention with a stellate incision into the hymen is necessary. In the absence of a hymenal bulge, this is likely a transverse vaginal septum. Referral to a specialist in pediatric and adolescent gynecology may be appropriate for successful resolution.

Ultrasound for both imperforate hymen and transverse vaginal septum demonstrates a central pelvic mass, and may also demonstrate a hematometra as well as hematocolpos.

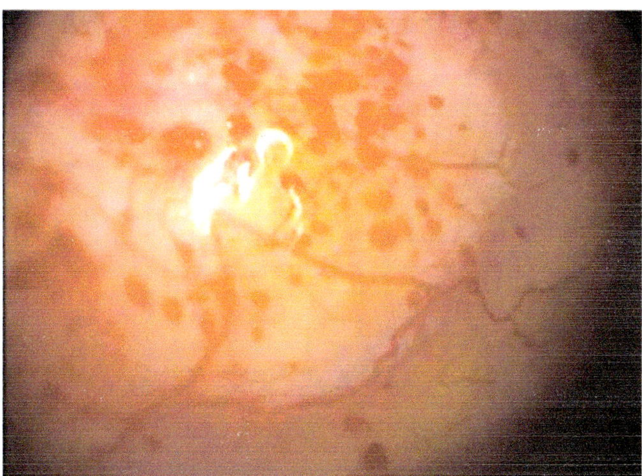

Fig. 12.5: Endometriotic implants

Uterine Didelphys with Obstructed Hemivagina

In uterine didelphys with obstructed hemivagina menses occurs with drainage from one side, but accumulation on the other side causes increasing atypical dysmenorrhea, with pain worsening during menses and lasting beyond the end of the period. Ultrasound demonstrates a collection, often not recognized as a blood-filled vagina. An absent kidney on the same side is usually diagnostic. Excision of the vaginal septum using a vaginal approach relieves the obstruction.

Noncommunicating rudimentary uterine horn with an endometrial cavity causes cyclic pain due to retrograde menstrual loss from the noncommunicating uterine cavity. The other horn will be normally draining. Management is operative removal of the rudimentary horn.

NONGYNECOLOGIC CAUSES OF PELVIC PAIN

The review of systems is helpful in eliciting non-gynecologic causes for pelvic pain and should include the gastrointestinal, musculoskeletal and urogenital (discussed in chapter 11) systems, as well as the psychosocial aspect of history.

Gastrointestinal

Appendicitis

Appendicitis is the most common nongynecologic cause of acute pelvic pain. It presents with palpable tenderness found at McBurney's point (one-third of the way from the anterior superior iliac spine to the umbilicus) in the right lower quadrant. Patients with classical findings of nausea followed by anorexia, fever and right sided pain with laboratory corroboration should be taken directly to surgery.

Irritable Bowel Syndrome

Irritable bowel syndrome (IBS) is characterized by abdominal pain, bloating, urgency, diarrhea and constipation. Constipation is a frequent cause of chronic lower abdominal pain. The onset of IBS is associated with a change in stool frequency and form, and the pain of IBS is often relieved by defecation. IBS is associated with many gynecologic disorders and may be exacerbated during menstruation. The patient's history is crucial in its diagnosis since it is a symptom-based diagnosis.

Diverticula

Diverticula are herniations of mucosal and submucosal layers through a muscular defect in the colonic wall.

Diverticulitis should be suspected in a patient with left lower quadrant pain, fever and elevated white blood cell count. These patients require antibiotics and bowel rest.

Musculoskeletal

Myofascial Pain Syndrome

Myofascial pain syndrome is a musculoskeletal cause of pelvic pain in which the pain originates from tender "trigger" points in skeletal muscle. The muscles of the lower abdomen can be evaluated by having the patient flex her abdominal muscles by lifting her head and the shoulders off the examination table. The examiner can then press on the lower abdominal muscles with one finger in various points to elicit the trigger points. Once identified, trigger points can be injected with local anesthetics.

Abdominal Wall Hernias

Abdominal wall hernias are diagnosed based on their location and fascial defects. They should be suspected if the pain intensity is related to position (e.g. worse while sitting or standing but improved while lying), or abdominal tenderness increases when the abdominal wall is tensed.

Psychosocial

Effects of Previous Physical, Psychological or Sexual Abuse

Numerous studies have documented that 40 to 50% of women with chronic pelvic pain have a history of abuse. Some investigators have shown that pain thresholds are reduced in survivors of abuse. The clinician should be aware and ask about abuse in all cases of chronic pelvic pain and offer appropriate counseling.

BIBLIOGRAPHY

1. Grover S. Pelvic pain in the female adolescent patient. Australian Family Physician 2006;35(11):850-3.
2. Karnath B, Breitkopf D. Acute and chronic pelvic pain in women. Hospital Physician 2007;43(7):41-8.
3. Pelvic Pain. Approach to the Gynecologic Patient. Merck Manual Professional. Merck and Co. Inc, Whitehouse Station, NJ, USA. Retrieved May 22, 2009, from www.merck.com/mmpe/sec18/ ch242/ch242d.html?qt=pelvic pain&alt=sh.
4. Pelvic Pain (January 2006). ACOG Publication Pamphlet AP099. Retrieved May 22, 2009, from www.acog.org/publications/patient_education/bp099.cfm?
5. Tidy C. Pelvic Pain (2009, January 9). Retrieved May 22, 2009, from http://www.patient.co.uk/doctor/ Pelvic-Pain.htm.

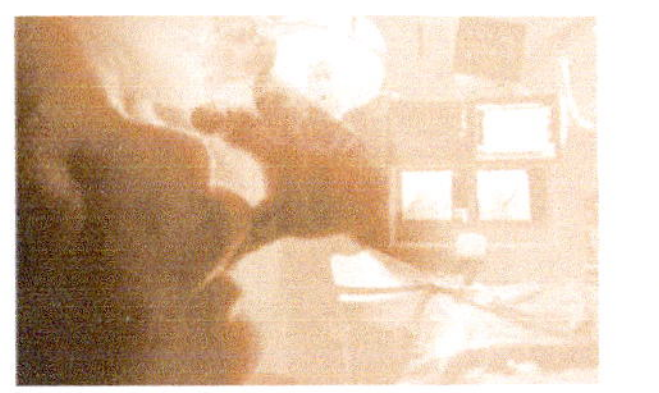

13 Gynecologic Tumors in Pediatric Patients

Franklin P Atencio, Julie Christine F Dimaano-De Torres

OVARIAN MASSSES

Fetal Ovarian Cysts

- Seen in 1 per 2,500 of pregnant women undergoing ultrasound examination
- Often diagnosed in the third trimester of pregnancy as shown in the Figure 13.1
- Etiology:
  - Conditions in the mother that increase secretion or placental transfer of B-Human chorionic gonadotropin (B-hCG). Stimulate fetal follicular cells and formation of ovarian cysts
    Examples:
    1. Rh isoimmunization
    2. Diabetes mellitus
    3. Gestational hypertension
  - Conditions in the fetus that cause nonspecific stimulation of the pituitary gland. Results in increase in follicle stimulating hormone (FSH) and luteinizing hormone (LH) drive follicular development
    Examples:
    1. Fetal hypothyroidism
    2. Fetal congenital adrenal hyperplasia
- Diagnosis is confirmed at birth
- Malignancy is very rare
- In 50–90% of the time, resolution is expected within 3 months after delivery
- Fetal ovarian cysts are not an indication for cesarean section

PHYSIOLOGIC CYSTS IN CHILDHOOD

A 12-year-old girl presented at the emergency room with severe abdominal pain. Ultrasound examination shows a unilocular cystic mass as shown in the Figures 13.2 and 13.3A and B.

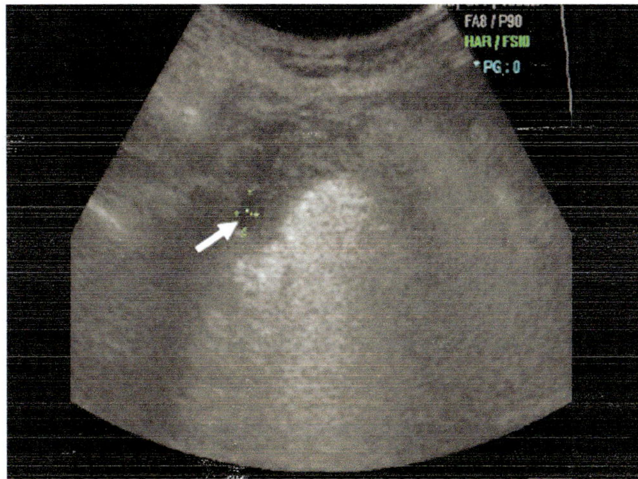

Fig. 13.1: One-month-old neonate with ovarian cyst (arrow) diagnosed at 35 weeks age of gestation and confirmed after birth

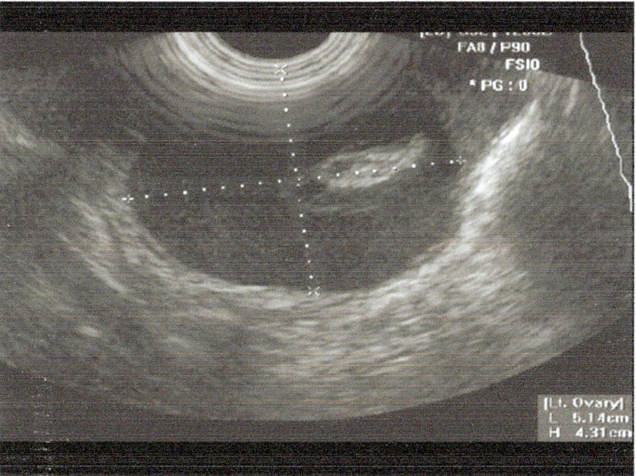

Fig. 13.2: Ultrasound examination shows a unilocular cystic mass at the left ovary with a hyperechoic nodule inside

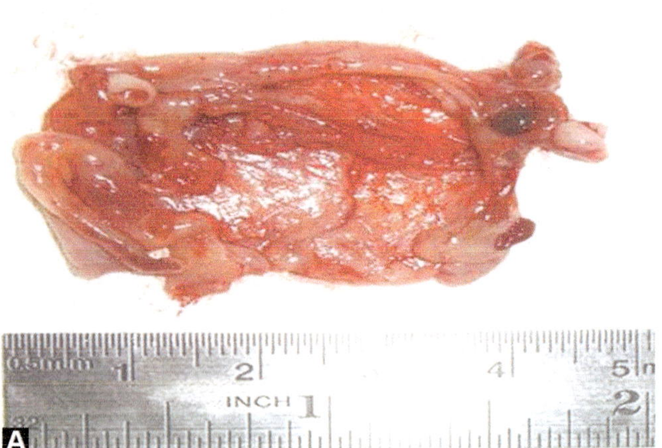

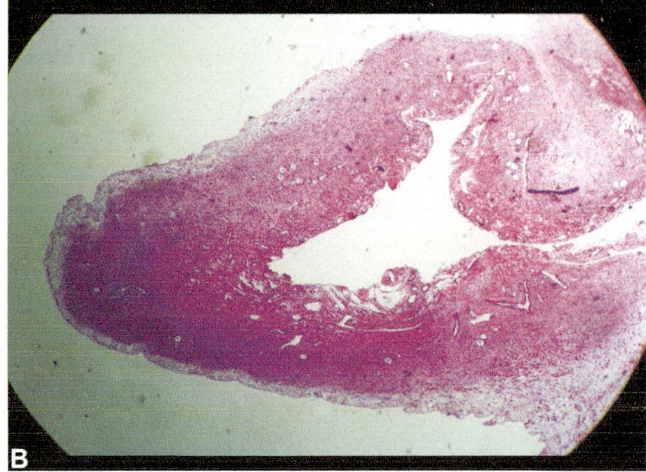

Figs 13.3A and B: (A) Ovarian cyst (cut section); (B) On exploratory laparotomy, a 5 cm x 5 cm thin-walled cyst with a 0.5 cm rupture is seen

Physiologic cyst in childhood:

- Rare because of the lack of estrogen in this age group
- Most tumors are asymptomatic and only noted incidentally on ultrasound
- Symptoms:
  - Relate to mass effect like torsion
  - Hormone production causing vaginal bleeding or breast enlargement
  - Palpable abdominal mass
- Malignancy is rare. If present, children usually would have germ cell neoplasm.

Types of Physiologic Cysts in Children

- Follicular cysts (Fig. 13.4)
- Theca lutein cysts
- Corpus luteum cysts (Figs 13.5 and 13.6).

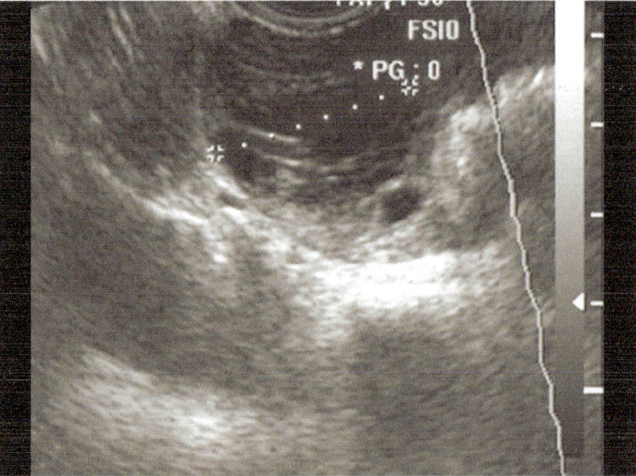

Fig. 13.5: Ultrasound picture. Corpus luteum cyst of the right ovary in a 13-year-old girl with abdominal pain

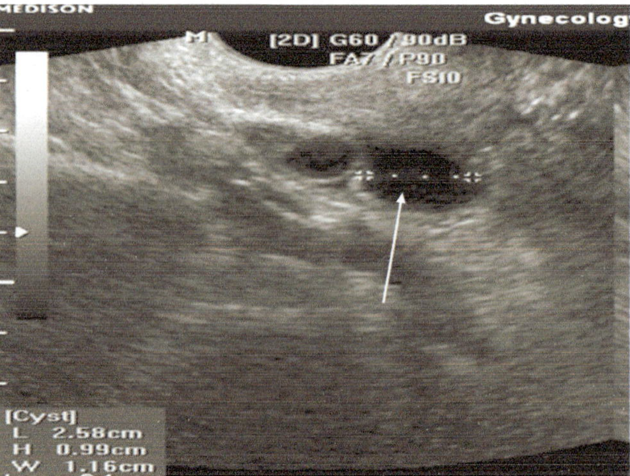

Fig. 13.4: A small follicular cyst (arrow) of the right ovary in a 15-year-old girl presenting with irregular menses

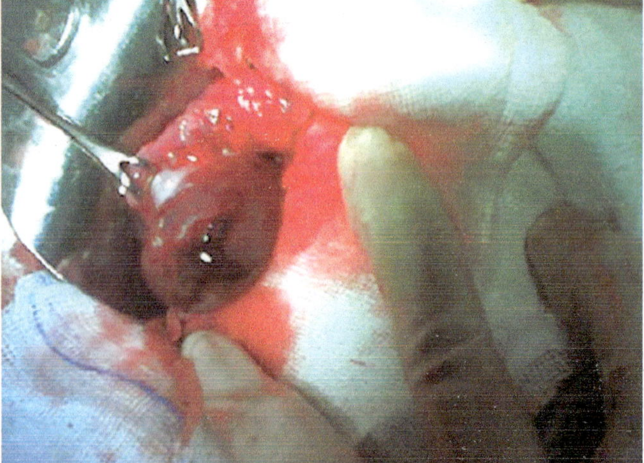

Fig. 13.6: Bleeding corpus luteum cyst on surgery

PATHOLOGIC OVARIAN CYSTS

Classification of ovarian tumors depends on their cell of origin, and can be epithelial, sex cord or germ cell types. Histology may show a benign, low malignant potential or a frankly malignant mass. Epithelial cell types are uncommon in children.

Pathologic cysts in children are mostly of the germ cell type as opposed to that in adults where epithelial tumors predominate. Some tumors in childhood may be associated with sexual precocity. Malignancy is not common in children and most malignant tumors are chemosensitive.

Classification of Ovarian Tumors

Ovarian tumors are classified into following types:

Germ Cell Type

- Dermoid cysts
- Immature teratoma
- Dysgerminoma
- Yolk sac tumor
- Embryonal tumors

Sex-cord Stromal Type

- Granulosa cell tumor
- Theca cell
- Sertoli and Sertoli-leydig cell
- Steroid cell tumors

Epithelial Cell Type

- Serous cystadenoma or cystadenocarcinoma (Fig. 13.7)
- Mucinous cystadenoma or cystadenocarcinoma
- Endometrioid
- Clear cell type
- Transitional cell type

A Case of Ovarian Mucinous Tumor in a 15-Year-Old Girl

A 15-year-old girl patient consulted for an abdominal mass, which she had first noted a month before the consult. The mass was progressively enlarging. Aside from constipation, she had no other remarkable symptoms like abdominal pain, nausea or vomiting, or urinary complaints. She had an excision of lipoma of the neck at 12 years of age. There was no family history of abdominal masses or cancer.

Physical examination of the chest, heart and lungs were normal. The abdomen was globular and enlarged by a cystic, slightly movable, nontender pelvoabdominal mass (Fig. 13.8) measuring 24 cm x 16 cm. Breasts were at Tanner stage 4. The external genitalia ware normal. The uterus and adnexa could not be assessed by rectoabdominal exam because of the huge pelvoabdominal mass.

On ultrasound, the left ovary (Figs 13.9 and 13.10) was converted to a 21.2 cm x 15.5 cm x 10.4 cm unilocular, thick-walled (0.5 cm) cystic mass with hyperechoic lines on an anechoic background. There was a mural nodule which measured 11.1 cm x 10.6 cm x 8.8 cm. On color flow Doppler, the resistance index (RI) was 0.89 while the pulsatility index (PI) was 1.74.

Serum CA-125 was 17.55 U/ml, while serum alpha-fetoprotein (AFP) was not elevated at 0.74 ng/mL. Serum lactate dehydrogenase (LDH) and B-HCG were also within normal limits. Other ancillary exams, like urinalysis, complete blood count (CBC) and chest X-ray, were all normal.

The patient underwent exploratory laparotomy. Intra-operatively, there was 20 cc of serosanguinous peritoneal fluid. The left ovary was cystic and enlarged to 22 cm x 18 cm

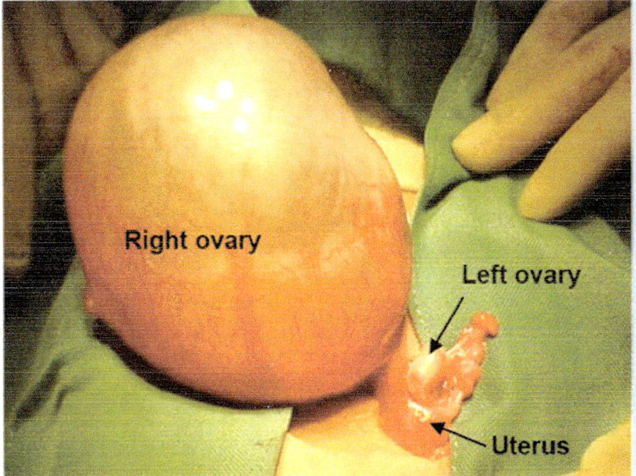

Fig. 13.7: Serous cystadenoma of the right ovary in an adolescent girl

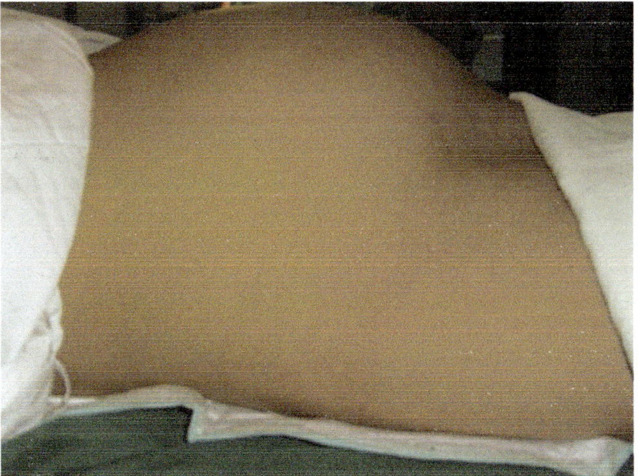

Fig. 13.8: Pelvoabdominal mass palpable on physical examination

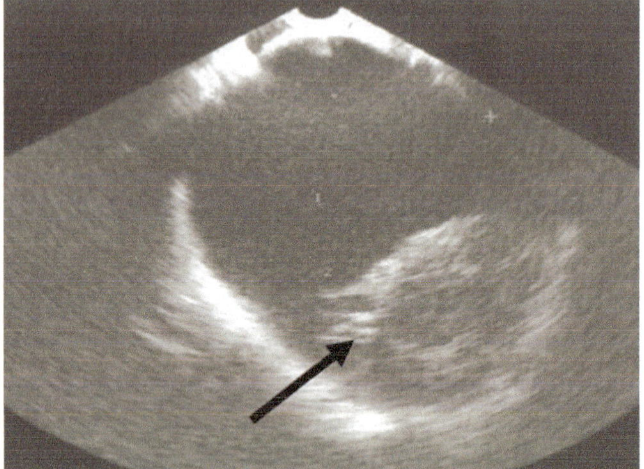

Fig. 13.9: Ultrasound of the left ovarian mass with mural nodule (arrow)

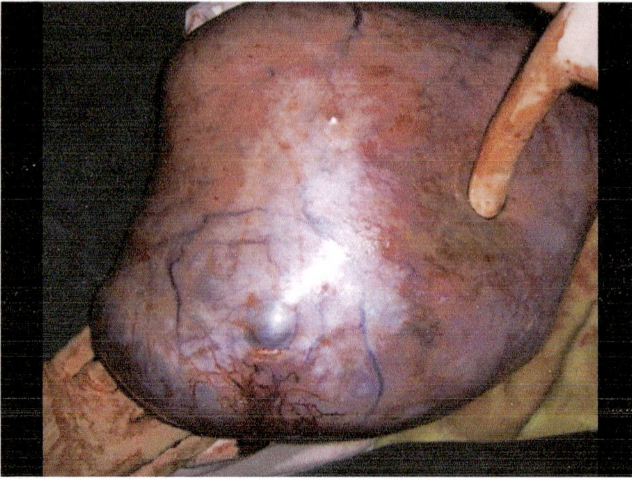

Fig. 13.11: On surgery, a huge mass on the left ovary was seen

with a smooth, intact capsule (Fig. 13.11). The left fallopian tube was 18 cm in length and was stretched out over the left ovary.

On cut section (Fig. 13.12), the mass was biloculated. The first locule exuded dark brown fluid; its inner walls were smooth. The second locule revealed a 10 cm x 8 cm solid area which, on cut section, showed a brain-like surface. The histopathology revealed a mucinous tumor of borderline malignant potential.

When they do appear in children and adolescents, serous and mucinous cystadenomas are usually associated with torsion. Borderline tumors (Figs 13.13A and B) are seen in the younger age group more often than epithelial cancer. There is still no consensus regarding the management of these tumors in young people in terms of preserving future fertility.

GERM CELL OVARIAN TUMORS

Dermoid Cysts

- Dermoid cysts (Figs 13.14A to C) is the most common benign ovarian tumor in children
- Bilateral 15 to 20% of the time
- May present with abdominal pain because of torsion
- Cystectomy, whether through a laparotomy approach or a laparoscopic approach, is the treatment of choice.

Microscopic examination of mature cystic teratomas shows mature cells originating from the three germ layers. These tumors arise from primitive germ cells and most commonly have elements of the three primitive germ layers, the most predominant of which are skin and neural elements.

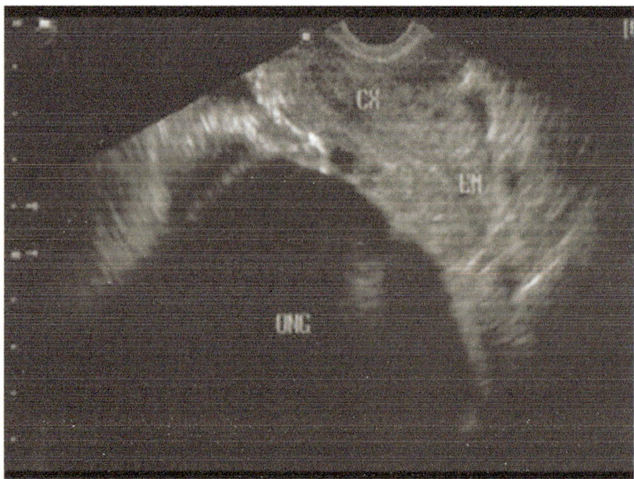

Fig. 13.10: The pelvoabdominal mass in relation to the uterus and cervix

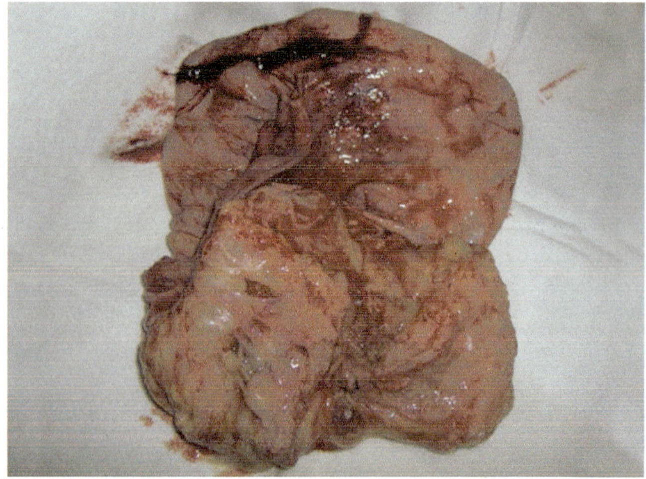

Fig. 13.12: The left ovarian mass on cut section

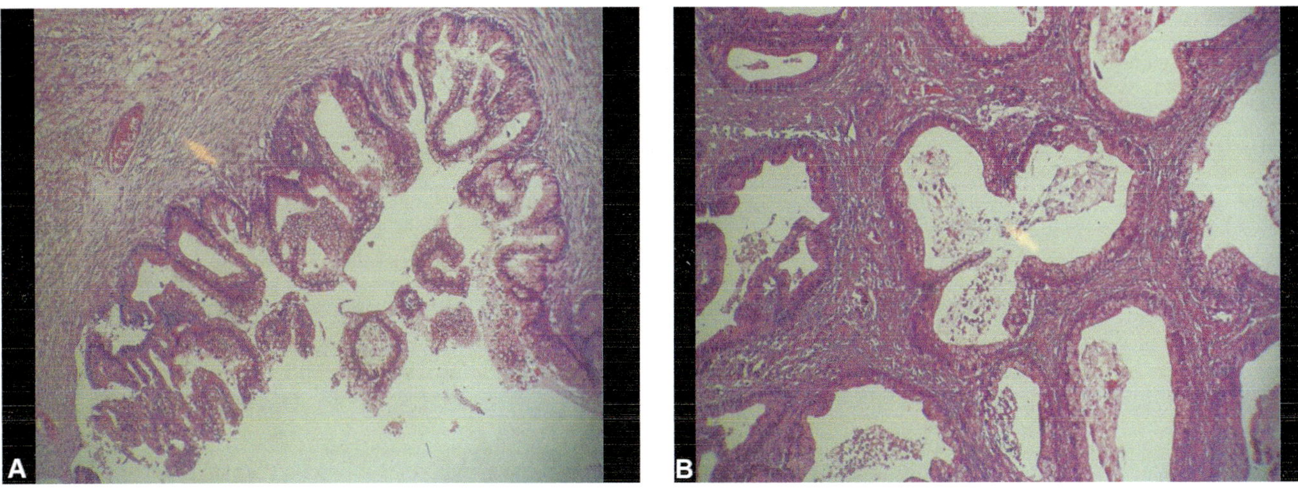

Figs 13.13A and B: Histopathology result revealed that the mass is a mucinous tumor of the borderline malignant potential

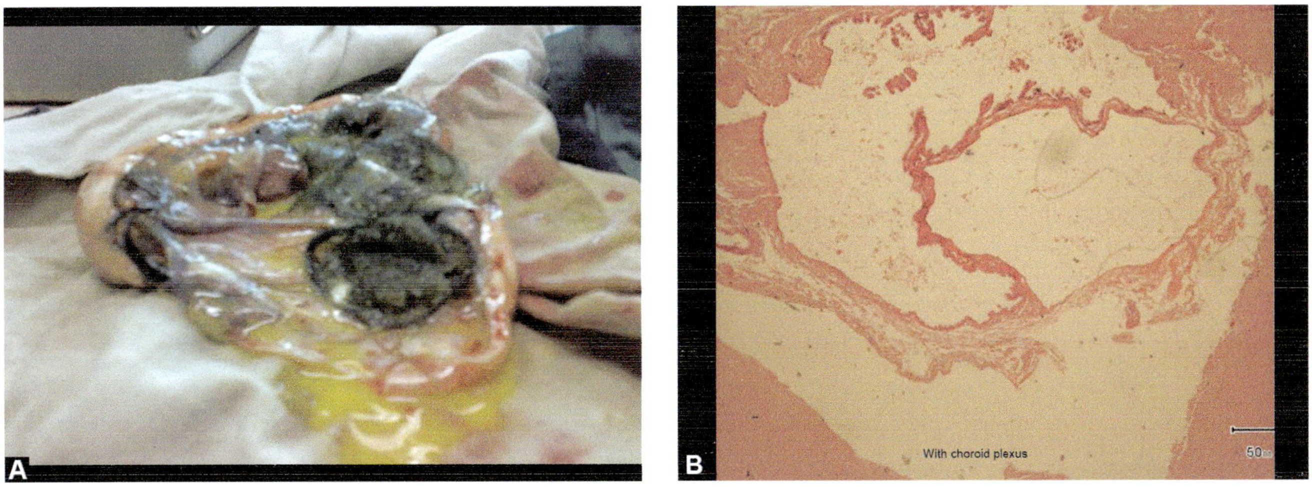

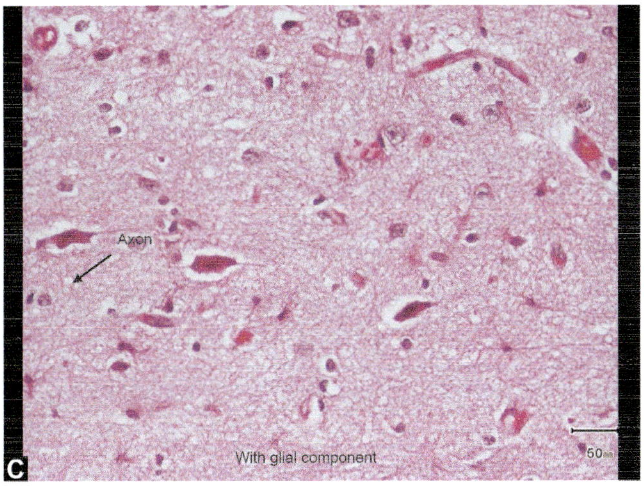

Figs 13.14A to C: Dermoid cyst in a 12-year-old girl patient presenting with on and off abdominal pain. Histopathology show cells from the ectodermal germ layer

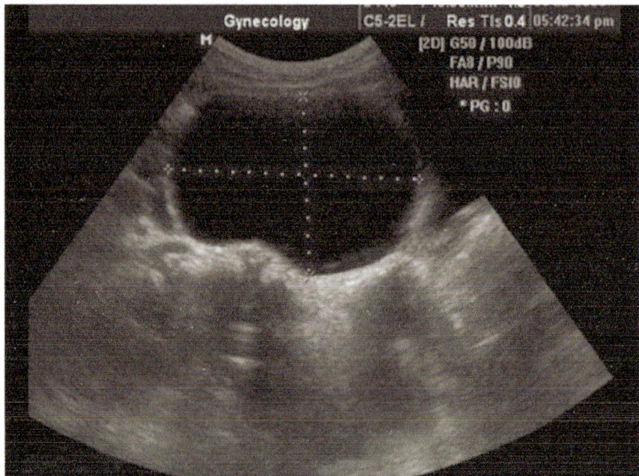

Fig. 13.15: A unilocular cystic mass at the left ovary which measured 8 x 6 cm

A Case of Dermoid Cyst in a Child

A case of a 10-year-old premenarcheal girl, who presented with on and off left lower quadrant abdominal pain of 1 month duration. On rectoabdominal exam, there was an 8 x 7 cystic movable nontender mass at the hypogastric area (Figs 13.15 to 13.19).

The patient underwent left oophorocystectomy. Intraoperatively, there was a 7 cm x 6 cm cystic mass with yellowish fluid within. Hair and cartilage (Figs 13.20 and 13.21) were noted on the pole of the cyst. Approximately 3 cm x 1 cm of normal ovarian tissue was noted.

IMMATURE OVARIAN TERATOMAS

- Immature ovarian teratomas (Figs 13.22 and 13.23) are less common than mature teratomas

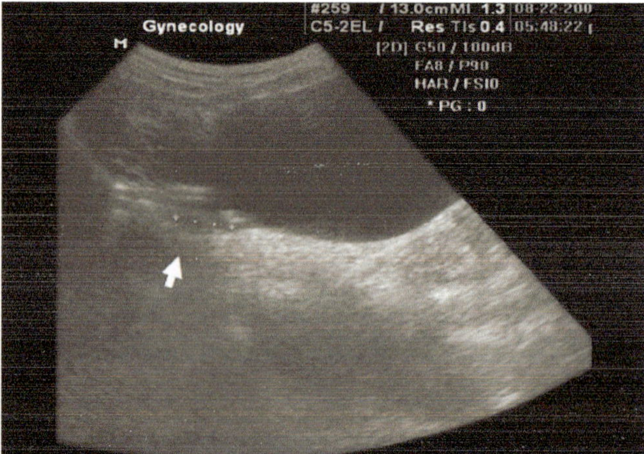

Fig. 3.16: Normal ovarian tissue was appreciated adjacent to the mass (arrow)

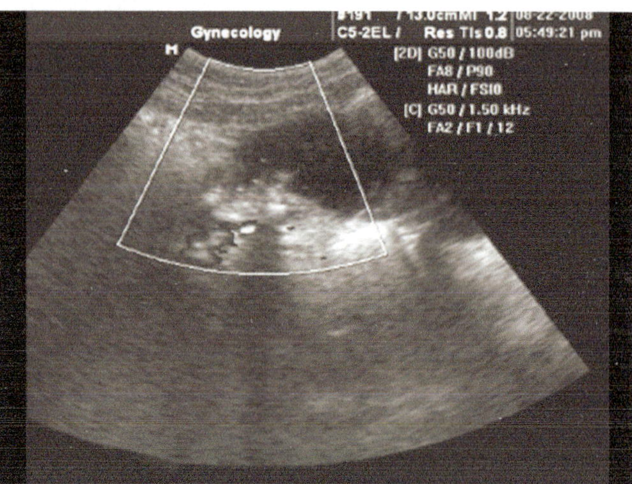

Fig. 13.17: Doppler studies revealed no significant vascular flow on the mass

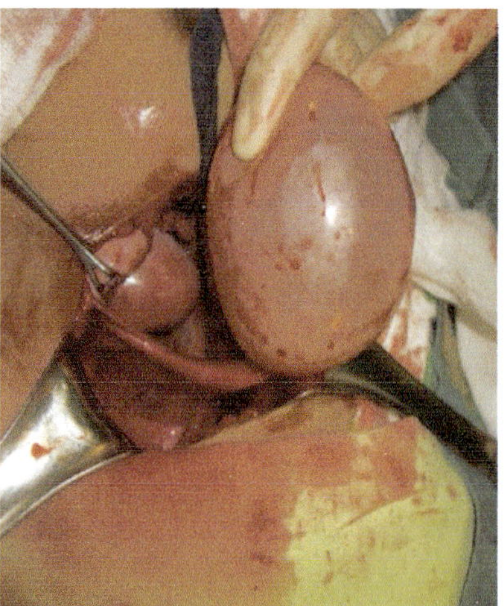

Fig. 13.18: Left ovarian cyst

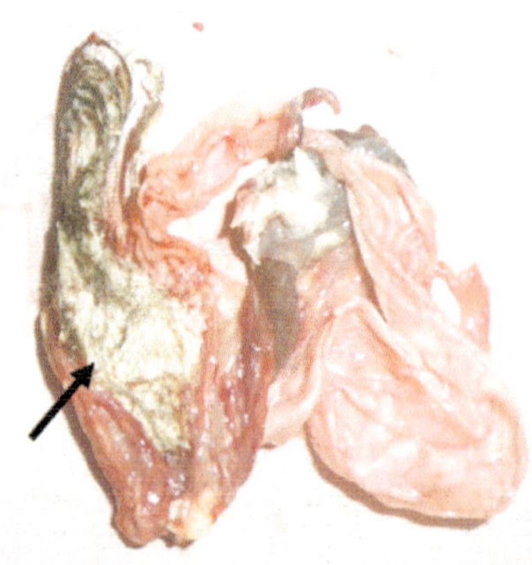

Fig. 13.19: Dermoid cyst, cut section. Note the tufts of hair mixed with sebum (arrow)

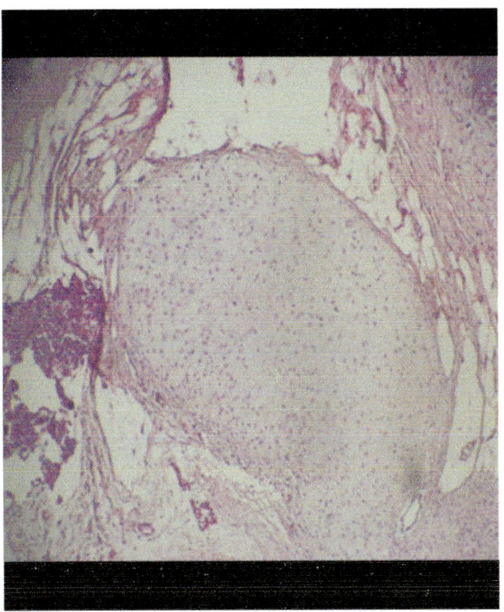

Fig. 13.20: Cartilage cells

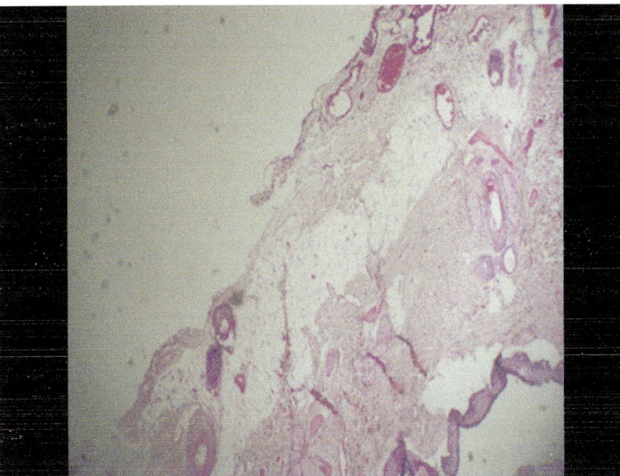

Fig. 13.21: Hair follicles and fat tissues

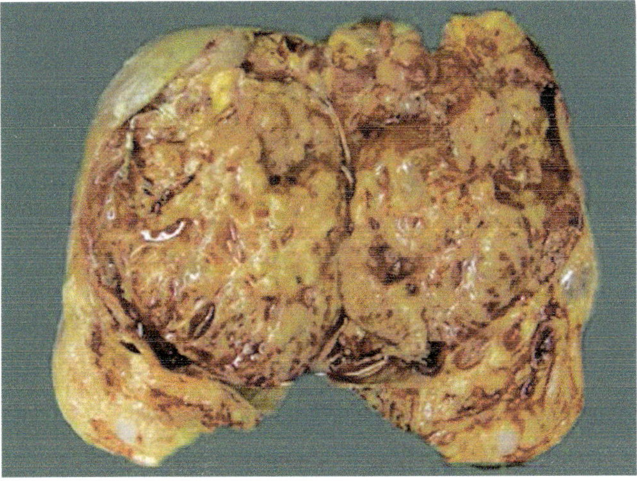

Fig. 13.22: Gross picture of immature teratoma

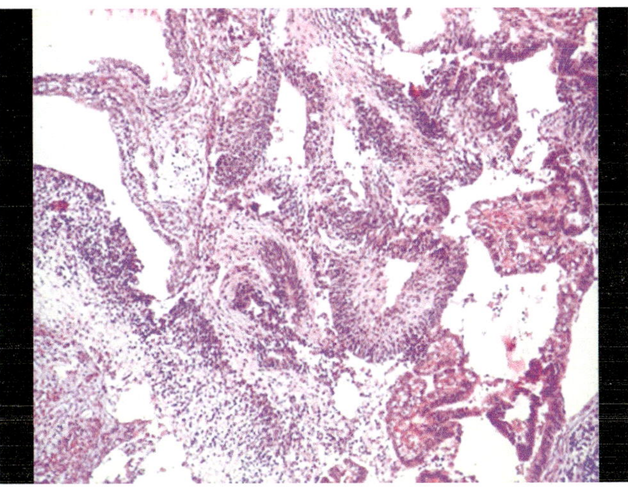

Fig. 13.23: Immature teratoma, histopathology

- Immature elements of the different cell lineages in the body is the hallmark feature
- Degree of the immaturity of the tissues correlates with the degree of malignancy
- Sometimes, may be admixed with other germ cell tumor elements like dysgerminoma, endodermal sinus (yolk sac) tumor, embryonal tumors or trophoblastic tumors.

GRANULOSA CELL TUMOR

Shown in the Figures 13.24 and 13.25.

Malignant Ovarian Masses in Children

Different tumor markers are listed in the Table 13.1.

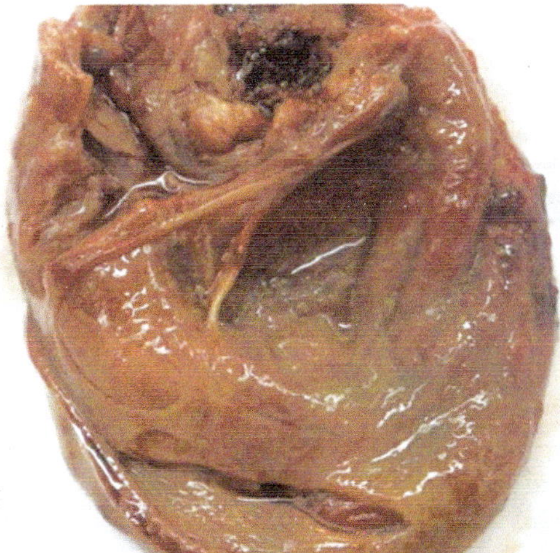

Fig. 13.24: Gross picture of granulosa cell tumor in 12-year-old girl patient presenting with acute abdominal pain. Note the presence of cystic and solid elements. Areas of hemorrhage are also present

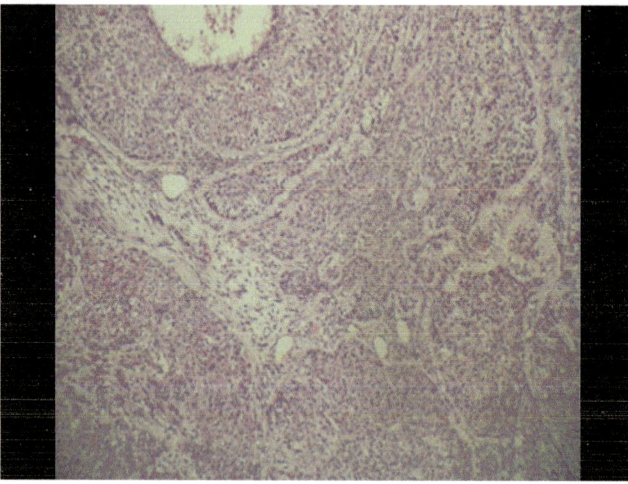

Fig. 13.25: Histopathologic picture of juvenile granulosa cell tumor. Unlike the adult type, Call-Exner bodies are not a usual component of the juvenile type

Malignant Ovarian Tumors in Children

Dysgerminoma

- Usually associated with abnormal sexual development and chromosomal abnormalities
- Some present with virilization and sexual precocity
- As a bilateral tumors in 10% of the patients
- Histologic feature: there are infiltration of plasma cells and lymphocytes among sheets and nests of cells.

Yolk Sac Tumor (Endodermal Sinus Tumor)

- Often unilateral and present with necrosis and hemorrhage
- On histopathology, hallmark feature are Schiller Duvall bodies
- Stain positive for AFP.

Embryonal Carcinoma

- Rare tumor, often mixed with other germ cell tumors
- Occurs in prepubertal patients 50% of the time
- Unilateral, rapidly growing, but responsive to chemotherapy
- Stains positive to PLAP, HCG, AFP and cytokeratin.

Ovarian Sex Cord Tumors (Granulosa, Sex cord Stromal)

- Commonly associated with abnormal endocrine manifestation due to estrogen and/or androgen secretion
- Elements of sex cord derived cells as well as ovarian stromal cells
- Often present in children as feminizing tumors causing isosexual precocious puberty
- Virilization effects may be seen in a females in cases of sertoli cell or sertoli-leydig cell tumors.

OVARIAN MASSES IN CHILDREN: 11-YEAR REVIEW, 1995–2006

By Catherine Canonizado-Donato

Age Distribution, Presenting Symptoms, Diagnosis and Management

Eleven year review of ovarian masses in children, their age distribution, presenting symptoms, diagnosis and management are listed in the Table 13.2.

Table 13.1:

Tumor markers for malignant ovarian masses in children

	Alpha-fetoprotein (AFP)	*B-Human chorionic gonadotropin (B-HCG)*	*CA-125*	*Lactate dehydrogenase (LDH)*	*Inhibin*	*Androgen*
Epithelial tumor	N	N	E/N	N	N	N
Immature teratoma	N	N	N	N	N	N
Dysgerminoma	N	E/N	E/N	E/N	N	N
Yolk sac tumor (Endodermal sinus tumor)	E	N	E/N	E/N	N	N
Embryonal carcinoma	E/N	E/N	N	N	N	N
Granulosa cell tumor	N	N	N	N	E	E/N
Sertoli-Leydig cell tumor	N	N	N	N	E/N	E

Key: E, elevated; N, not elevated

Table 13.2:
Age distribution of ovarian tumors, their surgical management and physician performing the procedure

	Age (Years)			
	Mean	*N*	*Range*	*Management*
Functional cyst				
Corpus luteum cyst	14	1	(–)	Oophorectomy(1)-pediatric surgeon
Hemorrhagic cyst	5.6	6	(0–10)	Salpingoophorectomy(6)-pediatric surgeon
Simple cyst	5.5	2	(0–11)	Salpingoophorectomy(1)-pediatric surgeon Oophorocystectomy(1)-PAG specialist
Epithelial				
Serous cystadenoma	11.3	3	(10–13)	Oophorocystectomy(1)-pediatric surgeon Salpingoophorectomy(1)-pediatric surgeon
Mucinous cystadenoma	14	2	(13–15)	Salpingoophorectomy(2)-PAG specialist
Germ cell tumor				
Mature teratoma	7.8	21	(0–19)	Oophorectomy, Salpingoophorectomy(12)-pediatric surgeon Oophorectomy, Salpingoophorectomy(2)-PAG specialist Oophorocystectomy(8)-PAG specialist
Immature teratoma	11	1	(–)	Salpingoophorectomy with omentectomy(1)-pediatric surgeon
Immature teratoma with yolk sac components	8	1	(–)	Salpingoophorectomy(1)- pediatric surgeon
Endodermal sinus tumor	4	2	(1–4)	Salpingoophorectomy(2)-pediatric surgeon Salpingoophorectomy, infracolic omentectomy, peritoneal fluid cytology, lymph node palpation(1)-PAG specialist
Endometrial cyst	17.5	2	(16–19)	Oophorocystectomy(2)-PAG specialist
Metastasis	1	1	(–)	Oophorectomy(1)-pediatric surgeon

Pediatric ovarian tumors differ from adult ovarian tumors in presentation, histology and biological behavior and mandate a different therapeutic approach. In adults, ovarian mass is usually discovered on a routine examination of an asymptomatic female. In children and adolescents, because they are not subjected to routine pelvic examination, they may present with acute abdominal pain and signs of peritonitis that can be difficult to distinguish from acute appendicitis. They may present with a large pelvoabdominal mass (Figs 13.26A to C) and concerns of malignancy. Young patients may also present with precocious puberty, masculinization and other signs of endocrine disturbances. Some patients with enlarged ovary experience ureteral compression and hydronephrosis, bowel obstruction or respiratory insufficiency. Rarely, some may present with vaginal bleeding.

Pelvic sonogram is a dependable method for determining the site of origin of a pelvic mass and can even suggest the specific diagnosis (Table 13.3) in pediatric patients with ovarian pathology. The use of sonography helps to avoid unnecessary surgery.

For benign tumors, surgical management should be conservative and mainly consists of cystectomy or excision of the ovarian lesion. Although it is technically difficult, the procedure minimizes the risk of subsequent infertility and helps conserve as much ovarian tissue as possible to maintain stable reproductive and endocrine function.

In the rare patient with malignant ovarian tumor confirmed by frozen section or tumor markers, complete

Table 13.3:
Ultrasound findings and histopathologic diagnosis

Ultrasound findings			*N*	*Histopathologic diagnosis*
Simple (%)	*Complex (%)*	*Solid (%)*		
3 (15%)	14 (70%)	3 (15%)	20	Mature teratoma, Immature teratoma
1 (100%)	–	–	1	Simple cyst
1 (25%)	3 (75%)	–	4	Hemorrhagic Infarction
–	2 (100%)	–	2	Endometrial cyst
2 (100%)	–	–	2	Serous cyst
–	1 (100%)	–	1	Mucinous cyst
–	2 (100%)	–	2	Endodermal sinus tumor

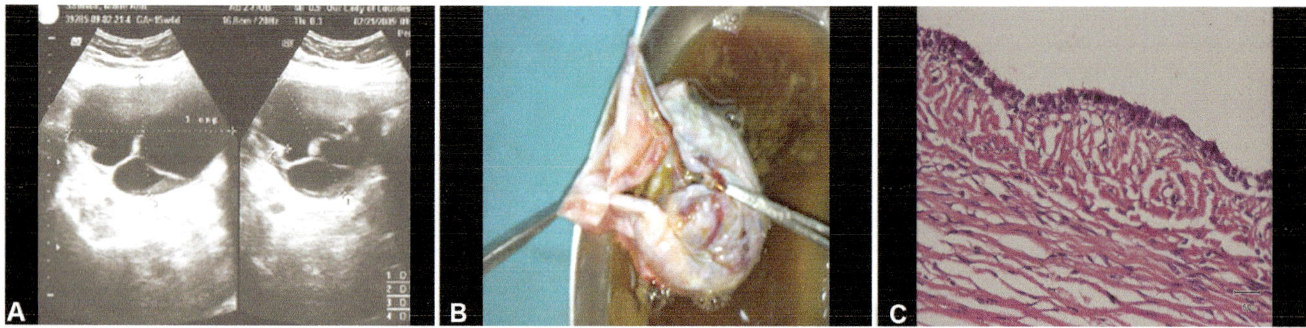

Figs 13.26A to C: (A) Ultrasound picture in a child presenting with a palpable ovarian mass; (B) Laparotomy reveals a multicystic serous cyst; (C) Histopathologic picture of serous cyst

surgical staging and resection of the tumor should be done. These patients should be followed up regarding the adverse effects of chemotherapeutic drugs, their fertility status and tumor recurrence (Table 13.4).

Table 13.4:
Presenting symptoms

Presenting symptoms	*N*
Abdominal pain	16/14
Abdominal mass	12/41
Abdominal enlargement	7/14
Weight loss	2/41
Incidental finding on antenatal ultrasound	2/41
Vomitting	1/41
Urinary frequency	1/41
Dysmenorrhea	1/41
Dysuria	1/41
Inguinal mass	1/41

VULVOVAGINAL TUMORS IN CHILDREN AND ADOLESCENTS

Skin Tag

Anxious parents may seek consult because of perineal skin tag. The two pictures show a perineal mass in an 8-month-old (Fig. 13.27) and a 1-month-old infant (Fig. 13.28). Pathogenesis is unknown.

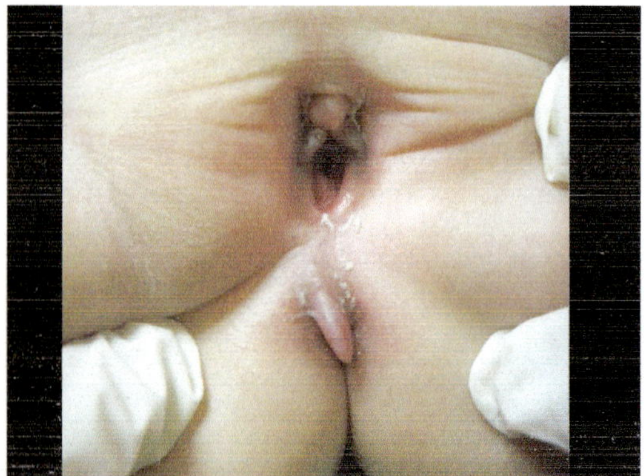

Fig. 13.27: Perineal mass in an 8-month-old child

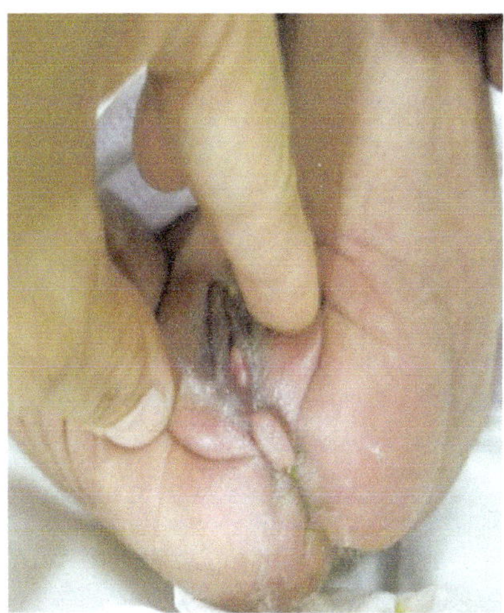

Fig. 13.28: Perineal mass in a 1-month-old child

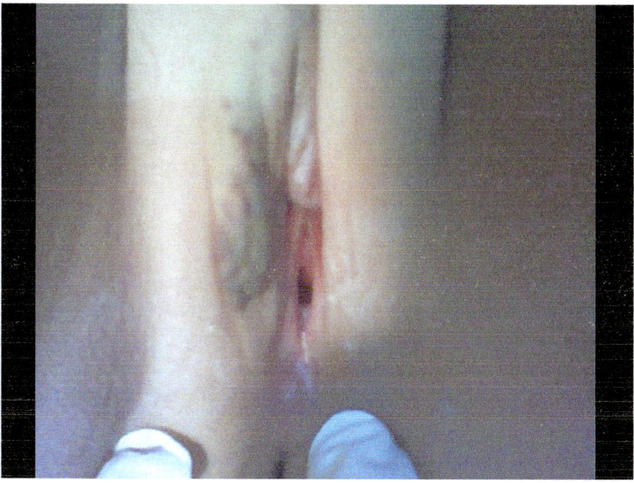

Fig. 13.30: Right labial hemangioma

In some literature, these skin tags have been renamed infantile perianal pyramidal protrusion. They have been associated with and have been believed to be an early manifestation of lichen sclerosus. They have also been seen in children with recurrent urinary tract infections, dysuria or painful defecation.

Excision and biopsy may be done, if these lesions become problematic, but observation may also be an option. Hymenal tags may also be a concern and may be excised if they cause obstruction or irritation (Fig. 13.29).

LABIAL HEMANGIOMA

One of the most complicated areas a hemangioma can develop in is the urogenital area or anogenital area (Fig. 13.30). These lesions, commonly called diaper area hemangiomas, are associated with pain, bleeding, recurring infection and ulceration.

Ulceration of hemangiomas (Fig. 13.31) occurs in 10% of all lesions during the growth period. As the hemangioma grows, the skin cannot keep up. The elasticity of the skin is reduced it then splits and opens. Because the skin over a hemangioma is compromised, it is not unusual for it to split after just a slight bump. Ulcerated hemangiomas are at great risk for infection. Perianal and urogenital lesions are at increased risk for infection because of urine and feces.

GENITAL PROLAPSED

Genital prolapsed (Fig. 13.32) in neonates is an uncommon condition. Its cause is uncertain; however, it has been associated with congenital anomalies that affect the musculature of the

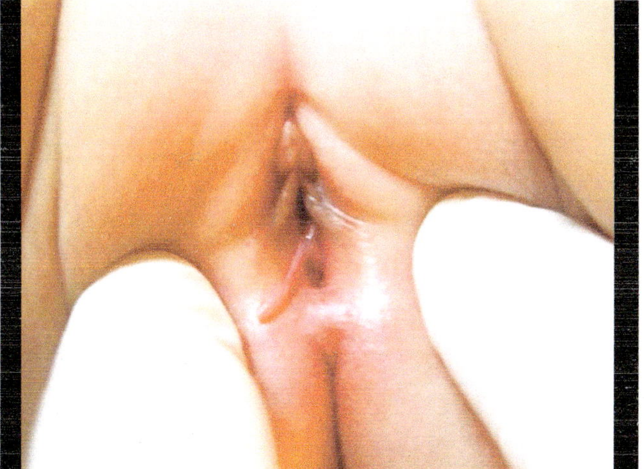

Fig. 13.29: An infant with a hymenal tag. This is a benign condition. Excision may be done if the lesion results in obstruction or irritation

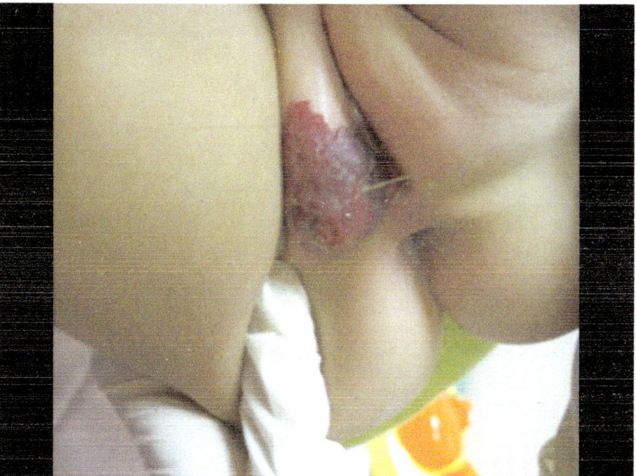

Fig. 13.31: Ulcerated labial hemangioma in an infant

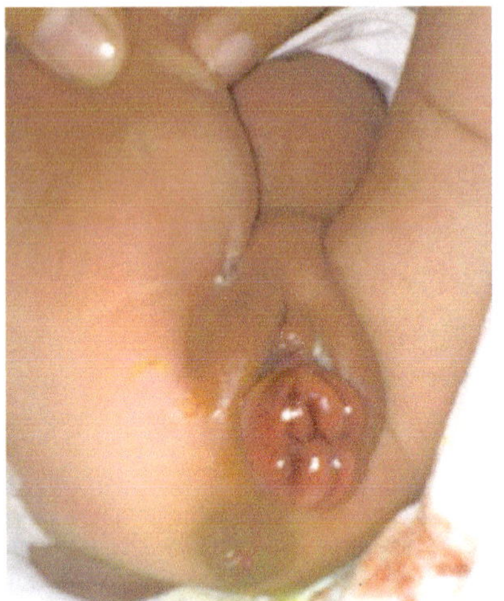

Fig. 13.32: Genital prolapsed in a newborn infant with lumbosacral meningocele

pelvic floor, primarily, neural tube defects. Other predisposing factors include increased intra-abdominal pressure, fetal maldevelopment and intrapartum trauma.

Although prenatal diagnosis may be difficult, there has been a documented case where targeted ultrasound examination is used to detect genital prolapse while the fetus is in-utero.

SQUAMOUS PAPILLOMA OF THE VULVA

Squamous papillomas are common benign tumors of the vulva. A 16-year-old girl presented with a slowly growing labial mass (Figs 13.33A and B). She underwent excision-biopsy of the mass (Fig. 13.34). Histopathology shows squamous papilloma (Fig. 13.35).

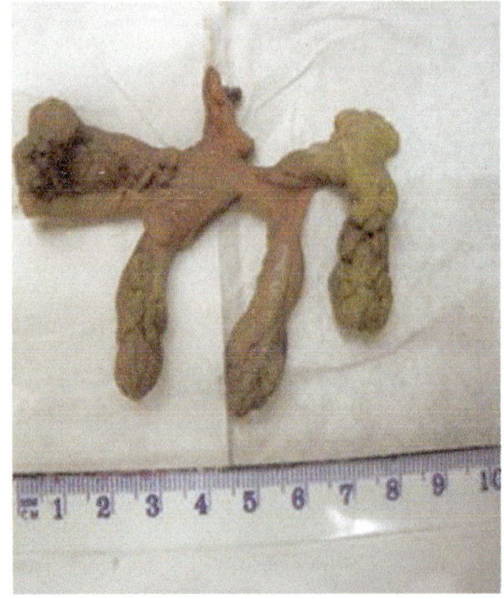

Fig. 13.34: Same patient as shown in the Figures 13.33A and B underwent excision-biopsy of the mass

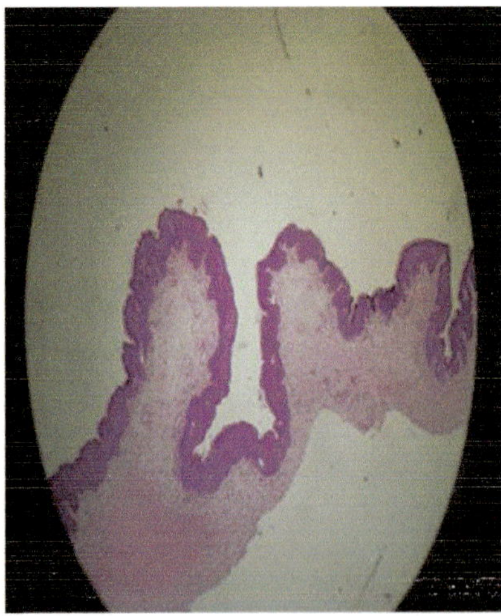

Fig. 13.35: Histopathology shows squamous papilloma

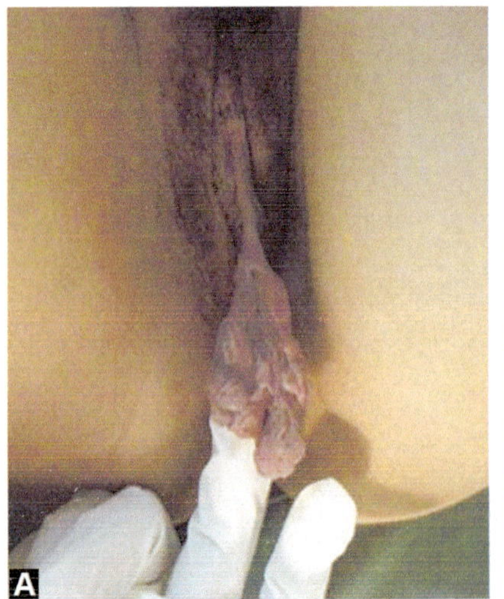

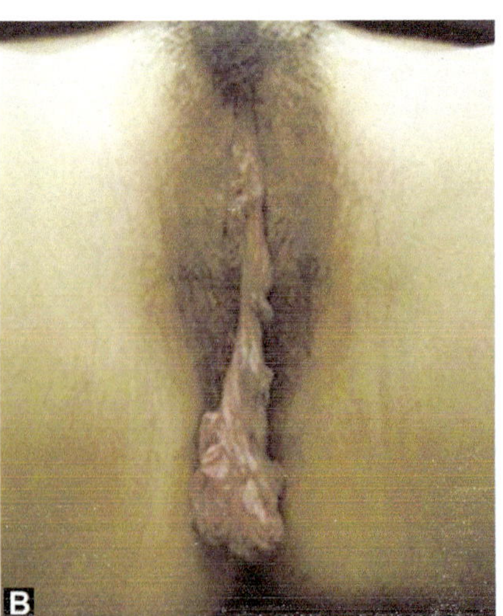

Figs 13.33A and B: A 16-year-old girl presented with slowly growing labial mass

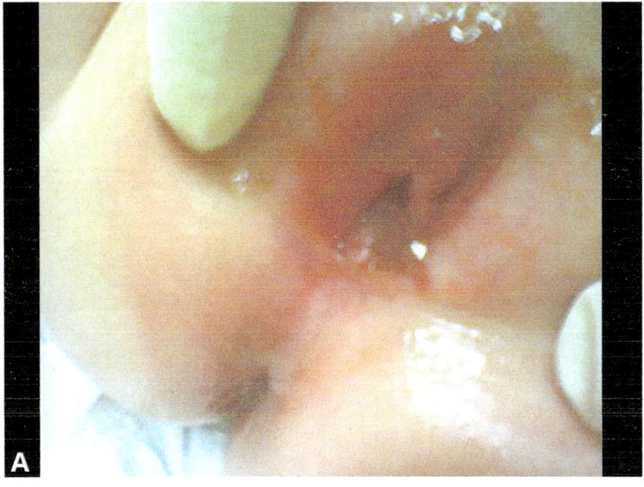

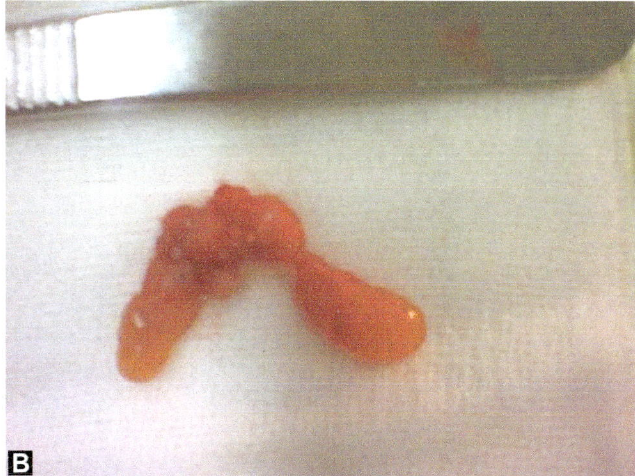

Figs 13.36A and B: Endodermal sinus tumor of the vagina preoperatively and the specimen, postoperatively

ENDODERMAL SINUS TUMOR OF THE VAGINA

This infant presented with vaginal bleeding and a vaginal mass. Excision of the mass is done and histopath reveals endodermal sinus tumor (EST) of the vagina (Figs 13.36A and B). Only 8% of EST (also known as yolk sac tumor) occurs in the vagina. This is a germ cell tumor that is derived from the embryonic remnants of the mesonephric duct.

NONGYNECOLOGIC TUMORS PRESENTING AS VULVAR MASS

Urethral Prolapse

Urethral prolapse in a 6-year-old girl presenting with bleeding are shown in the Figures 13.37A and B.

Etiology

- Uncertain, but genetic factors may play a role
- Estrogen lack may also be a factor since urethral prolapse is rare in women of child-bearing age.

Presentation

- The prolapse usually follows straining due to coughing or constipation
- Causes painless bleeding; may be associated with dysuria or vulvar pain
- Inspection of the vulva shows a tumor which is typically described as a reddish blue, donut-shaped mass.

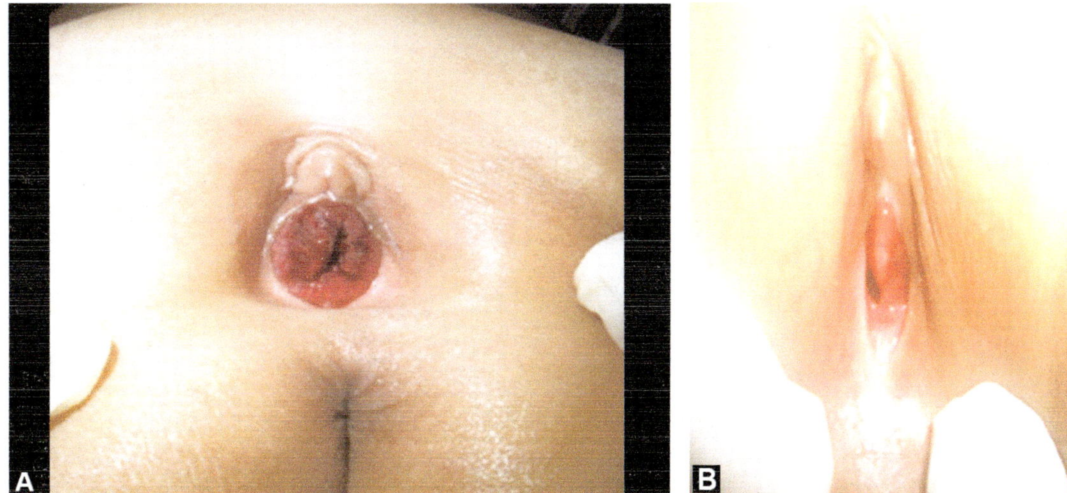

Figs 13.37A and B: Urethral prolapsed in a 6-year-old girl presenting with vaginal bleeding. (A) Before treatment with topical estrogen; (B) After treatment

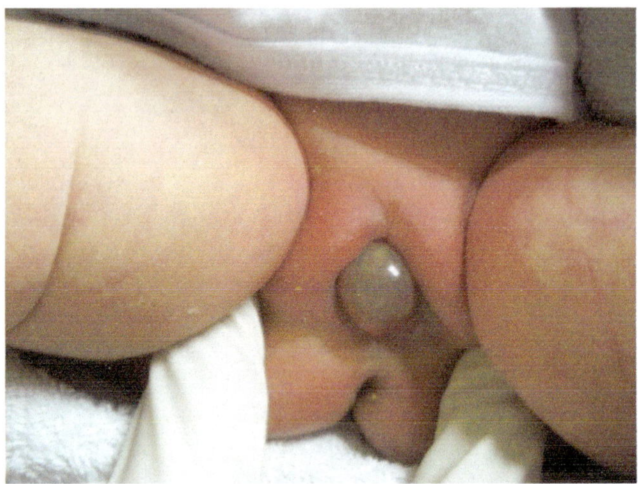

Fig. 13.38: Prolapse of ureterocele and its appearance as a vulvar mass

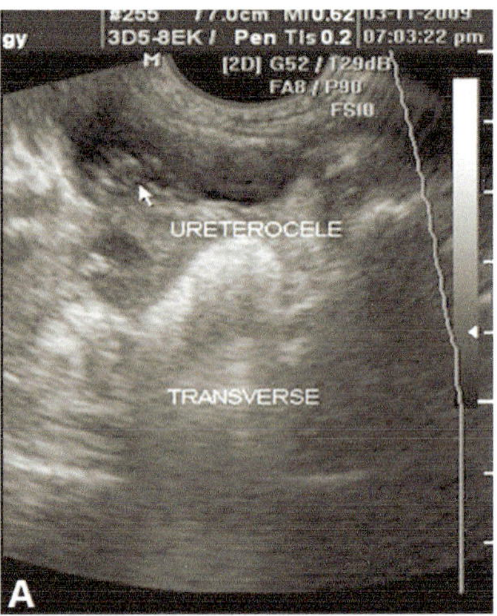

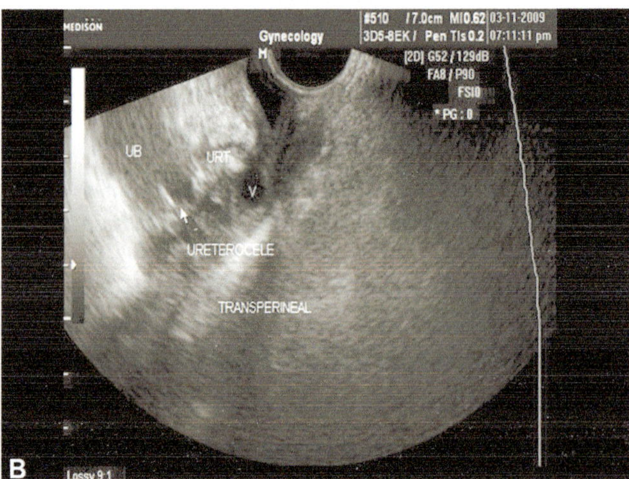

Figs 13.39A and B: Ultrasonography confirms a cystic mass inside the bladder that is continuous with the prolapsed vulvar mass

Management

- Conservative treatment
  - Local application of steroid and antibiotic
  - Application of estrogen cream on the prolapsed mucosa
- Surgical excision, if medical management fails.

PROLAPSED EXTRAVESICAL URETEROCELE

Prolapse of a ureterocele (Fig. 13.38) and its appearance as a vulvar mass is a rare condition. This may occur because of weakness in the distal ureteral wall. Diagnosis can be made by ultrasonography (Figs 13.39A and B) with the demonstration of a cystic mass inside the bladder that is continuous with the prolapsed vulvar mass.

BIBLIOGRAPHY

1. Allen L, Fleming NA, Strickland J. Adnexal masses in the neonate, child and adolescent. In: San FilippoJ, Lara-Torre E, Edmonds K, Templeman C (Eds). Clinical Pediatric and Adolecent Gynecology. New York: Informa Healthcare 2009; pp. 417-30.
2. Archana A, Ashma R, Gurung G. Ovarian tumors in childhood and adolescents: our eight years experiences. Nepal J of Obstet Gynecol 2008;3:39-42.
3. Boyd LR, Khush M, Kurtin JP. Management of ovarian cysts in the adolescent and young adult. In: Altchek A, Deligdisch L (Eds). Pediatric, Adolescent and Young Adult Gynecology. West Sussex, UK: Blackwell Publishing 2009; pp. 159-70.
4. Chatterjee U, et al. Endodermal sinus tumor of the vagina. J Indian Assoc Pediatr Surg 2003;8:235-8.
5. Cheng PJ, Shaw SW, Cheuh HY, et al. Prenatal diagnosis of fetal genital prolapse. Ultrasound Obstet Gynecol 2005; 26:204-6.
6. Donato CD, Almirante CY, De Guia B. Ovarian masses in children: an 11-year review at the Philippine Children's Medical Center. Journal of the Philippine Medical Women's Association 2006;43:17-32.
7. Hall K. Diaper area hemangiomas: a unique set of concerns. Hemangioma Newsline. [Online] MSN website. Available from: hemangnews@msn.com [Accessed March, 2009].
8. Hamel-Teillac D. Vulvo-vaginal disorders. In: Sultan C (Ed). Pediatric and Adolescent Gynecology: Evidence-Based Clinical Practice. Basel, Switzerland: Karger 2004; pp. 43-4.
9. Hanprasertpong J, Chandeying V. Gynecologic tumors during childhood and adolescence. J Med Assoc Thai 2006;89(Suppl 4):S192-8.
10. Ilica AT, Kocaoğlu M, Bulakbaşi N, et al. Prolapsing ectopic ureterocele presenting as vulval mass in a newborn girl. Diagn Interv Radiol 2008;14:33-4.
11. Jones HE, Fisher HJ. Urethral prolapse in girls. Arch Dis Child 1971;46:107-8.

12. Kumar VJ, Pushpa Kinil, Deepti Vepakomma, et al. Vaginal endodermal sinus tumor. Indian Journal of Pediatrics 2005;72:797-8.
13. Lacour M, Syed S, Linward J, et al. Role of pulsed dye laser in the management of ulcerated capillary hemangiomas. Archives of Disease in Childhood 1996;74:161-3.
14. Lang ME, Darwish A, Long AM. Vaginal bleeding in the prepubertal child. Canadian Med Assoc J 2005;172:1289-90.
15. Metz BJ, Rubenstein MC, Levy ML, et al. Response of ulcerated perineal hemangiomas of infancy to Blecaplermin Gel, a recombinant human platelet-derived growth factor. Arch Dermatol 2004;140:867-70.
16. Nussbaum AR, Lebowitz RL. Interlabial Masses in little girls: review and imaging recommendations. American J Roengen 1983;141:65-71.
17. Shawis RN, Gohary AEL, Cook RCM. Ovarian cysts and tumours in infancy and childhood. Annals of the Royal College of Surgeons of England 1985;67:17-9.
18. Templeman CL, Hertweck SP, Scheetz JP, et al. The management of mature cystic teratomas in children and adolescents: a retrospective analysis. Human Reproduction 2000;15:2669-72.

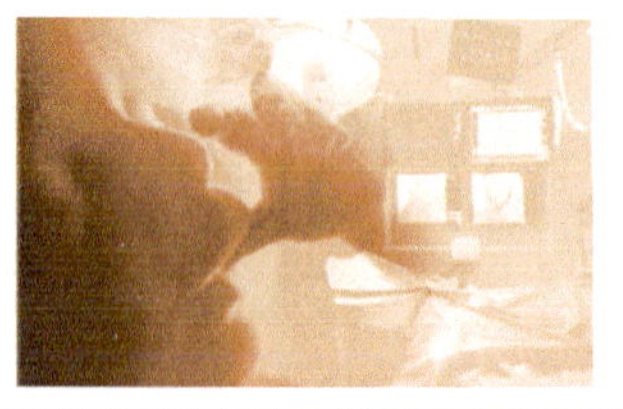

14 Adolescent Sexuality and Teenage Pregnancy

Alicia Berbano-Tamesis, Rosa Maria Hipolito-Nancho

ADOLESCENT SEXUALITY

Rosa Maria Hipolito-Nancho

DEFINITIONS

Adolescent sexuality is the totality of being a person according to the Sex Information and Education Council of the United States (SIECUS). It reflects human character and the way humans interact with each other. It has multidimensional concepts including ethical, psychological, biological and cultural dimensions. In a broader definition, sexuality refers to a range of issues including comfort with physical changes and interpersonal relationships, as well as gender roles, identity and sexual orientation. It encompasses one's attitudes, beliefs, sexual knowledge, behaviors, and includes physiologic responses like thoughts, feelings and relationships.

Gender identity: Internal acknowledgment of being either a male or a female.

Gender role: Outward expression of being male or female. It is the public expression of gender identity.

Sexual orientation: Physical and emotional attraction or arousal to another person. It describes one's attraction to the same sex or the opposite sex, or both. Heterosexual individuals are attracted to the opposite sex. Homosexual individuals are attracted to the same sex. Bisexual individuals are attracted to both sexes.

FILIPINO ADOLESCENT SEXUALITY

A survey on Filipino adolescent sexuality are listed in the Tables 14.1 to 14.4.

Table 14.1:
Demography of Filipino adolescent sexuality

Total Population
23% 10–19 years of age
20% 15–24 years of age
Sex ratio: 100.3 for age group 15–19; 99.3 for age group 20–24
(Sex ratio is the number of males per 100 females in the population)
Educational or Employment Status
85% reached high school status (2002, Raymundo et al.)
6 out of 10 finished high school or vocational training
12 million of the youth are employed or actively looking for employment
Marriage and Live-in Arrangements
According to the Young Adult Fertility Survey [YAFS (2002)]:

Contd...

Contd...

- There is a decrease in proportion of those who are formally married among the young people ages 15–24 (from 12% in 1994 to 9.6% in 2002)
- The proportion of living-in or common-law marriages rose from 4.7% to 6.0% (according to the National Statistics Office)

Growth and Development

Menarche: Mean age: 13.32 (1994) and 13.44 (1995)

Nutrition: 33 out of 100 adolescents 10–19 years of age were underweight (FNRI-DOST)

Fertility:

- Total fertility rate (TFR) declined from 5.97 (1970) to 3.73 (1996)
- TFR among young adult mothers increased from 27% (1980) to 30% (1996)
- Birth among 20 years old and below accounted for 36.3% of the total live births (1992) and 35.1% in 1992

Sexual Experiences

Homosexual experience: Prevalence rates

YAFS II (1994)	5.1% - Males; 1.8% - Females
YAFS III (2002)	4.7% - Males; 0.6% - Females
Sexual debut:	Age of first sexual encounter
YAFS I (1980)	21 years old for males; 18 years old for females
YAFS II (1994)	18 years old for both sexes
YAFS III (2002)	17 years old for males; 18 years old for females
Premarital sex:	% in population (Fig. 14.1)
YAFS I (1980)	12%
YAFS II (1994)	18% (2.2 million)
YAFS III (2002)	23.1% of respondents, more among males (31.3%) than females (15.7%)
SWS-NYC Survey (1996):	13% of youth ages 15–30 (2.7 million) engaged in premarital sex

Multiple sex partners:

YAFS III—34% males versus 9% females admitted having more than 1 partner

Commercial sex:

YAFS II versus YAFS III (data only in males)

More males in the ages 20–24 have paid for sex than in the younger age 15–19 years

More males who pay for sex are protecting themselves although at moderate levels only (48.35–56.1%)

Sexual Practices

Venue for first encounter (Fig. 14.2):

Partner or friend's house	48%
Hotel or motel	16%
Own house	14%

Use of contraceptive methods (Fig. 14.3):

YAFS II—21.7% versus YAFS III—21.0%

Practiced contraception in last premarital sex—24.7% in 1994 versus 24.8% in 2002

More females are becoming more proactive in the use of contraception

The younger age group (15–19 years old) is using contraception more in 2002 than in 1994

Condom users:

There is a doubling level in condom use with 19% in 1994 and 38.2% in 2002

Abortion

Young pregnancies account for 16.5% of abortion cases and 6.2% of spontaneous abortion in the Philippines, according to the latest report by World Health Organization

Table 14.2:
Sexual health among Filipino youth

YAFS III–Health care utilization: 21% males and 18% females sought consult for reproductive health complaints
HIV/AIDS–The Philippines has a low infection rate to HIV/AIDS
According to the Health Action Information Network (HAIN), five groups have been identified as most susceptible to HIV: women, young adults, men having sex with men, sex workers and overseas Filipino workers (OFWs)
Knowledge and awareness of HIV is high at 95% (YAFS II and YAFS III). But in the YAFS III Survey, about one-third of them believe that HIV/AIDS is curable (doubled from 12.5% to 27.8% in a span of 8 years).
73.4% of sexually active adolescents said they have no chance of getting AIDS.
Reproductive health complaints:
Females: Most common complaint of dysmenorrhea
Males: Most common complaint of painful urination

Table 14.3:
HIV/AIDS health profile in the Philippines

Total population*	91.1 million (mid-2007)
Estimated population Living with HIV/AIDS**	12,000 (7,300–20,000) (end 2005)
Adult HIV prevalence**	< 0.1% (< 0.2%) (end 2005)
HIV prevalence in most-at-risk populations**	IDUs: 1% (Cebu City) (2005); MSM: 1-3% (2001) (Cebu City and Quezon); Sex workers: 0.16% (2005) (Cebu City)
Percentage of HIV-infected people receiving antiretroviral therapy***	10% (end 2006)

*US Census Bureau
**UNAIDS
***WHO/UNAIDS/UNICEF toward Universal Access, April 2007

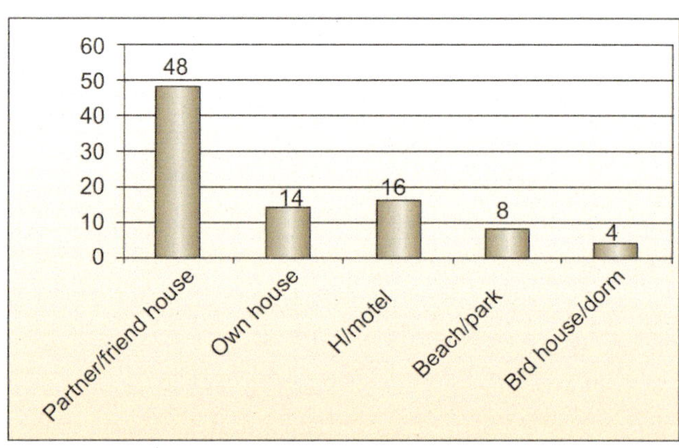

Fig. 14.2: The different venues where first premarital sex experience occurs

First Premarital Sex Experience

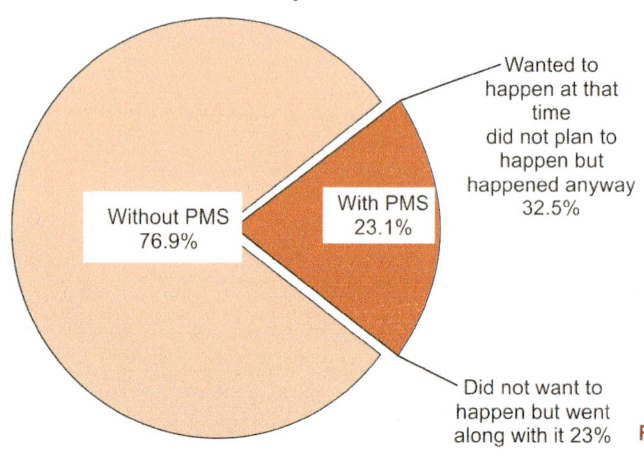

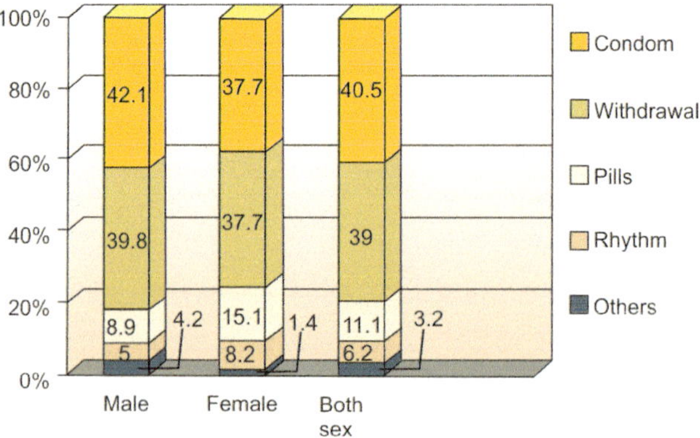

Fig. 14.3: Graph showing contraceptive methods use during the premarital sex experience

Fig. 14.1: Graph showing incidence of premarital sex

Reasons for Initiating Sexual Activity

- Curiosity
- Grown up feeling
- Partner pressure
- Friends having sex (younger adolescent)
- Being in love
- Physical attraction
- Feeling romantic
- Partner being high on drug or alcohol (older adolescent)

ADOLESCENT CONCERN AND NEEDS

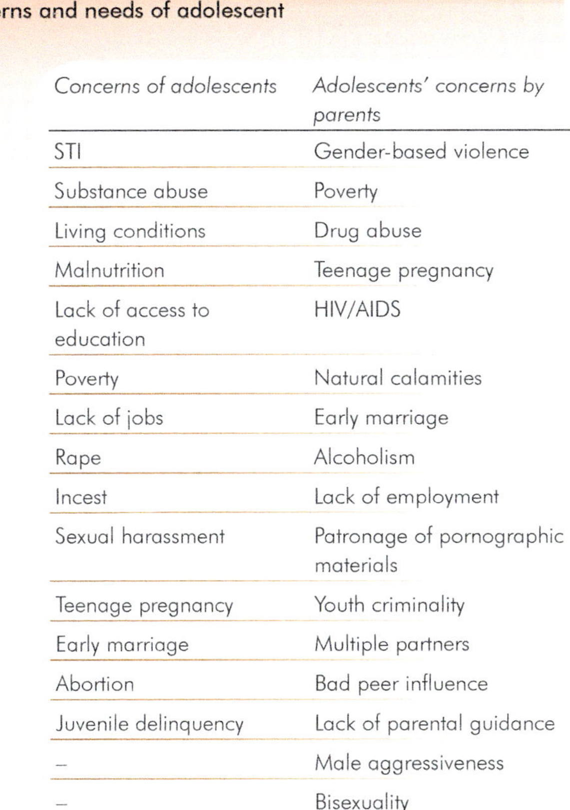

Table 14.4:

Concerns and needs of adolescent

Concerns of adolescents	*Adolescents' concerns by parents*
STI	Gender-based violence
Substance abuse	Poverty
Living conditions	Drug abuse
Malnutrition	Teenage pregnancy
Lack of access to education	HIV/AIDS
Poverty	Natural calamities
Lack of jobs	Early marriage
Rape	Alcoholism
Incest	Lack of employment
Sexual harassment	Patronage of pornographic materials
Teenage pregnancy	Youth criminality
Early marriage	Multiple partners
Abortion	Bad peer influence
Juvenile delinquency	Lack of parental guidance
–	Male aggressiveness
–	Bisexuality
–	Homosexuality

RISK BEHAVIOR AND SEXUAL HEALTH

Experience with Sex and Violence

In 10% of cases who had premarital sex said their first sexual experience happened without consent.

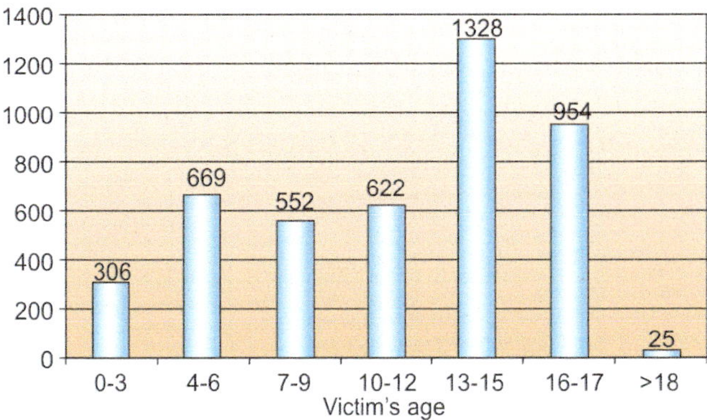

Fig. 14.4: Child abuse cases from all member CPUs treated in 2007 by age of the victim

In YAFS III, 4% said they had sex against their will while about 1% of men had same experience.

1997 SWS-NYC—6.8% (1.4 million) of Filipino youth had sex without their will; while 3.0% (0.6 million) reported forcing somebody to have sex with them.

Substance use: YAFS III (2002) reported increasing risk behaviors like smoking, drinking and drug experimentation among women. The gender gap is narrowing as more Filipinas are engaging in risky experimentation. Filipinas appear to have better judgment than men by not continuously engaging in risky behaviors.

Figures 14.4 and 14.5 show that CPU cases show a higher incidence of abuse among adolescents in various forms (physical, sexual, physical with sexual, neglect) among adolescents. This is likely due to their higher vulnerability as a consequence of risk-taking behaviors, the discovery of their burgeoning sexuality, and increasing exposure to the environment.

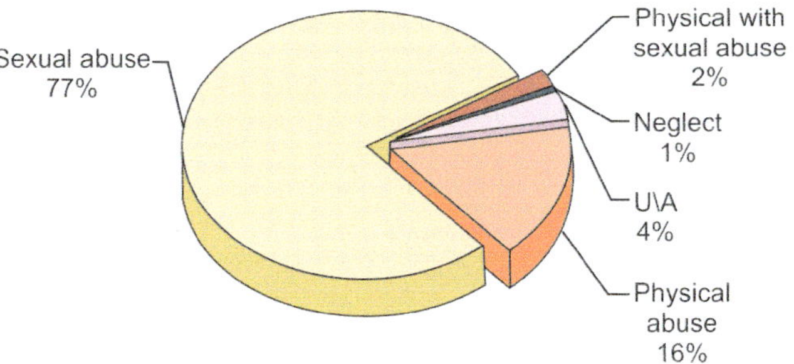

Fig. 14.5: Cases from all member CPUs treated in 2007 by Type (n = 4456)

MANY FACETS OF ADOLESCENT SEXUALITY

Alicia Berbano-Tamesis

THE CHALLENGE

1. Discussion of adolescent sexuality leads us to a different perspective or science into which it should be viewed.
2. Sexuality is not only in reference to gender, to reproductive function, to sexual urge, sexual instinct, but also the use of all of these in man's participation in the Divine plan.

The different perspectives into which sexuality should be viewed are as follows:

Anthropology: Science that deals with origins, physical and cultural development, biological features, social customs and beliefs of mankind. In other words, it is the study of man.

Sociology: Science or study of human society.

Theology: Study of divine things or of religious truths.

Metaphysics: Branch of Philosophy that deals with the question of knowledge and existence of man.

Philosophy: Study of truths and principles of existence, knowledge and conduct.

BIOPHYSICAL PERSPECTIVE

Sexuality, by means of which man and woman who give themselves to one another through acts which are proper and exclusive to spouses, is by no means purely biological. It concerns the innermost being of the human person. Procreation is therefore the continuation of creation.

Biophysics (Fig. 14.6) can furnish precise information about human sexuality. Knowledge about the dignity of the human body and sex can be obtained from the very Word of God going back to the beginning of the creation. Young men and women should therefore have great respect for their own bodies and for those of others.

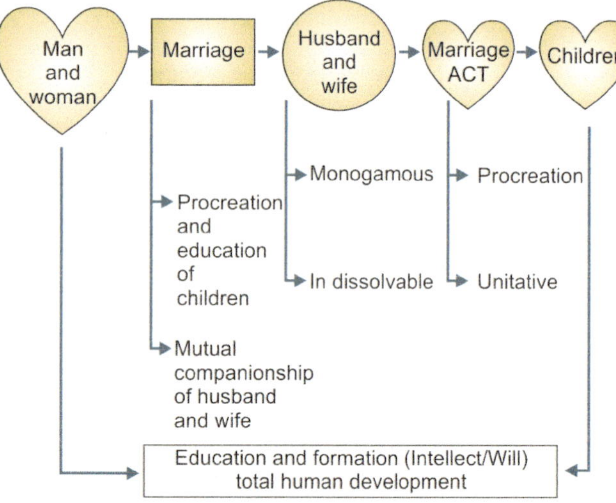

Fig. 14.6: Biophysics furnishes precise information about human sexuality

Man is a Sexual Being

By nature, man is a sexual being. Animal sex life is different from man's sex life in that it is natural and instinctive, as opposed to man's sex life which is more of a personal and moral level. Sexuality is the natural route by which human beings begin to exist.

PHYSIOLOGICAL OR ANATOMICAL FACTS THAT AFFECT ADOLESCENT SEXUALITY

Teen brain: The amygdala, which is the seat of emotion, is stimulated as the frontal lobe (seat of logic and reasoning) begins to mature during period of late adolescence.

Vaginal pH: It is different from that of adults and this makes adolescents more susceptible to sexually transmitted diseases and HIV.

The Brain

The brain (Fig. 14.7) is an organ of behavior. Both overt behavior and consciousness are manifestations of the work of the brain. Different regions of the brain regulate different functions. Thoughts, behavior and emotions are a result of how different parts of the brain work together to process information and memories.

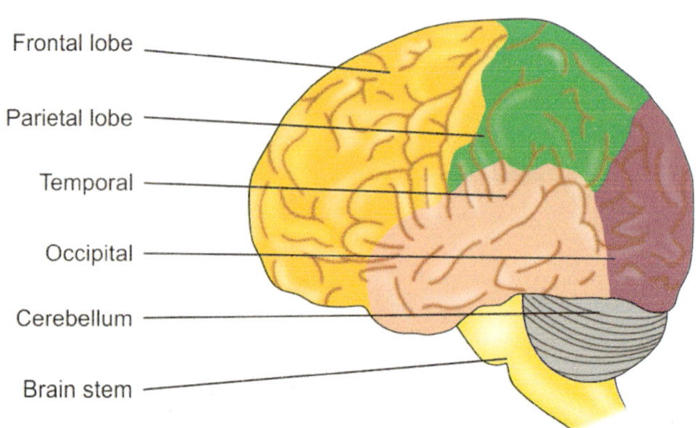

Fig. 14.7: Brain structure

Sexual Experience

Dating is becoming more a venue for sexual intimacies and activity than for socialization among the youth. The average age of sexual debut is 18 years old. The number of young adults engaging in premarital sex has steadily increased over the last decade (23% in 2002, or 4.9 million). Premarital sex experience initiates or accelerates the process of marriage. An estimated 34% of our youth have multiple sexual partners (1.6 million young people ages 15–27).

Young male adolescents have a higher rate of homosexual activity than females, e.g. 5.1% vis-a-vis 1.8%. About 4.6% of Filipino youth have been paid for sex. About 10% of girls with premarital sexual experience related that their first sexual experience happened without their consent.

Marriage

Filipino youth marry at an early age, usually before 20 years old.

Contraceptive Use

Contraceptive use is low among sexually active adolescents. About 74% (1.8 million) do not use any contraceptive method. Condoms are the most commonly used contraceptive method. Our youth have poor knowledge and low use of contraceptive methods. Only 27% think that the pill must be taken before or after sexual intercourse. Only 4% of young women can be considered knowledgeable on the subject of contraception and family planning.

Early Pregnancy

One-fourth of all women begin childbearing by age of 20 years. Less educated women are more likely to bear children in their teenage years than their better-educated counterparts.

Related Issues

- Increasingly, females are trying risky sexual behaviors (17% in 1994 and 30% in 2002)
- Sex is learned from peers, media, X-rated films and parents
- Media is the most common source of information about sex
- Over 90% of adolescents aged 15–24 believe that the government should provide family planning services
- Adolescents are generally conservative toward pre-marital sex and majority disapproves of homosexual relations and abortion. Males are more open to pre-marital sex
- About 89.82% of males would like a virgin bride

Cultural Practices and Tradition

- Arranged, early and trial marriage among cultural minorities
- Circumcised clitoris among Africans
- Cordillera tribes

  Teenage pregnancy is less among these tribes because of the following:
  - Respect for parents
  - Respect for others, based on what is right or wrong, especially in relation to sexuality

Emerging Issues

- Commercial sex:
  - College students for tuition
  - Professional prostitutes
  - *Use of technology:* Young couple having sex captured in tapes, which are then sold; persons involved may or may not be aware that their actions are recorded
- Same-sex relationships
- Tomboys or gays confused with their genders
- Casual sex: no relationship, just mutual attraction.

Sexually Transmitted Infections (HIV/AIDS)

The prevalence rate of Gonorrhea and Chlamydia are higher among young people. Most cases of HIV infections among females happen at a younger age compared to males. About 47% of infected females are between 20 and 29 years of age. In 6% among 78% of sexually active male adolescents who have never used condoms admitted to buying commercial sex, and males are more likely to pay, and be paid, for sex. Majority of those engaged in commercial sex do not use condoms. Awareness of AIDS is high. About 95% of all Filipino youth stated that they have heard of AIDS. There is a misconception that AIDS can be cured (23% in 2002).

Other Issues

- Sexuality among the mentally retarded
- Psychotic patients
- Victims of sexual abuse—poor self-esteem among these adolescents lead to premarital sex
- Children in difficult situations.

Advocacy Program in Relation to Adolescent Sexuality

I am Strong Program: This is a leadership and values formation program for high school and university students, parents and teachers. Its premise is on acquiring qualities like fortitude, temperance, perseverance, prudence and social justice.

Program on sex respect: This program introduces truth about love measured by principles of healthy human relationships.

These programs are holistic programs that integrate character education and values-based education in human sexuality. Chastity education and character formation should therefore be integrated in advocacy actions for the youth.

CONCLUSIONS

- Awareness of the dignity of man should be the springboard of advocacy actions
- Operation of man has spiritual dimensions
- Man has a role in the divine plan.

TEENAGE PREGNANCY

Rosa Maria Hipolito-Nancho

THE COMPREHENSIVE TEEN PREGNANCY PREVENTION PROGRAM

The Comprehensive Teen Pregnancy Program (Flow chart 14.1) of the Philippine Children's Medical Center.

Teen pregnancy rates: 46 of 1,000 births are from girls 15–19 years old Teen pregnancy rate = 8% Teenage pregnancy increased from 7% in 1998 to 8% in 2003 - 2003 Philippine Health Statistics 1 out of 5 mothers aged 15–24 die during pregnancy or childbirth - Save the children (2007)

The "Teen Pregnancy Clinic" of the Teen Republic, Philippine Children's Medical Center, is a comprehensive program that provides personalized, confidential prenatal care to pregnant teenagers ranging 11–19 years of age. Teenage patients are seen by a selected group of physicians and health care providers with extensive experience for caring for adolescent patients.

Pregnant teenagers are scheduled on specific days of the week in an effort to optimize the educational and social support resources available to them as well as their obstetrical or medical care. Teens enrolled in this program are able to and are encouraged to pursue their education throughout pregnancy.

A series of educational discussions on various parenting issues to be organized at convenient times making sure they do not interfere with school hours. Topics include but are not limited to:

- Self-esteem
- First aid
- Labor signs
- Baby care and safety
- Breastfeeding and proper nutrition
- Secondary abstinence or contraception
- Preterm baby nursery tour
- Parenting skills
- Labor and delivery tours
- Immunizations
- Feminine hygiene

After delivery, the teen mother is enrolled to the— "Teen Pregnancy Prevention Program" (Flow chart 14.1) which ensures comprehensive post-delivery care to the teen mother and the newborn baby. This is a 6-month clinic based program wherein the teen mother comes in for follow-up together with her baby. The teen mother receives one-on-one confidential and personalized counseling on family planning and pregnancy prevention, although involvement of family members, partners and friends is encouraged. During this period, a group of highly trained personnel gauges the needs and identify the high risk teen mothers based on several criteria and interventions are planned based on this assessment. Key components of this intervention are the behavioral skills development, abstinence plus sexual education, STD or HIV education, cervical cancer screening and prevention, parenting and life skills development, values education and social support evaluation. At the same time, the teen mother brings their child for regular pediatric care and immunizations.

Objectives of the Program

- To provide comprehensive prenatal care to pregnant teenagers:
  - To teach the pregnant teen about prenatal care and delivery
  - To teach the pregnant teen about responsible parenthood, parenting skills and life coping skills after delivery
  - To teach the pregnant teen about the importance of continuing and completing education
  - To provide social support to the pregnant teens and link them to support groups

Flow chart 14.1: Referral system for teen pregnancy prevention program

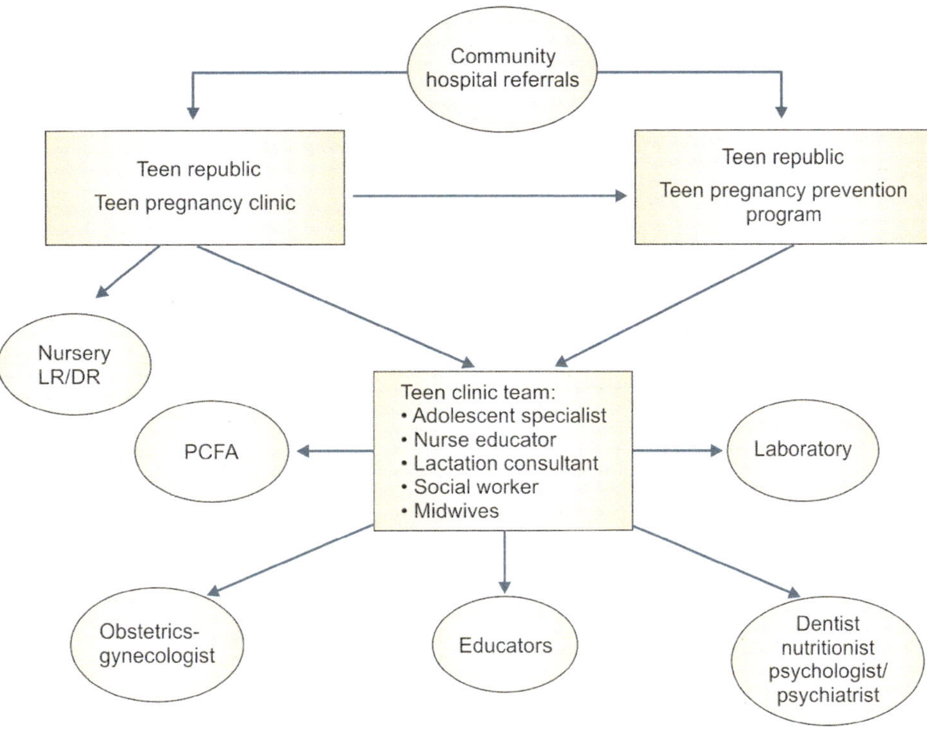

- To provide education and services for pregnancy prevention, STD and HIV education and on other risks related to teen pregnancy:
  - To encourage secondary abstinence as the only sure way of pregnancy prevention
  - To teach comprehensive sexual education and contraception
  - To counsel teens about STD, HIV testing and prevention of other health risks like smoking, substance abuse and sexual abuse.

The staff consists of highly trained physicians, experienced midwives, nurse educator or lactation consultant, a social worker and counselors. The obstetrics and gynecology staff is immediately accessible for referral and consultations. The dentists, the dietitian or nutritionist and psychiatrist or psychologist are also readily accessible in the clinic.

BIBLIOGRAPHY

1. Benson, Paul. Patient Information: Adolescent Sexuality. [Online] uptodate website. Available from www.uptodate.com [Accessed March, 2009].
2. Child Protection in the Philippines. [Online] Philippine Resource Network. Available from www.childprotection.org.ph [Accessed May, 2009]
3. Cuisia-Cruz, Erlinda. The Comprehensive Teen Pregnancy Prevention Program of the Philippine Children's Medical Center, 2008.
4. Feldmann J, Middleman B. Adolescent sexuality. Current Opinion in Obstetrics and Gynecology 2002;14:489-93.
5. Greydanus, Donald E Patel, Dilip R Pratt, et al. Essential Adolescent Medicine. New York: McGraw Hill Medical Publishers, 2006.
6. HIV/AIDS Health Profile. 2008. [Online] usaid website. Available from www.philippines.usaid. gov [Accessed September, 2008].
7. Ogena NB. How are the Filipino youth changing? The shifting lifestyles of our nation's young, 1970s and 1990s. Philippine Social Science Reviews 1999;56:83-106.
8. Raymundo C, Cruz G. Youth Sex and Risk Behaviors in the Philippines: A Report on a Nationwide Study, 2002 Young Adult Fertility and Sexuality Study (YAFS 3), 2004.
9. Sexual and Reproductive Health of Adolescents and Youth in the Philippines: A Review of Literature and Projects, 1995-2003. World Health Organization, Western Pacific Region, 2005.
10. Strasburger VC, Brown RT, et al. Adolescent Medicine: A Handbook for Primary Care. Philadelphia: Lippincott Williams and Wilkins, 2005.

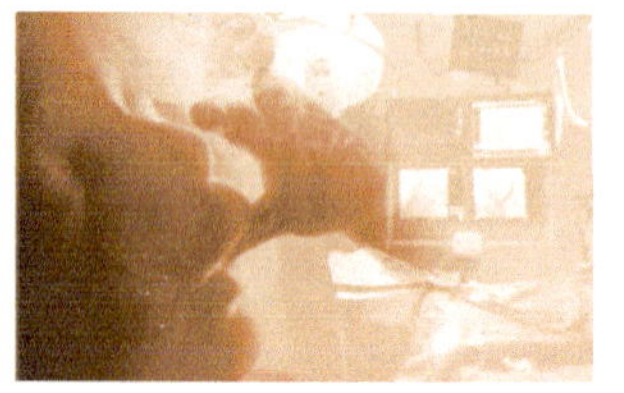

15 Immunization for Adolescents

Rosa Maria Hipolito-Nancho

Immunization for adolescents remains a challenge in the Philippines. Primarily, the government has not targeted adolescents in its immunization programs. Secondly, adolescents hardly come for preventive health services (Table 15.1). Many parents only realize that their children still need some boosters or catch-up immunizations when they are brought to a clinic or physician for consultation due to an illness. Because adolescents continue to be affected adversely by vaccine-preventable diseases like varicella, rubella, pertussis, hepatitis B and hepatitis A, it remains imperative to encourage parents to have their adolescents avail of immunizations.

To encourage immunizations in adolescents, it is important to establish a routine schedule for preventive health visits for teenager.

Recommendations for immunizations by the Society of Adolescent Medicine of the Philippines (SAMPI) are consistent with the recommendations of the Philippine Pediatric Society (PPS) Inc., the Philippine Infectious Disease Society of the Philippines (PIDSP), the Philippine Obstetrical and Gynecological Society (POGS) and the Philippine Foundation for Vaccination.

Table 15.1:

The Society of Adolescent Medicine of the Philippines recommends the following preventive series

Recommendations	*Early*	*Middle*	*Late*
Annual health screening	√	√	√
Risk assessment or screening	√	√	√
Growth monitoring and promotion	√	√	√
Physical examination	√	√	√
Developmental assessment	√	√	√
Anticipatory guidance or counseling	√	√	√
Immunizations update	√	√	√

SAMPI recommends the following:

1. Catch up immunizations should be given to all adolescents at every opportunity.
   Measles, Mumps and Rubella (MMR): A second dose is routinely given at 4–6 years of age or at ages 11–12 years, but may be given at any visit provided at least one month has elapsed from the first dose. Make sure that the adolescent is not pregnant and emphasize that she cannot be pregnant for at least 3 months thereafter.
2. *Tetanus Diphtheria Toxoid*: Should have 3 doses given at 0, 1, 6–12 months. Booster is given after 10 years. If a patient received DPT in childhood, a Td or Tdap booster is given at 11–12 years. If they missed the Td/Tdap booster at 11–12 years, it may still be given between 13–18 years.
   Acellular pertussis vaccine: The vaccine has been recently recommended by the PIDSP to be given in the form of a Tdap due to studies of recent increase in reported cases and because studies show that adolescents serve as reservoir of pertussis for infants and children. Adolescents aged 10–18 years should receive a single dose of Tdap instead of Td for booster immunization against tetanus, diphtheria, and pertussis, if they have completed the recommended childhood DTP/DTaP vaccination series and have not received Td or Tdap. Td booster is 10 years thereafter. An interval of at least 5 years between Td and Tdap is encouraged to reduce the risk for local and systemic reactions.
3. *Hepatitis B vaccine*: The adolescent should have received 3 doses during infancy. If they have not received

before, they should receive it in adolescence. Lapsed immunization does not entail repeating the entire series. Give dose at next visit as if usual interval had lapsed.

4. *Varicella vaccine*: First dose is given at 12 months old then second dose is given at 4–6 years. For catch-up, 2 doses are given. Varicella vaccine is given 3 months apart if the patient is less than 13 years old; If patient is more than13 years old, it may be given 4 weeks apart.
5. *Human papilloma virus vaccine (HPV)*: Given in 3 doses, it is now recommended in the Philippines for children 10 years and above. For the bivalent vaccine (HPV-16 and -18) it is given at a schedule of 0, 1 and 6 month schedule. For the quadrivalent vaccine (HPV-16, -18, -6 and -10) the schedule is 0, 2 and 6 months and can be given as early as 9 years.
6. *Influenza vaccine*: Given to immunocompromised patients like chronic cardiovascular conditions, chronic lung disease and renal disease. Influenza vaccine is recommended yearly.

BIBLIOGRAPHY

1. Immunization for Filipino Women 2007. Task force on immunization in women. Philippine Obstetrical and Gynecological Society (POGS), Inc.
2. Recommendations and Changes: Childhood Immunization Schedule 2009. Committee on Immunizations, Pediatric Infectious Disease Society of the Philippines.
3. Adolescent Immunizations, Society of Adolescent Medicine of the Philippines (SAMPI), Inc., (booklet) 2009.
4. Centers for Disease Control and Prevention. Immunization of adolescents: recommendations of the Advisory Committee on Immunization Practices, the American Academy of Pediatrics, the American Academy of Family Physicians, and the American Medical Association. MMWR 1996;45 (No. RR-13):[inclusive page numbers].

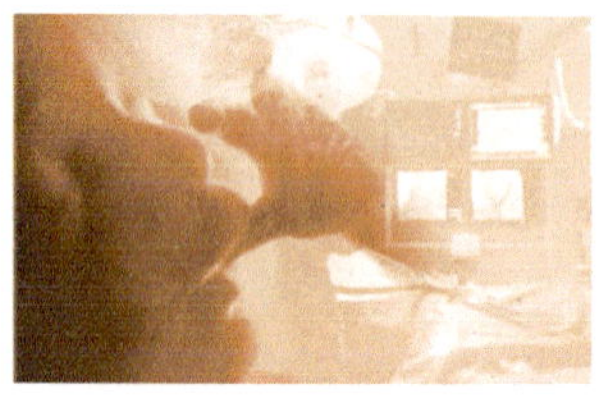

16 Sexual Abuse of Children and Adolescents

Bernadette J Madrid, Merle P Tan

PRESENTATION

The child or adolescent may be brought to the OB-Gynecologist for the following reasons:

1. The child or adolescent made a disclosure of sexual abuse.
2. The sexual abuse of the child may have been witnessed by another person.
3. The child or adolescent is referred by the police for a "medico-legal" evaluation.
4. The child or adolescent has a vaginal discharge.
5. The child or adolescent has a sexually transmitted infection.
6. The young adolescent is pregnant.
7. The adolescent got drunk or lost consciousness during a party or a date and the parents are worried that she might have been sexually abused.

MAKING THE DIAGNOSIS

Majority of the time when children and adolescents (the generic term, child, is used herein, to refer to both children and adolescent) are brought for medical evaluation, little or no history may be available except that provided by the child or adolescent. However, the medical diagnosis of child sexual abuse can be made on the basis of the child's history alone. Physical findings are present in less than 5% of cases. Even in cases where the perpetrator admits to penetration of the child's genitalia and where the adolescent is already pregnant, majority of genital findings are still normal. In one study of pregnant adolescents, only 2 out of 36 had evidence of penetration.

TYPES OF EXAMINATION

1. Acute evidentiary examination (within 72 hours of the incident) Forensic evidence collection may be appropriate (use rape kit).

   Body swabs collected in prepubertal children more than 24 hours after a sexual assault are unlikely to yield forensic evidence and most of the forensic evidence may be recovered from clothing and linen.
2. Non-acute examination (more than 72 hours).

   Forensic evidence collection with the use of a rape kit is not performed anymore. All examinations should not be traumatic to the child. Speculum and digital examination should not be performed on the prepubertal child unless under anesthesia and only for specific indications, e.g. for suspected foreign body. The hymenal orifice is not measured because it is not helpful in assessing the likelihood of abuse. The examination should be thorough from head to foot and not only centered on the genital area. The anal examination is an essential component.

CHILD MALTREATMENT MEDICO-LEGAL TERMINOLOGY AND INTERPRETATION OF MEDICAL FINDINGS IN CHILD

Sexual Abuse: A Consensus of Medical and Legal Child Protection Experts in the Philippines

Anogenital findings can be classified under the following categories:

Nonspecific findings: Findings that may be the result of sexual abuse depending on the timing of the examination with respect to the abuse, but which may also be due to other causes, or may be variants of normal.

Suggestive of abuse: Findings that have been noted in children with documented abuse and may be suggestive of abuse, but for which insufficient data exists to indicate that abuse is the only cause. History is crucial in determining overall significance.

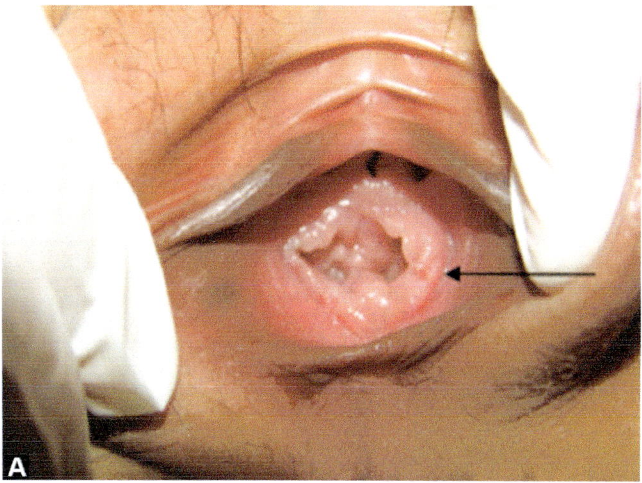

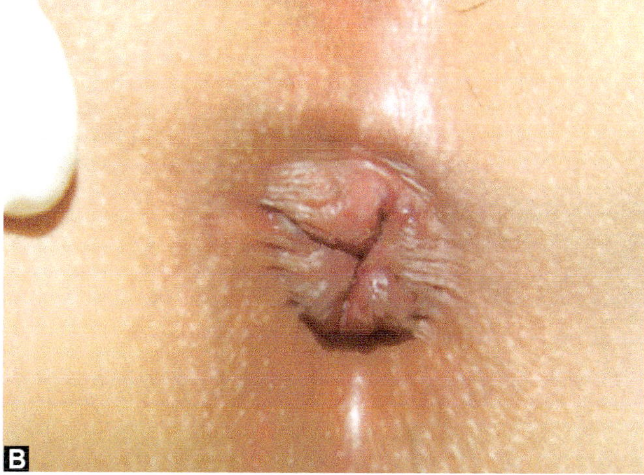

Figs 16.1A and B: (A) Petechiae at 3 o'clock; (B) Anal swelling and laceration at 5 o'clock

Clear evidence of blunt force or penetrating trauma: Findings which have no explanation other than trauma to the hymen or perianal tissues.

No evident injury at the time of examination: Findings are normal. The term "normal", "virgin state" or "intact hymen" is not used. The hymen of children heals very well. In fact, the hymen can grow back to "normal".

CLEAR EVIDENCE

Case 1

A case of sexually abused 15-year-old girl shown in the Figures 16.1A and B.

- A 15-year-old sexually abused girl with disclosure of penile—vaginal penetration
- Examined within 24 hours from the time of examination
- With genital and anal penetration

Case 2

A case of sexually abused 17-year-old pregnant teen shown in the Figures 16.2A and B.

SUGGESTIVE ABUSE

Case 1

A 15-year-old teen with disclosure of penile penetration by an acquaintance shown in the Figure 16.3.

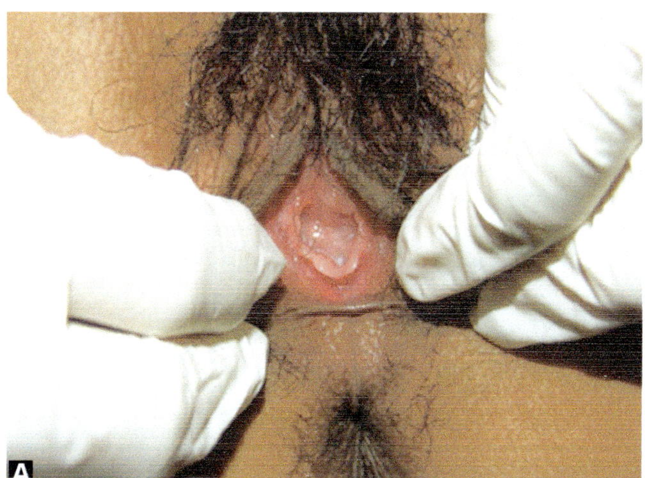

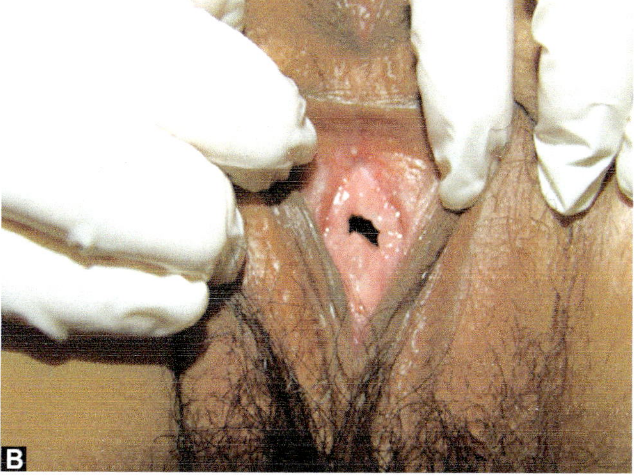

Figs 16.2A and B: (A) Supine position 17-year-old pregnant teen with normal anogenital findings; (B) Knee chest position. Fimbriated hymen, normal hymenal findings in a pregnant teen

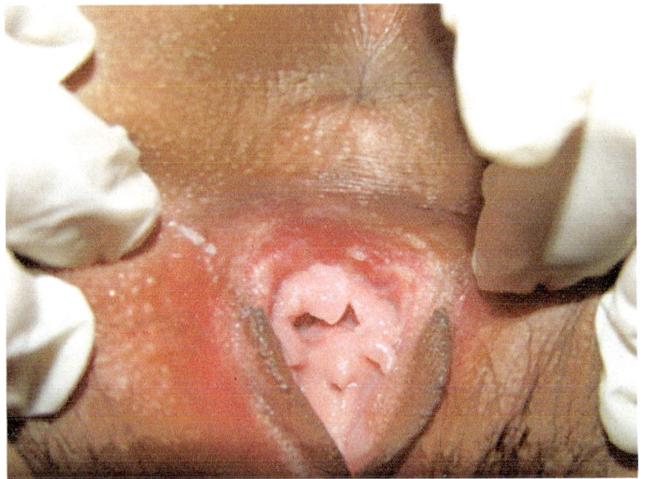

Fig. 16.3: Knee chest position. Deep notch at 7 o'clock

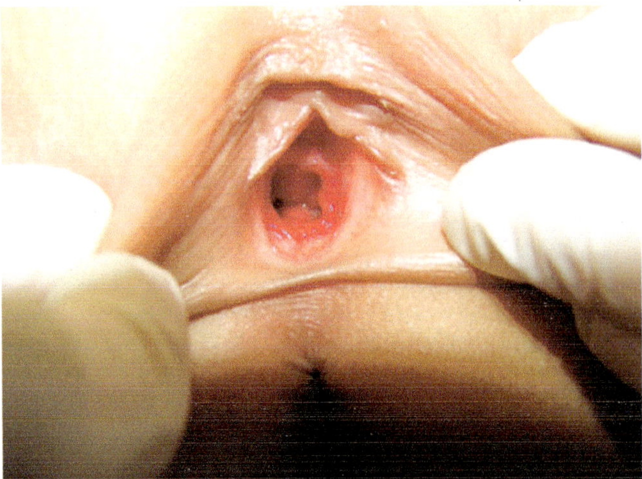

Fig. 16.4: Generalized redness of the hymen

NONSPECIFIC FINDINGS

Case 1

An 8-year-old girl with disclosure of penile penetration by a neighbor shown in the Figure 16.4. Examination done within 24 hours of incident.

NORMAL VARIANT

Case 1

A case with septate hymen is illustrated in Figures 16.5A and B.

Case 2

A 4-year-old girl child with chief complaint of vaginal discharge as shown in the Figures 16.6A and B. No disclosure of abuse.

NO EVIDENT INJURY

Case 1

A 7-year-old girl with disclosure of digital penetration shown in the Figure 16.7.

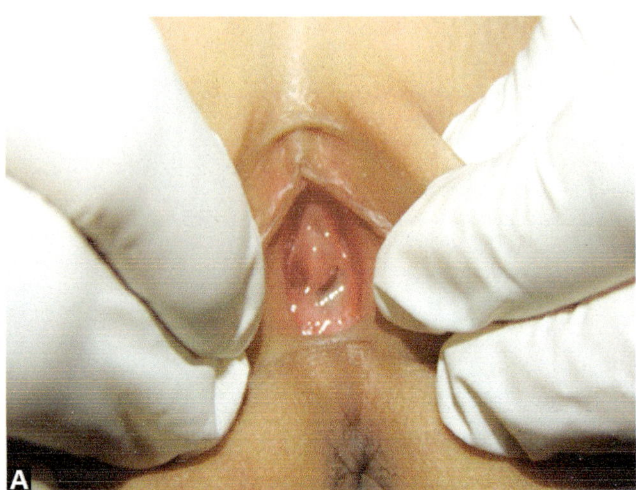

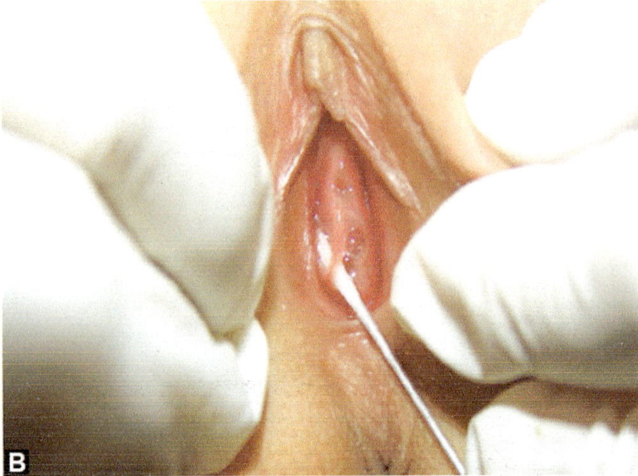

Figs 16.5A and B: (A) Septate hymen; (B) Septate hymen with cotton swab

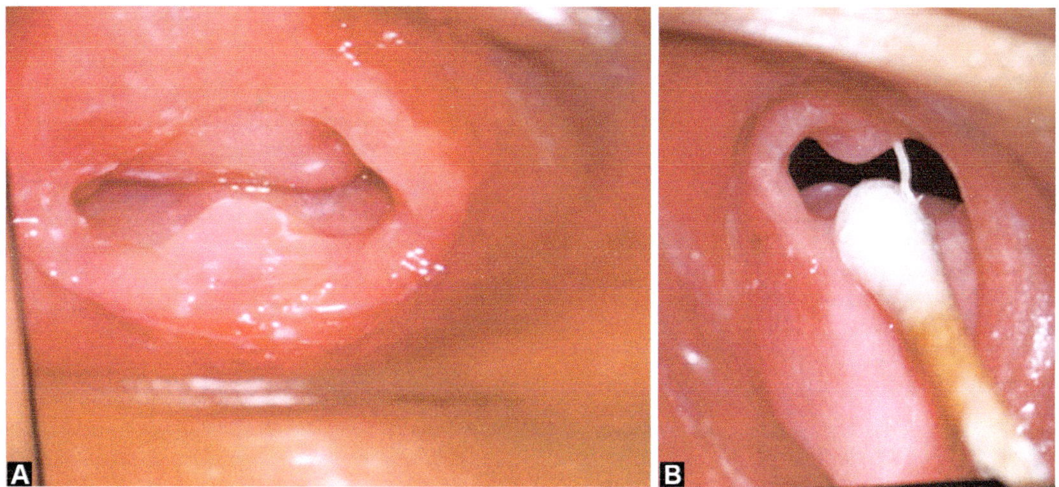

Figs 16.6A and B: (A) Supine position. Mound at 6 o'clock. Normal variant; (B) Knee chest position with pin worm

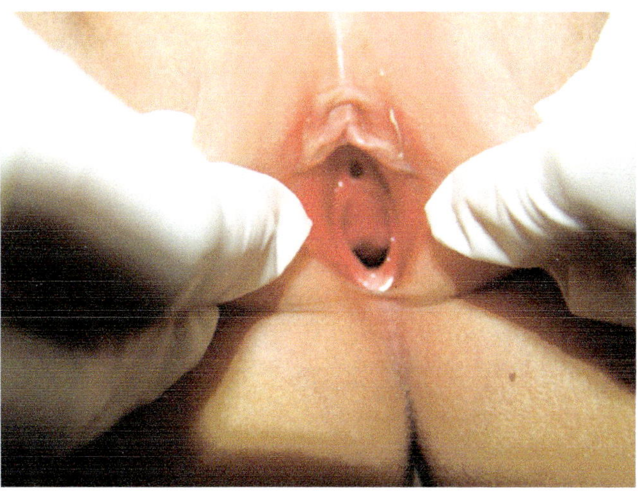

Fig. 16.7: Supine position. Annular hymen with no evident injury at the time of examination

BIBLIOGRAPHY

1. Heger A, Ticson L, Velasquez O, et al. Children referred for possible sexual abuse: a comparison of clinical history and medical findings in 2384 children. Child Abuse Negl 2002;26:645-59.
2. Kellog N, Menard S, Santos A. Genital anatomy in pregnant adolescents: "Normal" does not mean "Nothing Happened". Pediatrics 2004;113:67-9.
3. Christian C, Lavelle J, De Jong A, et al. Forensic evidence findings in prepubertal victims of sexual assault. Pediatrics 2000;106:100-4.
4. McCann J, Sheridan M, Boyle C, et al. Healing of hymenal injuries in prepubertal and adolescent girls: a descriptive study. Pediatrics 2007;119:1094-106.
5. Heppenstall-Heger A, McConnel G, Ticson L, et al. Healing patterns in anogenital injuries: a longitudinal study of injuries associated with sexual abuse, accidental injuries, or genital surgery in the preadolescent child. Pediatrics 2003;112:829-37.

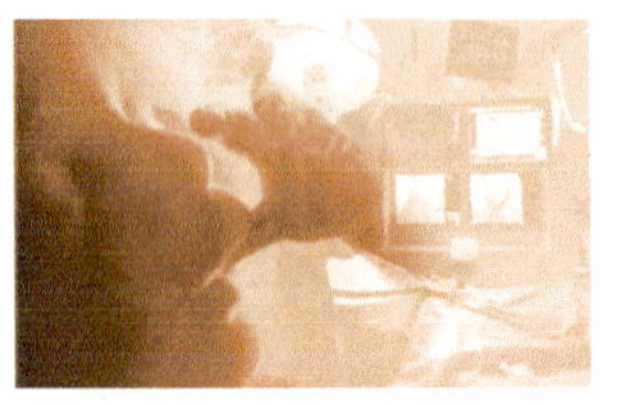

17 Genital Trauma in the Pediatric and Adolescent Female

Marietta S Sapaula

INTRODUCTION

Pain, swelling or bleeding in the genital area are the usual complaints of females who are likely to have genital trauma. Injuries can be intentional or accidental. Careful examination should be done to look for lesions not only externally but also the possibility of internal lesions should be considered especially, if patient is complaining of abdominal or low back pain. The exact prevalence and incidence of genital trauma is unknown. In adults, female genital trauma is primarily related to childbirth. In pediatrics, however, it is a common presentation of an accidental injury, like trauma, due to penetrating or nonpenetrating injuries. The injuries can be intentional like sexual abuse and female genital mutilation in countries like Africa and in some parts of Asia and the Middle East.

CAUSES OF GENITAL TRAUMA

Accidental Injuries

Accidental or unintentional genital trauma is seen as the most common presenting complaint in the pediatric emergency department. It has been noted that more than 80% of cases result from straddle injuries and 18.1% are from penetrating mechanisms, water jet injury and motor vehicle accidents. Other injuries that may cause genital trauma are bites and burns.

Straddle Injuries

Straddle injury occurs when the patient straddles an object during a fall, striking the urogenital area with the force of her body weight. Injury is caused by the compression of soft tissues against the bony margins of the pelvic outlet. Examples of objects that may cause these accidents are arms of chairs, countertops, ledges of pools and bathtubs, bicycle crossbars and ladder rungs. Manifestations may vary from abrasions to contusions, lacerations and most commonly, vulvar hematomas (Figs 17.1A and B and 17.2A and B). Typically these are nonpenetrating, unilateral and superficial, which usually involve the mons, clitoral hood and labia minora, anterior or lateral to the hymen. Straddle injury to the hymen or posterior fourchette is rare and should raise suspicion of sexual abuse.

A retrospective review of the cases of genital trauma at the Pediatric and Adolescent Gynecology Unit of the Philippine Children's Medical Center from 2002–2009 shows that the most common cause of accidental female genital trauma is a straddle injury (Table 17.1). Out of the 52 cases, only 1 was secondary to sexual abuse, the rest being due to straddle injuries.

Table 17.1: Genital trauma cases at the Pediatric and Adolescent Gynecology (PAG) unit of the Philippine Children's Medical Center (PCMC) from 2002-2009

Years	Total number of cases
2002	10
2003	9
2004	10
2005	2
2006	6
2007	6
2008	5
2009 (until June 2009)	4
Total	52

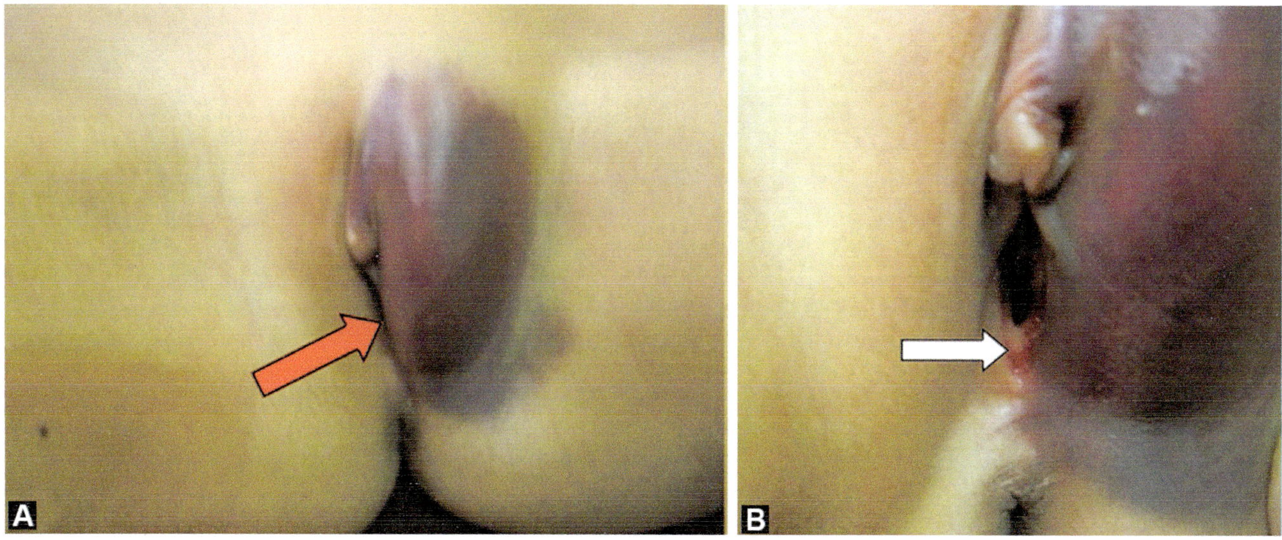

Figs 17.1A and B: A 6-year-old girl who straddled a chair during a fall, causing a 5 × 3 cm violaceous mass at the left labia majora (red arrow), with hymenal contusion at the 4 o'clock position (white arrow)

Animal and Human Bites

It is not uncommon to be bitten by animals especially a pet dog or a cat; but to be bitten in the genitalia, which is usually a covered area, is rare. The usual areas that may be affected are the extremities, but in children, bites may be seen on the face, neck and buttocks. Bites due to people are seen in all age groups. Small children may sometimes bite each other when they fight or an older sibling may bite the younger one because of jealousy. Young adults are frequently seen for bites in the genital area acquired during sexual foreplay.

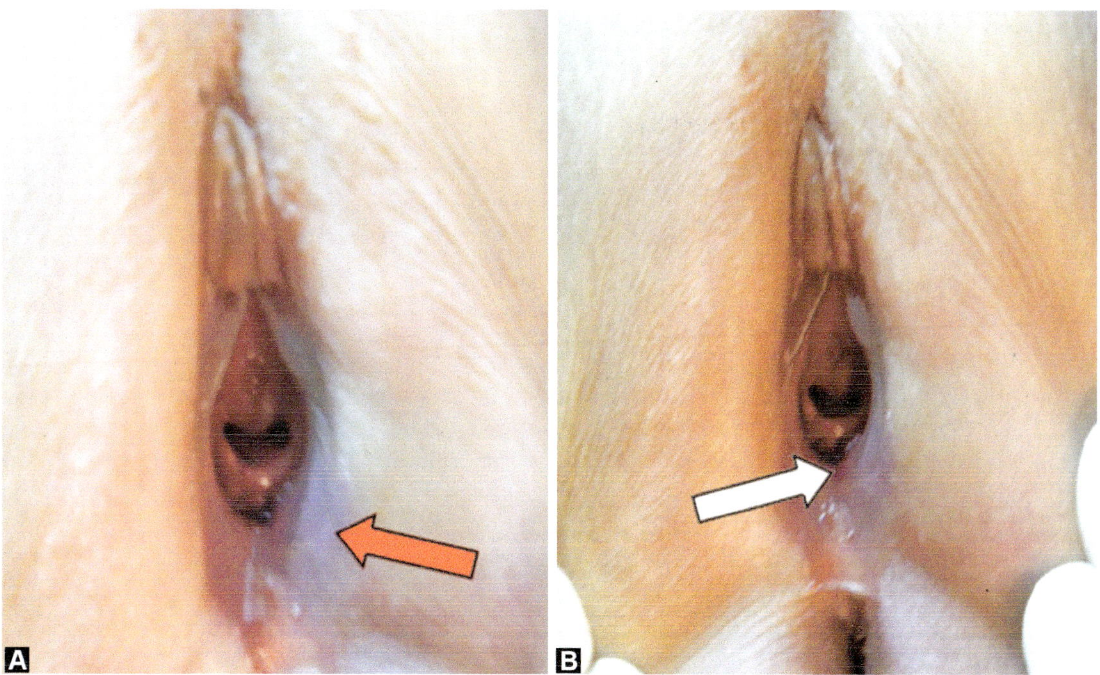

Figs 17.2A and B: A 7-year-old girl who presented with vaginal bleeding after she forcefully fell on a bicycle seat, causing posterior labia minora hematoma (red arrow), and a 0.75 cm perihymenal laceration at the posterior fourchette (white arrow)

Love bites qualify as human bites. By far the most common location of the human bite-related injury is on the hand. Treatment of a severe human bite should not be delayed. In addition to tissue trauma, infection from the biting organism's oral flora is a major concern. Animal bites may result in transmission of rabies infection. Human bites can theoretically transmit rabies, hepatitis and HIV. Screening for hepatitis or HIV is recommended if the attacker is known or suspected to be seropositive.

Thermal and Chemical Burns

Many burns in childhood are accidental. These are usually due to the negligence of the caretaker. Genital injuries due to burns are uncommon because the thighs provide protection to the perineum except in situations in which more than 30–50% of the total surface area is involved. In most studies, 78% of young children sustain thermal injuries due to their own actions, 20% are innocent bystanders, and 2% are victims of child abuse. The most common injury is scald burn, constituting about 70% of all thermal injuries in young children. Scald burns usually occur in the kitchen, primarily due to hot liquid spills and mainly affect the upper part of the body. Some may occur while the child is being bathed. Accidental burns can be in a splash pattern with irregular margins and non-uniform depth. Non-accidental burns often have very specific pattern such as burns consistent with immersion or dunking. Only children with deliberate immersion sustain deep burns of the buttocks and/or the area between the anus and the genitals. This gives a characteristic doughnut pattern in the buttocks which has a regular edge, with uniform depth.

Contact burns may be caused by flames or hot solid objects. Cigarette and iron burns are the most frequent types of these injuries. Purposely inflicted "branding" injuries usually mirror the objects that caused the burn. The object will have partial impression on the child's body if it is accidental in nature. Multiple cigarette burns are distinctively characteristic of child abuse. Trauma from a lighted cigarette can produce a lesion that can be difficult to distinguish from Varicella or impetigo.

Foreign Object Impalement

Ambulatory children can sustain accidental perineal impalement injuries and severe internal injuries may accompany minor external findings. Sometimes the physical findings may appear minimal, but on close observation, the patient may have a serious underlying injury. Usual objects that may cause impalement are sharp or pointed objects like in-lawn sprinklers, pails, pipes, fencepost, and furniture like chair tops, bedposts or leg of stools. These sharp or pointed objects can pierce the vagina, urethra, bladder, anus, rectum and peritoneal cavity. Accidents like these may be mistaken for sexual assault. The medical history should be congruent with an eyewitness story. The object that caused the trauma may be presented or the place where the accident happened may also be visited.

Vaginal Insufflation Injuries

Vaginal injuries due to high-pressure douche have been associated with water-skiing, jet-skiing and water slides. As pressurized water enters the vagina, the walls may over-distend and tear. Significant blood loss may occur. Such injuries may produce no sign of external genital trauma and only careful vaginal examination will reveal source of bleeding and true extent of the injury.

Pelvic Fractures

Fractures may be sustained as a result of motor vehicle accidents, falls or collapse of a building. Bone fragments from a fractured pelvis may cause penetration and laceration of the vagina, lower urinary tract or rectum.

Penetrating injuries of the vagina can lead to urological trauma. Up to 30% of patients with pelvic fractures can have bladder injury. The most common signs and symptoms are gross hematuria, abdominal tenderness, inability to void, abdominal distention and suprapubic bruising. Extravasations of urine may result in swelling in the perineum and/or anterior abdominal wall. Urine and blood coming out of the vagina are the manifestations of urethral injury. Management includes catheter drainage only for extra peritoneal ruptures; open surgery, if there is bladder neck involvement and presence of bone fragments in the bladder wall; and immediate surgical repair for intra peritoneal rupture.

Injury to the urethra in females may also be incurred in penetrating injuries but it is rare compared to males. The combination of straddle fractures with diastases of the sacroiliac joint has the highest risk of urethral injury. Injuries can vary from simple stretching to partial rupture to complete disruption. The most common presentation of urethral disruption is blood at the introitus, vagina, or urethral meatus, hematuria, the inability to void or labial edema. Retrograde urethrography is the gold standard for evaluation.

Non-accidental Injuries

The causes of non-accidental injuries resulting to genital trauma include childbirth, sexual assault and female genital cutting or circumcision.

Childbirth

Traumatic injury to the genital tract may occur during childbirth. A surgical procedure, like an episiotomy, is made to allow delivery of a child. Uncontrolled delivery or interventions involving use of instrumentation (e.g. forceps delivery, vacuum extraction) may cause injury to the perineum and anus, and/or the clitoris and anterior structures. Complications of these may be wound infection and if there is extension of the midline tear to the anal sphincter, this may result in a rectovaginal fistula.

Consensual or Nonconsensual Intercourse

Consensual or nonconsensual intercourse should be considered in the differential diagnosis of vaginal trauma. Coital injuries should always be considered as a differential diagnosis in all cases of abnormal vaginal bleeding particularly in children and adolescents. Thorough history taking and physical examination should be exercised. Inadequate information may be given because patient may be too embarrassed or distressed to give an accurate account of how the injury occurred. The diagnosis may be wrongly attributed to a hymenal tear or menstrual bleeding, and the diagnosis of a more serious injury may be overlooked or delayed unless a proper pelvic exam is done to evaluate the vaginal bleeding. Minor vaginal lacerations are not uncommon with initial coitus; however, deep vaginal lacerations may be sustained and may present with intense vaginal pain, profuse or prolonged vaginal bleeding and shock. A study by Bakers and Sommers showed that adolescents are at increased risk for sustaining more genital injuries than older females, and the expected number of injuries increases as the age decreases. Predisposing factors for coital injury include coitarche, clumsiness and rough coitus in unconventional positions, penovaginal disproportion, substance use by either or both partners, surgical alteration of the vagina, puerperium, insertion of foreign bodies, and physical and emotional unpreparedness of the victim like in sexual assault. Patients with vaginal agenesis may sustain deep lacerations and forceful penetration (Fig. 17.3) may lead to urethral intercourse.

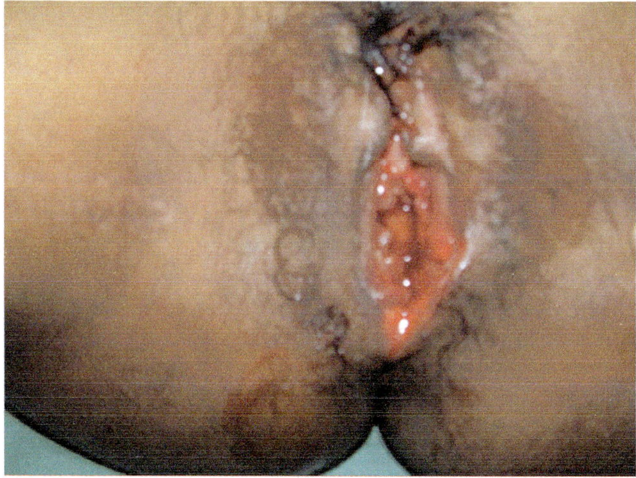

Fig. 17.3: Perineal laceration in a sexual assault

Female Genital Mutilation or Cutting

Female genital mutilation or cutting (FGM/C) (Figs 17.4A to D) comprises all procedures that involve partial or total removal of the external female genitalia, or other injury to the female genital organs for nonmedical reasons. An estimated 92 million girls have been subjected to FGM/C in Africa. They are also increasingly found in Europe, Australia, Canada and in the USA, primarily from immigrants from Africa and Southwestern Asia. Traditional birth attendants or trained midwives perform this on children and adolescents between 4 and 14 years old and as early as less than a year old in some countries like Ethiopia. The girls suffer complications leading to death through conditions like hemorrhagic shock from severe bleeding, neurogenic shock due to severe pain and trauma and septicemia due to overwhelming infection. Others enter into a state of shock induced by severe pain, psychological trauma and exhaustion from screaming.

Reasons for doing these are:

Sexual: Control or reduce female sexuality.

Sociological: Initiation of girls into womanhood, social integration and the maintenance of social cohesion.

Hygiene and aesthetic reasons: Where it is believed that the female genitalia are dirty and unsightly.

Health: Belief that it enhances fertility and child survival.

Religious reasons: Mistaken belief that it is a religious requirement.

The WHO, the International Council of Nurses (ICN), the International Confederation of Midwives (ICM) and the International Federation of Gynecologists and Obstetricians (FIGO) have openly condemned this practice of willful damage to healthy organs for nontherapeutic reasons.

World Health Organization categorization of female genital mutilation:

Type I: Removal or splitting of the clitoral hood, termed "hoodectomy" (or "clitorodotomy"), with or without excision of the clitoris (Fig. 17.4B). The clitoral hood is homologous to the foreskin of the penis, which is removed during circumcision.

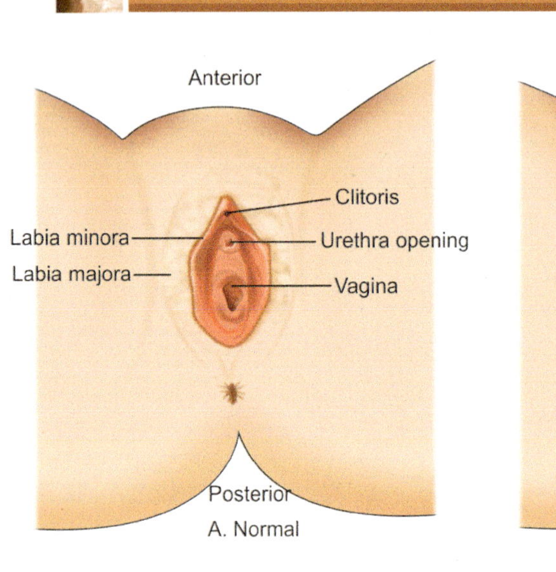

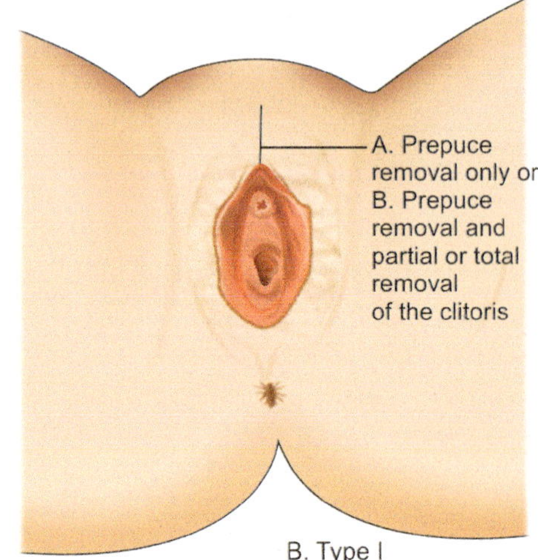

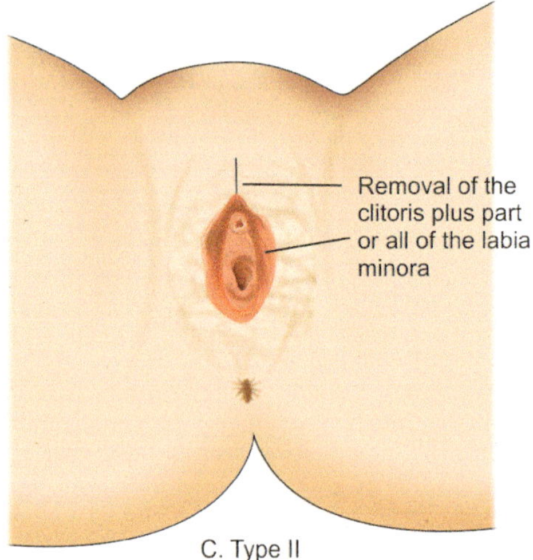

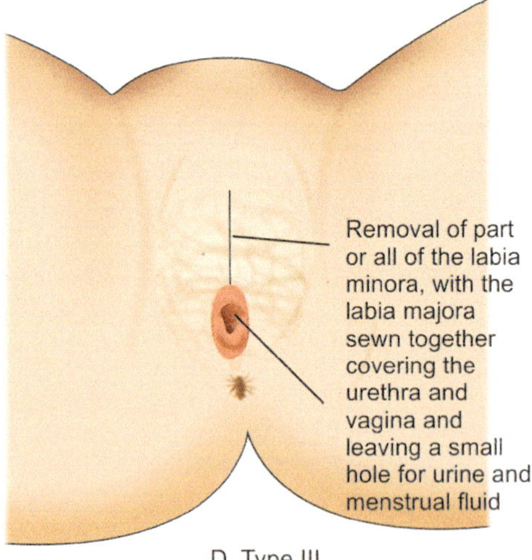

Figs 17.4A to D: (A) Normal female anatomy; (B to D) The different types of FGM/C according to WHO categorization

Type II: Excision of the clitoris with partial or total excision of the labia minora (Fig. 17.4C); the most common type accounting for about 80% of all cases.

Type III: Excision of part or all of the external genitalia and stitching/narrowing of the vaginal opening (infibulations) (Fig. 17.4D). It is the most extreme form and accounts for about 15% of all FGM/C procedures. Infibulation is also known as "pharaonic circumcision".

Type IV (Other types): There are other forms that are collectively referred to as Type IV and may not involve any tissue removal at all. This includes a diverse range of practices, including pricking the clitoris with needles, burning or scarring the genitals as well as ripping or tearing of the vagina or introducing herbs into the vagina to cause bleeding and a narrowed vaginal opening. Type IV is found primarily among isolated ethnic groups as well as in combination with other types.

HISTORY AND PHYSICAL EXAMINATION

In pediatric and adolescent age groups, patient history has been shown to be as important as physical examination in determining the cause of the trauma. The physician should be astute in determining whether the history is compatible with the physical findings. Discrepancies between the history and physical findings should arouse suspicion of sexual assault or abuse.

Initial evaluation of the patient should reveal whether she is in distress or unstable. The thorough history and physical examination should be delayed until patient is adequately resuscitated. Initial vital signs should be noted. A complete examination is indicated, with particular attention to cardiovascular status and to the abdominal and genital examinations. Extra genital injuries help to support or refute the history or mechanism of injuries. Young or virginal patients feel a great deal of anxiety about the genital and internal examination. The physician should aim to establish rapport and give assurance that the examination will be as comfortable as possible. Verbal consent is obtained before proceeding with the examination and a female nurse chaperone should be present. Every part of the physical examination process must be explained.

If sexual abuse, nonconsensual coitus, or excessive brutality is suspected, utmost care should be maintained to avoid any additional trauma to the victim. A trained specialist in assessing victims of sexual violence should be consulted.

Evaluation of a pediatric or an adolescent patient is very much different from the examination of an adult. An understanding of variations in normal anogenital anatomy is essential, as is an understanding of the physical findings that can mimic signs of trauma or sexual abuse. There are positions and techniques that may facilitate examination of a young patient. For prepubertal children, positions include: supine frog-leg, prone knee-chest or on lateral decubitus. Labial separation and traction should be done to further aid visualization (Fig. 17.5). A speculum exam is usually not necessary; however, if undertaken, anesthesia should be given. Pubertal and postpubertal adolescents can be examined in a lithotomy position; the use of a speculum may be helpful in the examination of the internal structures.

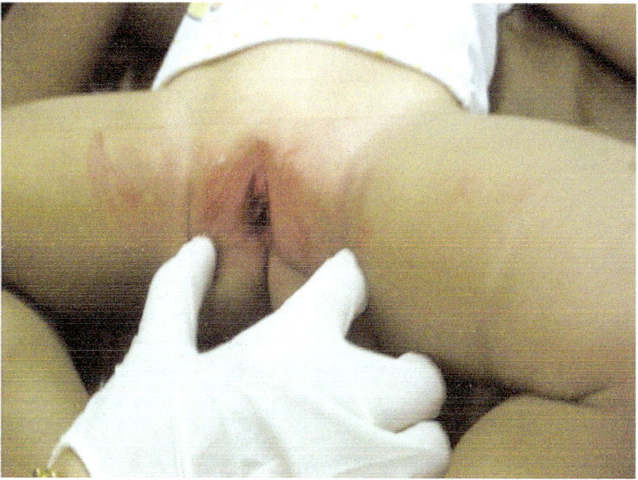

Fig. 17.5: Labial separation done on a frog-leg position

Photodocumentation is the standard of care for evaluation of child sexual abuse cases. Colposcopy provides the vehicle for peer review, research that can be reviewed and replicated, and most importantly it prevents repeated examination of the victim. Vaginoscopy is helpful in the diagnosis of vaginal laceration or foreign bodies. The use of a hysteroscope provides fluid distention allowing adequate visualization of the vaginal vault. Laparotomy or laparoscopy is indicated if there are signs of peritoneal irritation or ongoing hemodynamic instability.

Physical findings may range from normal findings to lesions like abrasions, minor lacerations and hematoma. It is important to note that a normal exam does not exclude the possibility of sexual abuse. In one study presenting as perineal bleeding, the most common injury (79%) sustained after a straddle injury is laceration or abrasion of the labia minora or majora. Lacerations of the posterior fourchette and vulvar hematoma represent 16% and 13% respectively. The study revealed that hymenal and vaginal injuries are almost exclusively due to penetrating type mechanism. Another study revealed that the labia minora is the most commonly injured by blunt perineal trauma. Injuries tended to be found in either posterior or anterior, but not both. One patient has noted to have hymenal injury to the hymen caused by a fall in a splits-type position. These studies suggest that simple blunt trauma is not often associated with evidence of injury to the hymen or vaginal mucosa. Such injury is highly suspected for penetrative mechanism and sexual abuse. Injuries from penile penetration may present as hymenal tears in the posterior fourchette.

MANAGEMENT

A child with minor genital trauma should be kept inactive except for toilet privileges for the first 24 hours after injury. Small vulvar hematomas or minor lacerations may be managed conservatively and resolve spontaneously (Figs 17.6A and B). Ice pack is recommended during the first 12–24 hours after the injury to reduce edema. Sitz baths may keep the wound clean and may facilitate voiding in girls with mild urinary symptoms. Analgesics may be given for pain.

If urination becomes a problem, an in-dwelling catheter is inserted and progression of the hematoma is determined. Surgical intervention may be necessary if there is vast expansion of the hematoma and hematocrit is falling. Evacuation of an enlarging hematoma will reduce the pain, hasten recovery and prevent necrosis, tissue loss, and secondary infection. Incision is made on the medial aspect near the vaginal orifice. If there is a lot of bleeding from the vaginal lacerations, surgical repair of the wound should be done to approximate the tissues and obtain hemostasis.

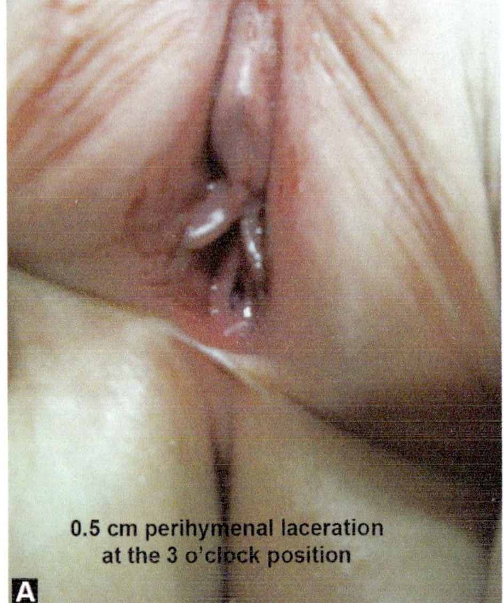

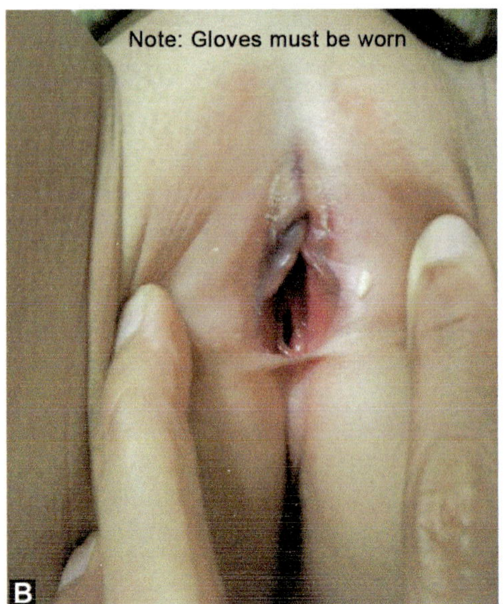

Figs 17.6A and B: A toddler who presented with vaginal bleeding after straddling on her bike. (A) Abrasions on the labia majora, contusion on the labia minora and clitoral hood and a 0.5 cm perihymenal laceration at the 3 o'clock position are noted; (B) Treatment with ice pack on the perineal area, pain reliever and antibiotics results in decrease of redness and resolution of vaginal bleeding after 2 days

Antibiotic therapy and application of estrogen cream for 3–7 days would be appropriate.

Genital trauma can also be catastrophic. The laceration may extend to the vaginal vault if the upper vagina has been penetrated directly by a sharp object. The cervix may be avulsed from its attachment to the vagina and the tear may extend along the vagina and enter the peritoneal cavity. Such condition may necessitate exploratory laparotomy to rule this out. Bowel and bladder involvement must be confirmed by catheterization and rectal palpation. If difficulty is encountered in assessing an injury above the hymen, complete examination must be done under general anesthesia.

Figure 17.7 shows the distribution of the management of cases of genital trauma at the Pediatric and Adolescent Gynecology Unit of PCMC since its inception. Of the 52 cases, 10 (19%) warranted surgery. Nine (17%) of them are due to straddle injuries, where evacuation of vulvar hematoma, repair of vulvar and perineal lacerations are done. One case is due to sexual abuse necessitating repair of perineal laceration.

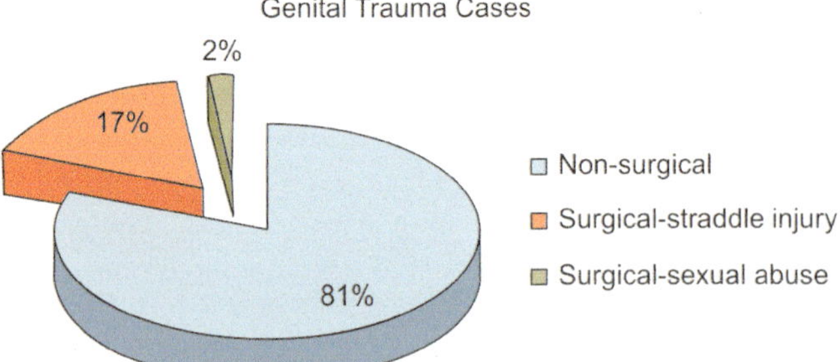

Fig. 17.7: Distribution of management of genital trauma cases at the PAG Unit in PCMC, 2002-2009

After Care for Trauma Victims

Whatever circumstance, whether physical or emotional injury or sexual assault, the experience always leave an indelible mark in the heart and mind of the trauma victims. It is not very easy to go through the journey of recovery especially for those who are sexually abused. There are flashbacks, nightmares, mood swings and guilt feelings, and sometimes attempts of suicide. It is most appropriate that the victim should be allowed to go through process of coping. Specific interventions, such as pain assessment and management, psychological evaluation and support, should be initiated at once. Family support is likewise necessary.

BIBLIOGRAPHY

1. Abasiattai A, Etuk S, Bassey E, et al. Vaginal injuries during coitus in Calibar: a 10 year review. Niger Pos Grad Med J 2005;12(2):140-4.
2. Anate M. Vaginal trauma at sexual intercourse in Llorin, Nigeria. An analysis of 36 cases, West Afr J Med 1989;8(3): 217-22.

3. Annual Reports (2002–2008). Pediatric and Adolescent Gynecology Unit. Philippine Children's Medical Center.
4. Atiyeh B, Rubeiz M, Ghanimeh G, et al. Management of pediatric burns. Ann of Burns and Fire Disasters 2000; 13(3):136-42.
5. Baker R, Sommers M. Relationship of genital injuries and age in adolescent and young adult rape survivors. JOGNN 2008;(37):282-9.
6. Benjamins LJ. Genital trauma in pediatric and adolescent females. J Pediatr Adolesc Gynecol 2009;22:129-33.
7. Berkoff MC, Zolotor AJ, Markoroff KL, et al. Has this prepubertal girl been sexually abused. JAMA 2008;300(23): 2779-92.
8. Burns injuries in child abuse, US Department of Justice, Office of Justice Progams, Office of Juvenile Justice and Delinquency Prevention.
9. Daniels RV, McCusky C. Abnormal vaginal bleeding in nonpregnant patient. Emerg Med Clin N Am 2003;21(3) 751-72.
10. Djakovic N, Lynch T, Martinez-Pineiro Y, et al. Guidelines on urological trauma. Eur Urol. 2005;47:1-15.
11. Female genital mutilation. World Health Organization Fact sheet # 241. [Online] WHO website. Available from www.who.int/mediacentre/factsheets.
12. http://en.wikipedia.org/wiki/File:FGC_Types.jpg. [Accessed September 1, 2009].
13. Kellog ND, Menard SW, Santos A. Genital anatomy in pregnant adolescents: "normal" does not mean "nothing". Pediatrics 2004;113(1 Pt 1):e67-9.
14. Lacy J, Brennand E, Ornstein M, et al. Vaginal injury from a pressure jet in a prepubescent girl. Pediatr Emerg Care 2007;232:112-4.
15. Legano L, McHugh MT, Palusci VJ. Child abuse and neglect. Curr Probl Pediatr adolesc Health Care 2009;31:1-26.
16. Mendez DR. "Straddle Injuries" Up To Date. [Online] uptodate website. Available from http://www.uptodate [Accessed 2009].
17. Merritt DF. Genital trauma in children and adolescents. Clin Obstet Gynecol 2008;51:237-48.
18. Merritt DF. Genital trauma. In: Altchek A, Deligdisch L (Eds). Pediatric, Adolescent and Young Adult Gynecology. West Sussex, UK: Blackwell Publishing 2009; pp. 97-110.
19. Muram D. Round table discussion: the medical evaluation of sexually abused children. J Pediatr Adolesc Gynecol 2003;16(1):5-14.
20. Onen A, Ozturk H, Yayla M, et al. Genital trauma in children: classification and management. Urology 2005;65:986.
21. Rossenberger E. Treatment of human bites. [Online] helium website. Available from www.helium.com/item/936816 [Accessed 2011].
22. Spitzer RF. Unintentional pediatric female genital trauma. Pediatric Emergency Care 2008;24:831-5.
23. UNICEF. Child protection from violence, exploitation and abuse. Fact Sheet. [Online] unicef website. Available from www.unicef.org/protection.

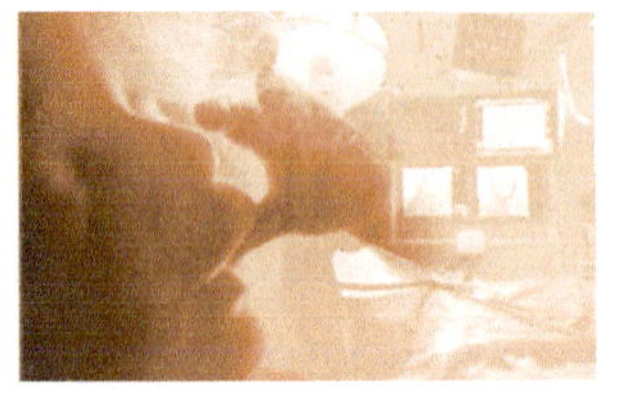

18 Endoscopy in Pediatric and Adolescent Gynecology

Blanca C De Guia, Maria Therese Beriña-Mallen

Gynecologic endoscopy is fast becoming a popular alternative to the conventional laparotomy in managing surgical gynecologic cases. Its use is likewise being explored as the possible first line of treatment among pediatric and adolescent patients, with majority of diseases in these age groups being benign. Other than better cosmetic result, endoscopy presents with other significant advantages such as shorter hospital stay, earlier postoperative recovery and reduced postoperative pain. This chapter aims to review the important anatomic points of the pediatric female patient which ensure a safe endoscopic surgery thus avoid potential dangers intraoperatively. Basic concepts of gynecologic endoscopy will likewise be discussed.

LAPAROSCOPY

Indications

Indication for the laparoscopy is listed in the Table 18.1.

Anatomic Considerations

Following anatomic considerations are important while performing laparoscopy:

Table 18.1: Indication for the laparoscopy

Oophorocystectomy	*Ovarian detorsion*
Oophorectomy	Gonadal biopsy
Abscess drainage	Intersex exploration
Salpingostomy for ectopic pregnancy	Exploration for pelvic pain

1. The bladder of a child (Fig. 18.1) is an intraperitoneal organ; attention must be given not to injure it during surgery. This can be avoided by either of the following measures:
   - Foley catheter placement
   - Intraoperative crede maneuver
2. Inferior epigastric vessels:
   - Located lateral to the obliterated umbilical arteries (Fig. 18.2)
   - May be hit during placement of the lateral trocars
   - *Safety measures:*
     - Transillumination
     - Choose puncture site, which is medial to the obliterated umbilical arteries.
3. Umbilical incision:
   - The umbilicus is the thinnest part of the abdominal wall; it is where the peritoneum closely underlies the fascia

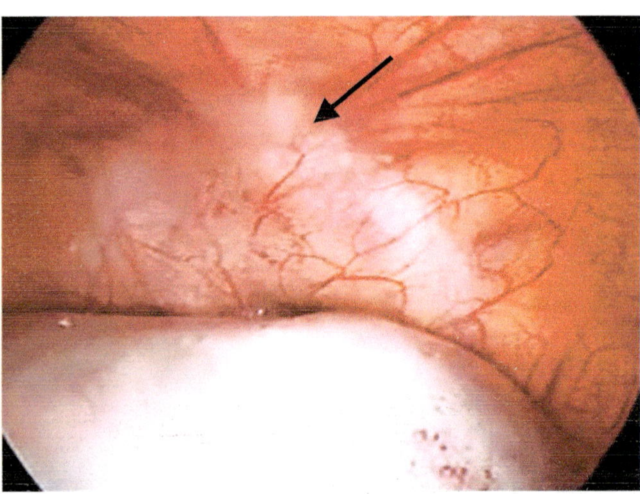

Fig. 18.1: Urinary bladder viewed laparoscopically

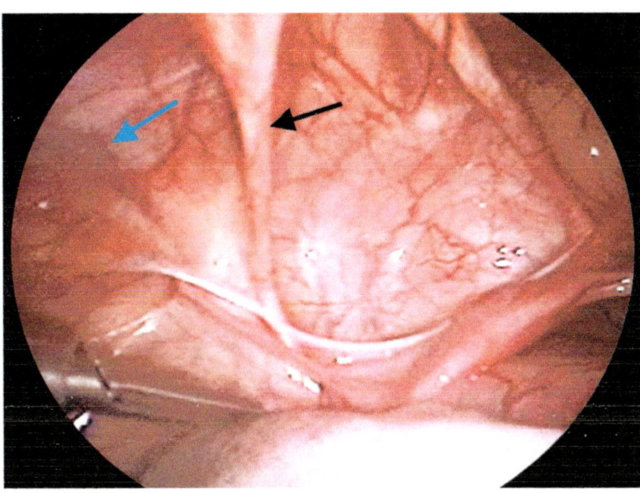

Fig. 18.2: Obliterated umbilical artery (black arrow) and inferior epigastric artery (blue arrow)

- *Safety measures*:
  - When making an umbilical incision, always lift the umbilicus using either your hands or using towel clips.

4. Children do not have well-developed fascia yet, making them more prone to herniation later on:
   - *Safety measures*:
     - Use small diameter trocars (2, 3 or 5 mm)
     - Leave valve open while withdrawing trocar to avoid negative intra-abdominal pressure
     - Leave the camera on to visualize the trocar as it is withdrawn.
5. Uterine manipulators or levators are usually not necessary among these age groups; the uterus is too small to obscure the operative field.

Anesthetic Considerations

1. Anesthetic risks are almost similar in children and in adults
2. Children have limited functional lung capacity thus raising concerns on the effect of intraperitoneal CO_2 under pressure
3. Prolonged fasting is not necessary:
   - Clear liquids may be administered up to 2-4 hours prior to surgery, with no increased risk of pulmonary aspiration.

Table 18.2:
Basic equipment used in laparoscopy

Laparoscope	Output monitor/ Screen	Instruments (forceps, graspers, scissors)
Light source	Video camera	Secondary trocars (2 mm, 3 mm, 5 mm)
Insufflator	Irrigation-aspiration system	Monopolar or bipolar electrocautery

Instrumentation

Basic equipment needed to perform laparoscopy is listed in the Table 18.2 and shown in the Figures 18.3A to H.

Technique

1. Establishment of pneumoperitomeum:
   - Umbilicus is the most ideal site of entry
   - A higher site of entry may be chosen in case of anticipated difficulty secondary to adhesions from previous surgery, or in case of huge masses (Fig. 18.4)
   - Entry is done either through the open technique or through use of the Veress needle (Fig. 18.5)
   - Confirm, if placement is intraperitoneal:
     - Drop of saline technique
     - Direct visualization (Open technique)
   - Insufflate CO_2:
     - In children, a low flow rate of 2 L/minute is appropriate (maximum 6 L/minute)
     - Insufflation pressure of 8–10 mm Hg is adequate; for infants less than 4 months old, it should be less than 6 mm Hg.
2. Placement of primary trocar:
   - Place a 5 mm trocar through the umbilical port, directing it toward the pelvic area
   - Pass the laparoscope through the trocar sleeve.
3. Placement of secondary trocars:
   - Place patient in Trendelenburg position; the force of gravity should allow the bowels to move out of the pelvic area
   - Under direct visualization, the lateral trocars are then inserted, directing them toward the cul-de-sac.
4. Inspect abdominal and pelvic organs
5. Perform desired procedure (oophorocystectomy, oophorectomy, etc.)
6. Closure of abdominal incisions:
   - Removal of lateral trocars should be done under direct visualization, with incisions examined internally for bleeding
   - Remove laparoscope

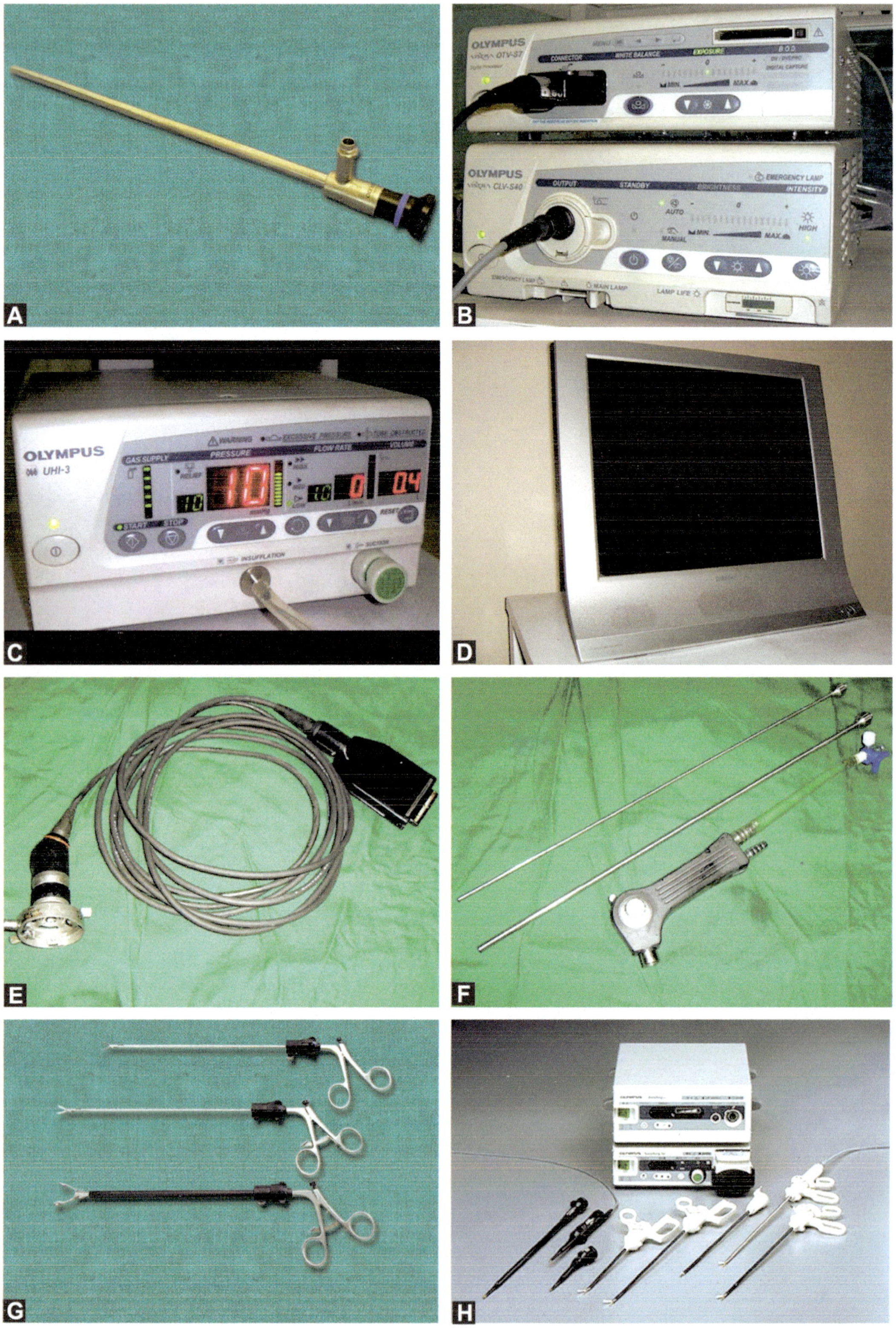

Figs 18.3A to H: (A) A 3 mm laparoscope; (B) Light source; (C) Insufflator; (D) Output monitor or screen; (E) Video camera; (F) Suction or irrigation system; (G) Scissors and grasping forceps; (H) Sonosurg

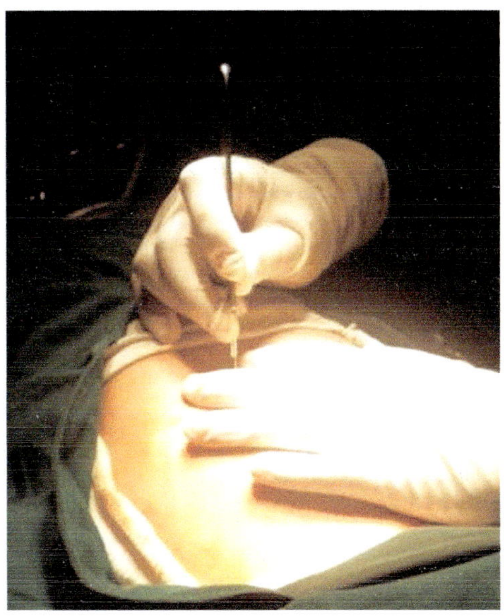

Fig. 18.4: Umbilical entry is not possible in the case of a huge ovarian mass; the laparoscope is instead placed 4 cm above the umbilicus

- Allow intra-abdominal gas to escape
- Facilitate decompression of pneumoperitoneum by taking patient out of Trendelenburg position.

Complications

1. Anesthesia-related:
   - Distension of the abdomen may compromise excursion of the diaphragm
   - CO_2 may be absorbed, especially if operating time is prolonged:
     - May manifest as cardiac arrhythmia

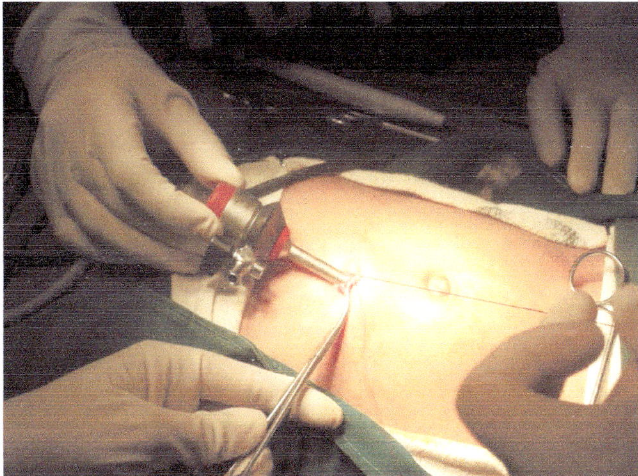

Fig. 18.5: Open technique

     - Measures which may reduce hypercarbia to a minimum
       - Constant monitoring by pulse oximetry
       - Endotracheal intubation and assisted ventilation.
2. Induction of pneumoperitoneum:
   - Extraperitoneal gas insufflations:
     - Caused by insufflation of gas before the peritoneal cavity has been entered
     - Diagnosed by palpation of crepitus under the skin.
   - Pneumothorax
     - Insufflation of gas into the pleural cavity
     - More common when a high site of insertion is chosen
     - Avoided by directing the needle or the trocars away from the diaphragm, toward the pelvic cavity
   - GIT injury
   - Blood vessel injury
     - Omental or mesenteric vessels (smaller vessels)
     - Major abdominal or pelvic vessels

   Prevented by lifting the abdominal wall and angling the needle or trocars toward the pelvis.
   - Gas embolism:
     - Intravascular insufflation of gas
     - Fatal especially when a large CO_2 embolus occludes the pulmonary artery
     - Suspect when there is decreased end-tidal CO_2, decreased O_2 saturation, (+) mill-wheel murmur and severe hypotension
     - Management: stop insufflation; place patient in left lateral decubitus position; give 100% O_2
       - If initial measure fails, cardiac puncture is done to release the gas.
3. Insertion of trocars (Fig. 18.6):
   - Injury to blood vessels in the abdominal wall:
     - Most commonly injured vessels:
       - Inferior epigastric artery
       - Located between the insertion of the round ligament at the inguinal canal and the obliterated umbilical artery
     - Superior epigastric artery
     - Superficial circumflex iliac artery

   Prevented by:

   Transilluminating the abdominal wall before insertion.

   Direct visualization laparoscopically:
   - How to manage bleeding:
     - Cautery
     - Suturing
     - Tamponade bleeding using Foley catheter balloon

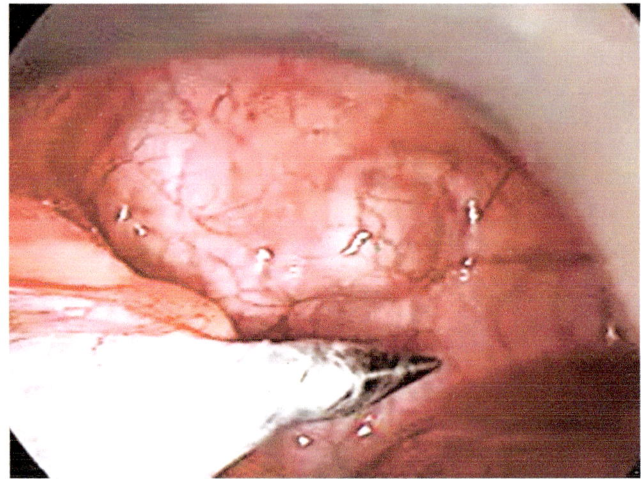

Fig. 18.6: Laproscopic visualization of lateral trocar insertion

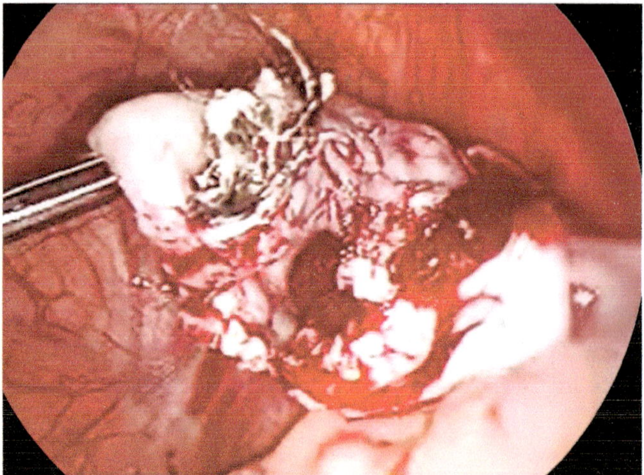

Fig. 18.7: Intraoperative spill of contents of a mature cystic

- Injury to intra-abdominal vessels:
  - Treatment:
    - Resuscitation
    - Laparotomy
    - Vascular repair or ligation, if necessary (when vitality of bowel segment has been compromised), bowel resection and anastomosis.

4. Thermal damage:
   - Results from passage of electric current from the electrode into the tissues that it comes into contact with
   - To prevent this, ensure that no other tissue is in contact with the electrode as electricity is being applied.
5. Other complications:
   - Shoulder pain
   - Results from conversion of CO_2 to carbonic acid, which is a peritoneal irritant
   - Shoulder pain is referred pain resulting from diaphragmatic peritoneal and phrenic nerve irritation
   - Incisional hernia:
     - Incisions greater than 7 mm should be closed in layers in order to prevent this
   - Nerve injuries:
     - Brachial plexus injury:
       - Preventive measures:
     - Keep the patient's arms tucked to her side
     - Avoid abducting arms to greater than 90°
     - Avoid Trendelenburg position with arms abducted
   - Injury to nerves of the left and hip and sacroiliac joints:
     - Results from prolonged periods in the lithotomy position, and may affect either of the following nerves: femoral, lateral femoral, common peroneal, obturator and sciatic
     - Avoided by minimizing extrinsic pressure on the hip and leg joints
     - Not common in the pediatric population because the lithotomy position is not commonly employed
   - Intraoperative spillage of cyst contents (Fig. 18.7):
     - Chemical peritonitis is suspected when there is postoperative fever and ileus
     - Managed by doing copious lavage with normal saline solution (Fig. 18.8).

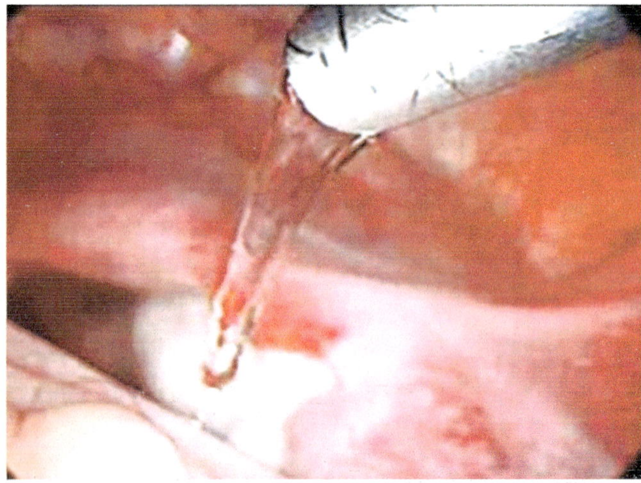

Fig. 18.8: Copious irrigation with NSS until lavage fluid is clear

SAMPLE CASES

Case 1

An 11-year-old girl was brought in due to intermittent hypogastric pain and dysuria. Urinalysis was normal. Abdominal ultrasound showed a 13x9x7 cm pelvoabdominal mass with septations (Figs 18.9A to F). Color flow was negative. On physical examination, a 13 x 9 cm cystic, slightly movable, non-tender mass was noted, the upper border of which was palpable at the level of the umbilicus. Serum tumor markers (B-hCG, LDH and AFP) were all within normal limits. Patient underwent laparoscopic oophorocystectomy. Histopatholgic report showed mature cystic teratoma of the ovary.

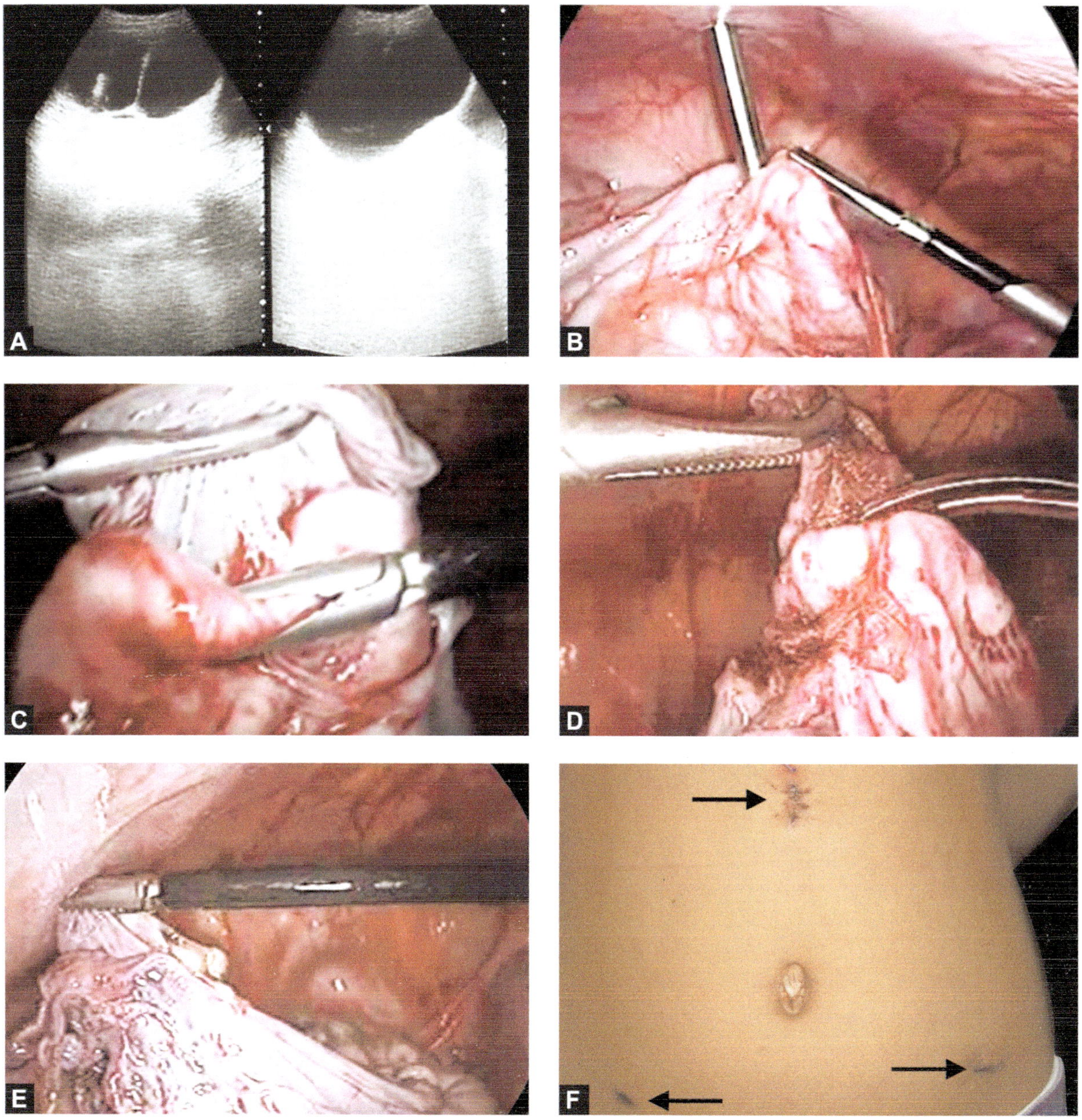

Figs 18.9A to F: (A) Ultrasound image of the patient showing a huge cystic mass with separations with no color flow; (B) Prior to cystectomy, the ovarian cyst was decompressed using the lateral trocar as the puncture instrument. Cyst fluid was then suctioned; (C and D) Cystectomy was then performed by initially cutting through the cyst wall plane, followed by blunt and sharp dissection until the cyst wall was dissected free from the remaining normal ovarian tissue; (E) Specimen retrieval was done through one of the lateral port entry sites; (F) Abdominal incisional scars 4 weeks postoperative (black arrow)

Case 2

A 10-year-old girl was brought in due to intermittent hypogastric pain, frequency and dysuria. Abdominal ultrasound showed an 8 x 7 x 5 cm cystic, anechoic, rounded mass with echogenic stippling, noted at the right adnexa, superior to the bladder (Figs 18.10A to H). Color flow was negative. Serum tumor markers (B-hCG, LDH and AFP) were all within normal limits. On physical examination, there was a 7 x 6 cm cystic, movable, non-tender, midline abdominal mass. Patient underwent laparoscopic oophorocystectomy. Histopathologic diagnosis was mature cystic teratoma of the ovary.

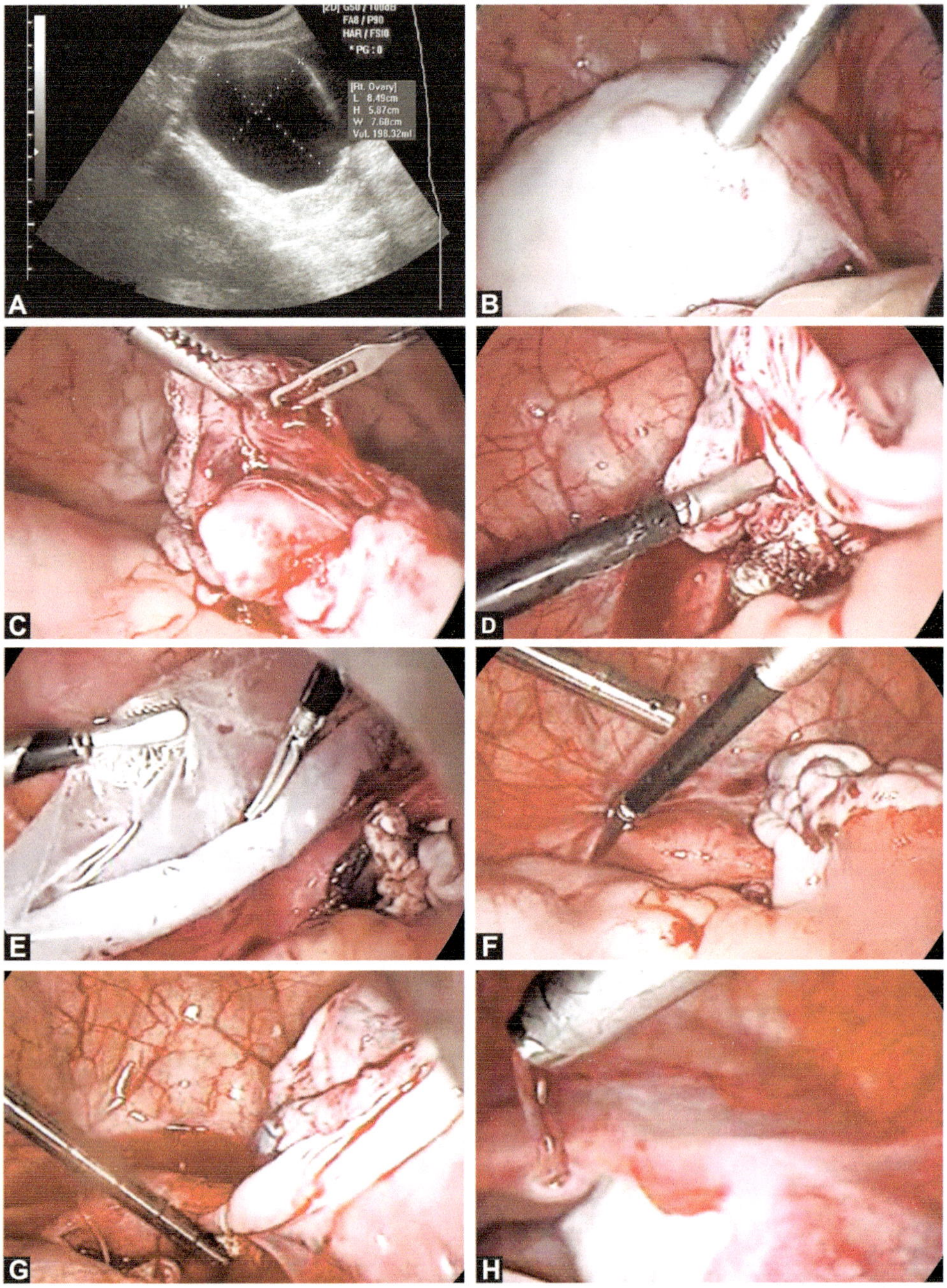

Figs 18.10A to H: (A) Ultrasound image showing an 8 x 7 x 5 cm cystic, anechoic, rounded mass, with echogenetic stippling; with negative color flow; (B) Decompression was achieved by suctioning intracystic fluid using one of the lateral trocars as puncture instrument; (C) Cystectomy was performed through blunt and sharp dissection; (D) Intraperitoneal spill of cystic contents after inadvertent rupture during dissection; (E) Specimen retrieval was achieved using a plastic bag as container, followed by delivery through the umbilical port; (F) The remaining normal ovarian tissue was left unsutured after cyst removal; (G and H) Intraoperative spill of cyst contents was managed by copious lavage with normal saline solution until the lavage fluid was clear

VAGINOSCOPY

Vaginoscopy is the visualization of the vaginal canal using an endoscope with irrigation properties (cystoscope, bronchoscope, hysteroscope, etc.). This is more commonly done to examine infants and children. Care should be taken not to damage the hymen during the procedure for cultural and forensic reasons. Visualization of the vaginal canal, the cervix and the fornices is achieved using a distension fluid, the most commonly used of which is normal saline solution.

Indications

- Persistent vaginal discharge
- Unexplained vaginal bleeding
- Abnormal appearance of the external genitalia
- Suspicion of vaginal foreign body
- Suspicion of vaginal tumor
- Diagnosis of certain Müllerian anomalies
- Blunt genital trauma with possible intravaginal extension.

Instrumentation

The following instruments are used in the vaginoscopy and are shown in the Figures 18.11A to D:

- A 4–5 mm endoscope (hysteroscope, cystoscope or bronchoscope)
- Continuous normal saline flow system
- Video camera
- Output monitor or screen
- Light source
- Instruments (scissors, forceps, cautery).

Technique

Different steps to see through the vaginoscope are given below and shown in the Figures 18.12A to D:

1. Induction of anesthesia

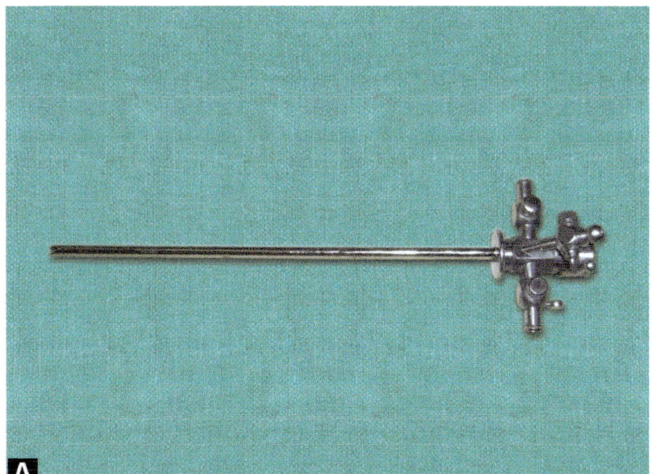

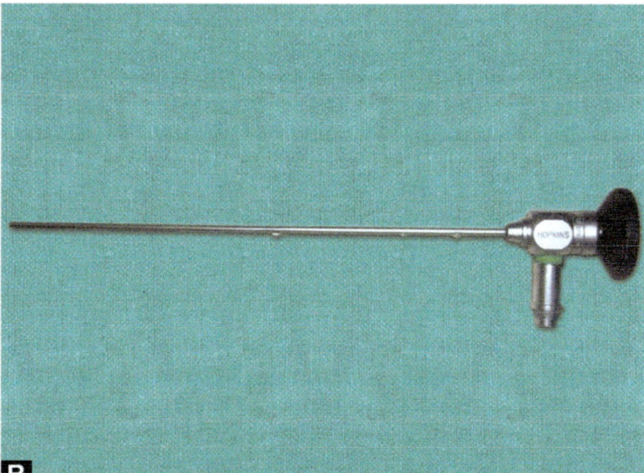

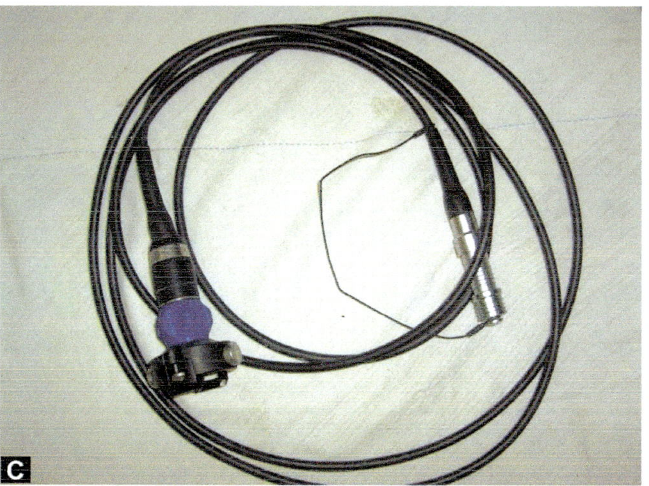

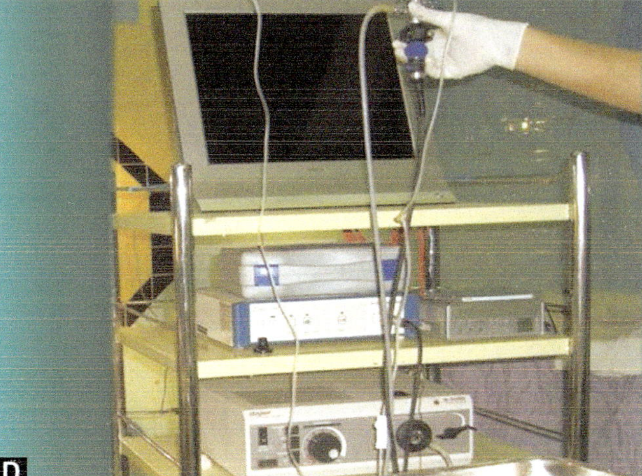

Figs 18.11A to D: (A) A 4–5 mm endoscope; (B) Video camera; (C) Light source cable; (D) Monitor and light source

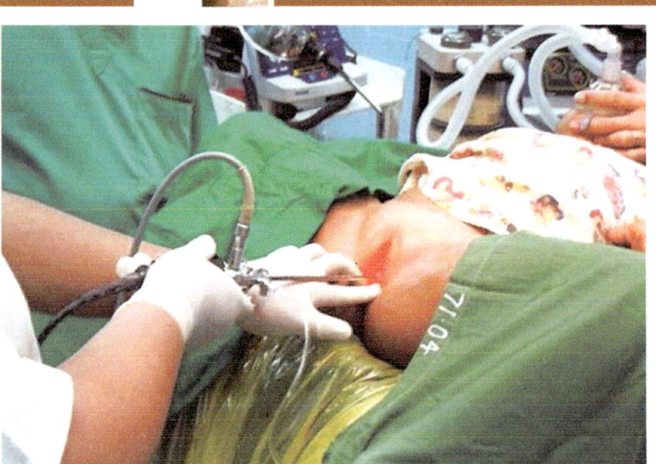
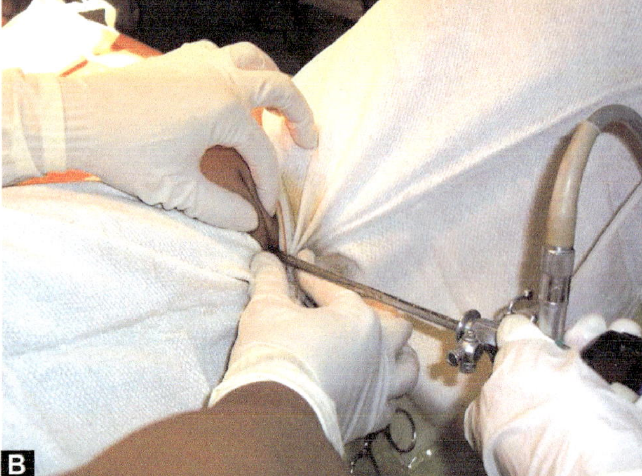
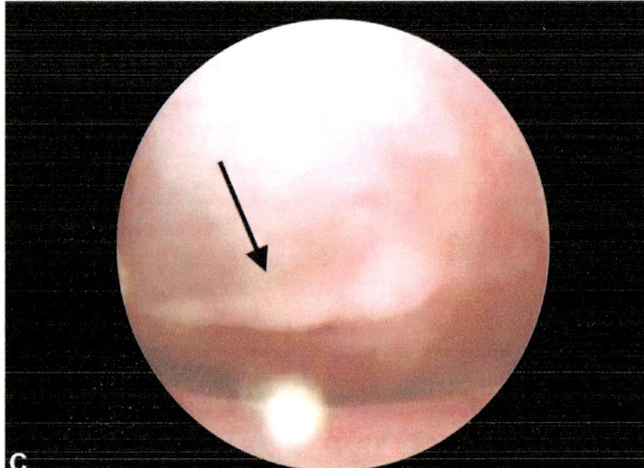
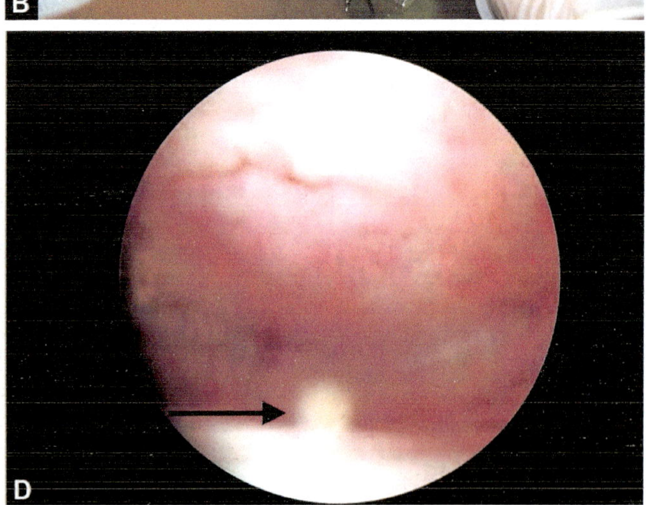

Figs 18.12A to D: (A) Patient supine position, with thighs and knees flexed, hips abducted; (B) Vaginoscope being inserted. Note how vulvar tissues are squeezed to prevent egress of fluid; (C) Slit-like cervix seen through the vaginoscope (black arrow); (D) Posterior fornix (black arrow)

2. Place patient in a supine position, with thighs and knees flexed and hips abducted
3. Asepsis and antisepsis
4. Empty bladder
5. Document the anatomic features of the hymen before inserting any instrument into vaginal introitus
6. Insert lubricated 2–5 mm hysteroscope (with attached continuous flow normal saline solution) through the vaginal orifice with one hand, while the other hand gently squeezes the vulvar tissues around the scope to prevent the egress of the distending fluid
7. Inspect the vaginal walls, cervix and fornices
8. Biopsy of vaginal tumors or masses and extraction of vaginal foreign bodies may be done using appropriate forceps. When bleeding is present, they may either be cauterized or sutured
9. Remove the instruments after the procedure.

Normal Findings

In prepubertal females, the characteristics of the hymen and vaginal mucosa are secondary to the "unestrogenized" state of the vaginal epithelium (Figs 18.13A to H).

Abnormal Findings

Abnormalities associated with vaginoscopy are presented in Figures 18.14A to G.

Complications

Uncommon; may include infections, hymenal ring damages.

LOCAL STATISTICS

Based on the annual reports of the Pediatric and Adolescent Gynecology Unit of the Philippine Children's Medical Center, there were 43 cases of vaginoscopy done from April

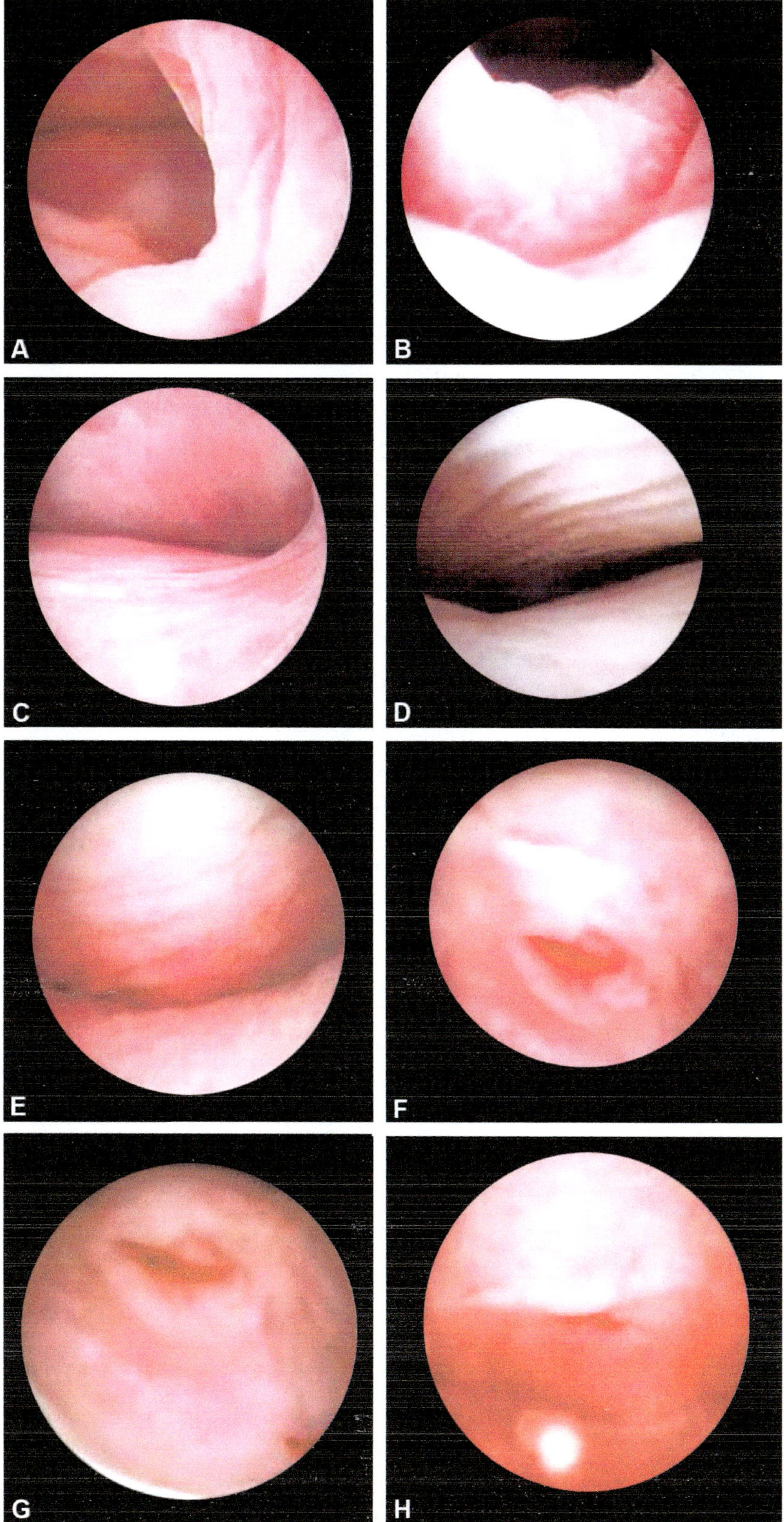

Figs 18.13A to H: (A and B) The hymen is thin and pink; (C) Vaginal mucosa is pink; (D and E) Vaginal side walls smooth, and almost free of rugae; (F to H) Cervix appears as a pink, doughnut-shaped structure, oftentimes flushed to the vaginal wall

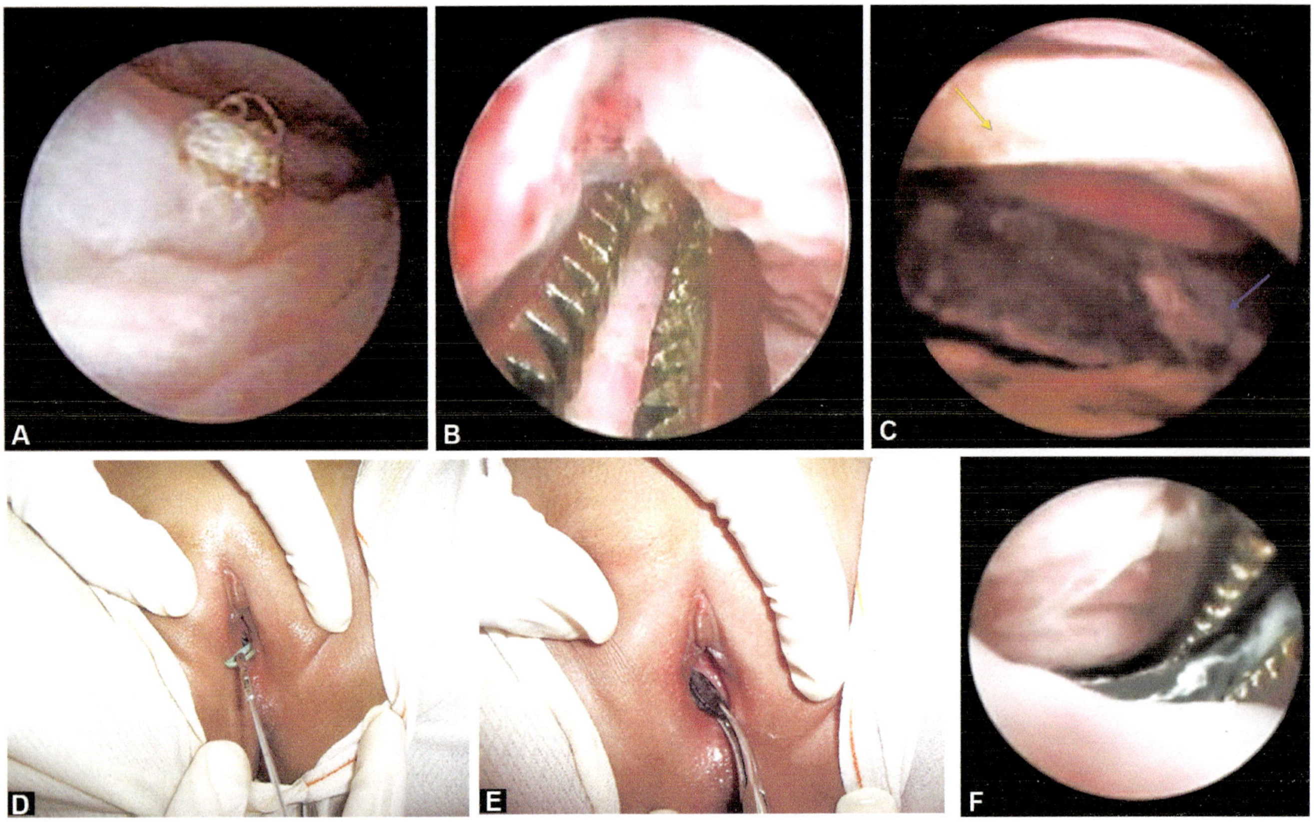

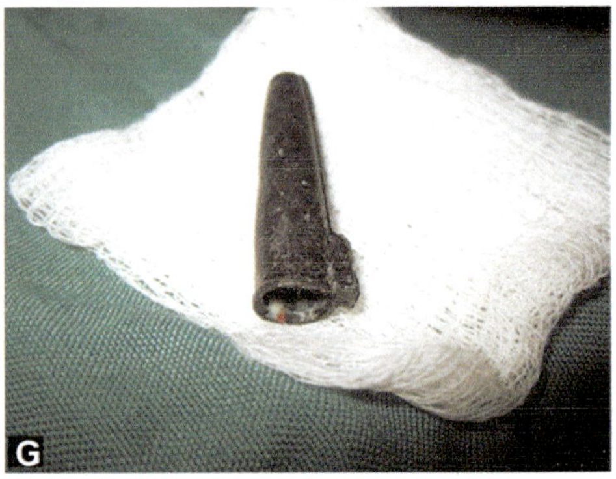

2005 to April 2009. During the period the statistics obtained are shown in the Figures 18.15 to 18.17.

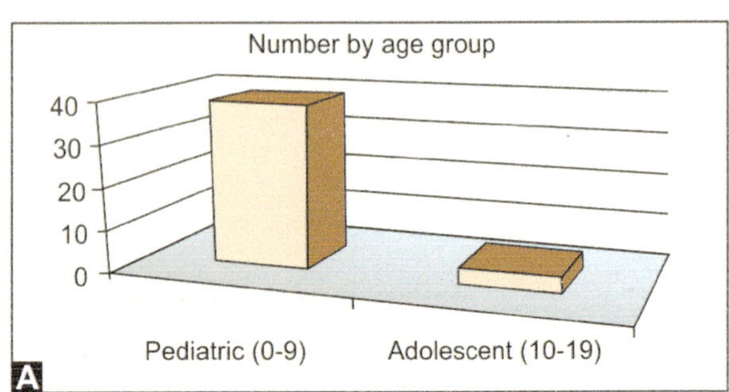

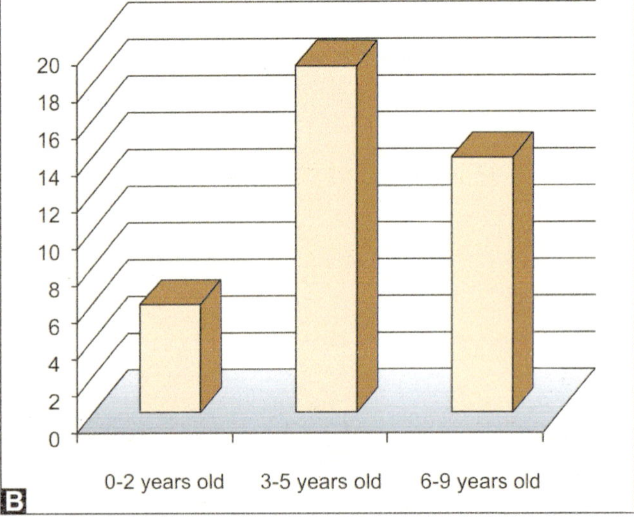

Figs 18.15A and B: Age group distribution of vaginoscopy cases done at a tertiary referral center for pediatric gynecologic cases

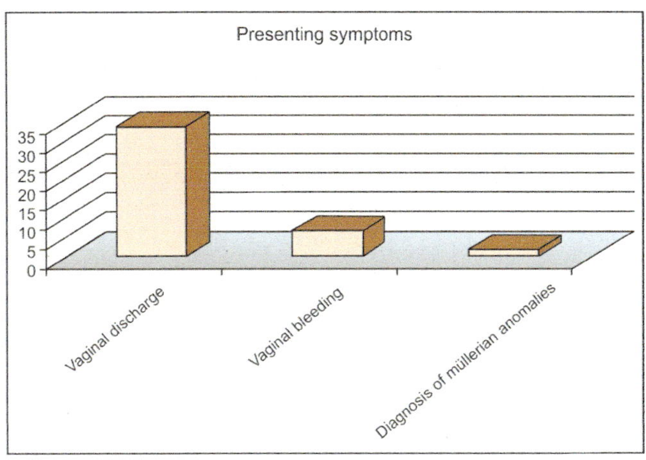

Fig. 18.16: Most common presenting symptoms of patients undergoing diagnostic vaginoscopy

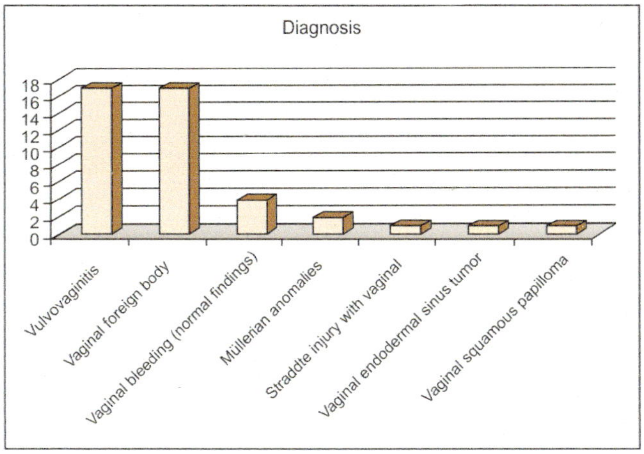

Fig. 18.17: Postoperative diagnoses of patients who underwent vaginoscopy

BIBLIOGRAPHY

1. Annual Reports (2002 to 2008). Pediatric and Adolescent Gynecology Unit, Philippine Children's Medical Center, Quezon City.
2. Golan A. Continuous flow vaginoscopy in children. Journal of Lower Genital Tract Disease 2000;5(2):85-6.
3. Howard S. Laparoscopy in children. Clinical Obstetrics and Gynecology 1997;40 (1):210-8.
4. Lobe T (Ed). Pediatric Laparoscopy. Georgetown, Texas, USA: Landes Bioscience, 2003.
5. Mann W, et al. Vaginoscopy. [Online] uptodate website. Available from www.uptodate.com [Accessed September, 2008].
6. Parker J, Hibbert ML, Dainty LD, et al. Microhydrovaginoscopy in examining children. Obstetrics and Gynecology 2000; 96:772-5.
7. Walker DM, Campana A (Eds). Practical training and research in gynecologic endoscopy for developing countries. Geneva Foundation for Medical Education and Research. Available from www.gfmer-ch/Books/Endoscopy_book.

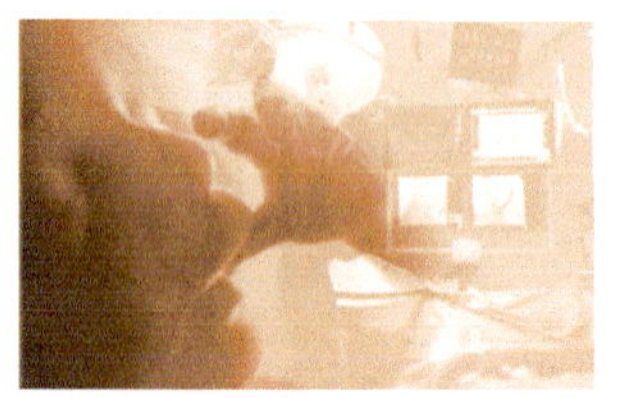

19 Pediatric and Adolescent Gynecology as a Subspecialty in the Philippines

Corazon Yabes-Almirante

Pediatric and Adolescent Gynecology as a field of specialty was the subject of the whole volume (volume 142) of the annals of the New York Academy of Sciences published in May 10, 1967. It was the first attempt according to Warren R Lang, consulting editor "to review attitudes, research and progress in the field of pediatric and adolescent gynecology". At that time, adequate vaginal examination of little girls was taboo.

Goldfarb claims that as late as 1996 it was not acceptable to look at the genitalia of pediatric and adolescent gynecology patients without gynecological complaints and without sexual experience when they are less than 18 years.

At the Philippine Children's Medical Center where the first Perinatal Center in a children's hospital was launched in 1988, children with gynecological problems were referred to the obstetrician-gynecologist or perinatologists (high risk pregnancy specialists) by the pediatricians. With increasing number of referrals, in 1996, author was asked by the hospital administrators to study the possibility of putting up services for pediatric and adolescent gynecology. An observation of the system at a center in the USA gave author the idea that the Children's Center was the best place to launch the specialty since it involved many specialists already in-house in the Center: obstetrician-gynecologists perinatologists, sonologists, reproductive endocrinologists, gynecological cancer specialists, pediatric urologists, adolescent medicine specialists, pediatric endocrinologists, pediatric psychiatrists, anethesiologists, ambulatory pediatricians, nurses and social workers experienced in dealing with children and their parents. It took more than 5 years to develop the core group of trainers and find the structure and facility to house the outpatient clinic, and get a slot at the pediatric operating room for gynecological surgeries. Getting the proper equipment and instruments took some time, but in April 22, 2002, the Pediatric and Adolescent Gynecology Services was opened at the Antepartum Unit of the Philippine Children's Medical Center. Fellowship training program started in 2002. Table 19.1 shows the

Table 19.1: Fellowship training program in pediatric and adolescent gynecology

The objective and scope of the training curriculum include the following

Objective

The main objective of fellowship training program is to develop a center for services, training and research in the specialty of pediatric and adolescent gynecology in a children's hospital, the Philippine Children's Medical Center.

Specific Objectives

1. To develop and implement a curriculum for a 2-year fellowship program in pediatric adolescent gynecology.
2. To establish a comprehensive referral center for pediatric and adolescent gynecological conditions.
3. To provide gynecological services to the pediatric age group of patients.
4. To supplement the needs of the women and child protection unit of the Philippine Children's Medical Center.

Contd...

Contd...

5. To do research on pediatric gynecologic conditions, basic and clinical.

Special Requirements for Training in Pediatric and Adolescent Gynecology
A graduate of a 4-year residency program in obstetrics and gynecology. Diplomate status is preferred, but not obligatory.
The Pediatric and Adolescent Gynecology Unit is committed to:

1. Provide service for the referral and transfer of patients with pediatric and adolescent gynecologic problems, in collaboration with other gynecologists within and outside the center.
2. Have an adequate clinical workload with a full range of gynecologic problems.
3. Have appropriate clinical facilities for investigation of above problems.
4. Collaborate with other consultant pediatrician or endocrinologist or surgeon and other staff who are also committed to the care of pediatric and adolescent gynecological disorders.
5. Have an adequate gynecological pathology service.
6. Have a research program in the subspecialty.

Fellowship
This program involves 2 years of clinical and surgical training with the last year also devoted to prospective research work.
Training Program

The following knowledge and skills should be acquired:

A. A basic knowledge of:
   1. Physiology and pharmacology of pediatric patients;
   2. Gross and microscopic pathology relating to gynecological cases.

B. An advanced knowledge of:
   1. Anatomy, and growth and development of the reproductive organs;
   2. Endocrine physiology and pharmacology of substances that regulate the reproductive system;
   3. The endocrine dynamics of the menstrual cycle;
   4. The physiology of conception;
   5. Immunology and genetics related to reproduction;
   6. Psychosocial aspects of pediatric and adolescent reproductive diseases (e.g. sexual abuse).

C. Clinical competence in the management of pediatric and adolescent gynecologic diseases:
   1. Diagnosis and management of diseases of the reproductive tract;
   2. Diagnosis of pituitary, central nervous system, thyroid and adrenal diseases related to reproduction;
   3. Expertise in surgical and endoscopic techniques related to reproductive problems;
   4. Expertise in ultrasound of the reproductive organs;
   5. Fertility control and family planning.

Contd...

Contd...

D. Experience and knowledge of:
   1. Administrative and management skills;
   2. Teaching;
   3. Legal and ethical issues;
   4. Epidemiology, statistics, research and audit.

E. Adolescent Health Care:
   1. Psychosocial history-taking;
   2. Family dynamics and inter-relationships;
   3. Detection of risky adolescent behavior;
   4. Reproductive health counseling;
   5. Sexually-transmitted diseases;
   6. Adolescent pregnancy.

Scope

1. Pediatric physiology (fluids and electrolytes) and pharmacology.
2. Ability to identify normal features of the pediatric and prepubertal genitalia including the breast.
3. Ability to diagnose common gynecologic disorders in children.
4. Thorough understanding of normal embryology and sexual differentiation.
5. Ability to recognize congenital malformations of the vagina, cervix and uterus and its reproductive implications and approach to management.
6. Understanding of the basic principles of genetics and its correlation with pediatric gynecological conditions.
7. Pediatric urogynecologic knowledge.
8. Pathology of genital tumors in children.
9. Importance of sonographic evaluation as an immediate tool for the evaluation of suspected pelvic pathology, gender identification and sexual development disorders.
10. Operative and reconstructive procedures.
11. Knowledge of biology, physiology, psychology, endocrinology, nutrition and sexuality of adolescents
12. Development of sensitivity in approaching psychological and sexual implications of genital malformations.
13. Knowledge of sexual abuse, demographic characteristics and prevalence, perpetrator characteristics and genital findings.
14. Pap smear interpretation.
15. Knowledge of breast disorders.
16. Knowledge of the management of gynecologic and gyne-endocrine disorders.
17. Special procedures: (A) Vaginoscopy, (B) Colposcopy, (C) Hysteroscopy, (D) Ultrasound diagnosis, (E) Pediatric laparoscopy.
18. Development of gender sensitivity.
19. Knowledge on adolescent sexuality-risk taking behavior.
20. Knowledge on the management of acute genital trauma in premenarcheal girls.
21. Knowledge on the basic concepts of molecular biology as applied to pediatrics.
22. Pediatric and adolescent gynecology office setting.
23. Research on STD's in the adolescent and sexually abused children.
24. Sex education.

Contd...

Contd...

Pediatric and Adolescent Gynecology Consultant Staff
Corazon Yabes-Almirante, MD (Head)
Franklin P Atencio, MD
Rosalinda B Arceo, MD
Jose S Baens, MD
Blanca C de Guia, MD (Training Officer)
Ma Socorro C Bernardino, MD
Marcela Dianalyn Sazon-Carlos, MD
Fellows: Marites M Butaran, MD, Maria Therese B Mallen, MD, Julie Christine Dimaano-de Torres, MD

Clinical Rotations
First Year
Ambulatory Pediatrics (3 months)
Adolescent Medicine (2 months)
Pediatric Urology (on call, within the 2 years of training)
Pediatric Surgery (2 months)
Ultrasound
Women and Child Protection Unit (on call, within 2 years of training)
Research Output—basic
Second Year
Community or Primary health care (3 months)
Pediatric Endocrinology (2 months)
Genetics/National Institute of Human Genetics (3 months)
Research Output—prospective clinical

Services
The Pediatric and Adolescent Gynecology Clinic is located at the Antepartum Unit, second floor of the Philippine Children's Medical Center front building from 8:00 am to 5:00 pm. Emergency and ward referrals are seen promptly by the Pediatric and Adolescent Gynecology Fellow on-call for 24 hours. Our services cater to gynecologic conditions in female patients' newborn to 19 years old.

Contd...

Contd...

Multidisciplinary Services Team Staff
Fusca Piczon, MD (Ambulatory Pediatrics)
Cecilia Gan, MD (Child Protection Unit)
Alicia Tamesis, MD (Adolescent Medicine)
Alvin Caballes, MD (Pediatric Surgery)
Jose Alcantara, MD (Pediatric Anesthesia)
David Bolong, MD (Pediatric Urology)
Lorna Abad, MD (Pediatric Endocrinology)
Carmencita Padilla, MD (Genetics)
Adoracion Tanega, MD (Child Psychiatry)
Bu Castro, MD (Forensic Medicine)

Out-Patient Services

1. Comprehensive gynecologic exam specifically for pediatric patients.
2. Pap smear and sexually transmitted disease screening
3. Colposcopy
4. Vaginoscopy
5. Ultrasound: transabdominal, transvaginal, transrectal and transperineal
6. Color Doppler and 3D ultrasound
7. Reproductive health counseling
8. Genetic counseling
9. Gynecologic evaluation of sexual and physical abuse with proper documentation and report for medico-legal purposes.
10. Sex Education

In-Patient Services

1. Acute and elective gynecologic surgery
2. Reconstructive surgery
3. Pelvic laparoscopy, hysteroscopy
4. Management of gyne-endocrinologic disorders
5. Management of congenital abnormalities of the female reproductive tract

Training program published in the Journal of Pediatric and Adolescent Gynecology (2005;18(2):145-7). Also available online at International Federation of Pediatric and Adolescent Gynecology (www.figij.org).

description of the 2 year fellowship training program in Pediatric and Adolescent Gynecology at the Philippine Children's Medical Center. The first graduate passed the IFEPAG exam in 2004. There were 9 IFEPAG fellows in the Philippines (2 passed in 2003, 6 passed in 2006). Table 19.2 shows the total number of IFEPAG fellows (161), also shown including the 32 countries where they come from. Table 19.3 shows the 20 accredited centers for training by FIGU. The Philippine Children's Medical Center was the first in Asia.

Table 19.2:

The following shows the current number of members of IFEPAG (passers of Certifying Examinations in Pediatric and Adolescent Gynecology):

Fellows by country		*Fellows by region*	
Argentina	23*	Asia	10
Australia	1	Europe	56
Brazil	14	Latin America	92
Chile	20	North America	3
Canada	3	**Total**	**161**
Colombia	8		
Cuba	1		
Czech Republic	8		
Finland	1		
Germany	10		
Greece	7		
Guatemala	1		
Hong Kong	1		
Hungary	12		
Israel	2		
Italy	6		
Latvia	1		
Lithuania	1		
Mexico	2		
Panama	2		
Paraguay	2		
Peru	4		
Philippines	9		
Poland	1		
Serbia	2		
Slovakia	1		
Spain	1		
Switzerland	1		
Ukraine	1		
Uruguay	7		
Venezuela	8		
Total	**161**		

Table 19.3

For fellowship training programs in pediatric and adolescent gynecology, the following centers are currently accredited by FIGIJ:

Accredited training center	*Contact person*	*Contact details*
Finnish Student Health Service	Dr D Apter	The Sexual Health Clinic, Family Federation of Finland, PO Box 849, 00101, Helsinki, Finland; Phone: +358-9-61622226; Fax: +358-9-645017; email: dan.apter@vaestoliitto.fi
University of Texas Medical Branch	Dr A Berenson	87 Galveston TX 77550 USA; Phone: 1.4097470366
University of Medical School of Debrecen	Prof A Borsos	PO Box 37, H-4012, Debrecen, Hungary; Phone/Fax: 36(52)417171
UO Ginecologia dell'Infanzia e dell' Adolescenza, University of Florence	Dir Prof V Bruni	V Morgagni 85 50134, Firenze, Italy; Phone: +39 055 7947551; Fax: +39 055 7947552; email: vbruni@unifi.it

Contd...

Contd...

Aretaieion Hospital, Department of Pediatric and Adolescent Gynecology and Reconstructive Surgery, University of Athens	Prof G Creatsas	9 Kanari Street, GR 10671, Athens, Greece; Phone: +30 210 7217835, +30 210 7286353; Fax: +30 210 7233330, +30 210 7286282; email: geocre@aretaieio.uoa.gr (Prof Creatsas), edeligeo@aretaieio.uoa.gr (Assoc Prof E Deligeoroglou)
University of Louisville School of Medicine	Dr S Paige Herweck	550 S Jackson Street, Louisville, KY, 40202, USA; Phone: 1.5028521365; Fax: 1.5028521911
The Charles University of Praha	Prof Jan Horejsi	Vuvalu 84, CZ 15006, Praha 5, Czech Republic, Phone: 420-2. 2443-4220; Fax: 00420-2-2443-4220; email: jan.horejsi@lfmotol.cuni.cz
Centro de Medicina Reproductiva y Desarrollo Integral del Adolescente, Facultad de Medecina, Universidad de Chile	Prof Dr Ramiro Molina, Prof Zanartu	Casilla 70011-7, Santiago, Chile; Phone: 562 9786484; Fax: 562 7356512; email: cemera@uchile.cl
Hospital for Sick Children, Pediatric and Adolescent Gynecology, Division of Endocrinology, University of Toronto	Dr Lisa M Allen	555 University Avenue, Toronto, Ontario, M5G 1X8, Canada; Phone: 1. 416 8136188; Fax: 1. 416 8137935
Post Graduate Medical University	Prof J Orley	1389 XIII Szabolcs U 35, Hungary: Phone: 3611358-308: Fax: 3611209086
Residencia de Postgrado Universitario de Ginecologia Infanto-Juvenil, Servico de Ginecologia Infanto Juvenil, Hospital de Ninos, JM delos Rios, Facultad Central de Venezuela	Dr Antonio Pereyra Perez, Dr Bestalia Sanchez dela Cruz	Telefax: 02.5747049: email: bestalia@yahoo.com
Hospital de Clinicas dela Universidad de Bs. As, Argentina, Seccion Ginecologia Infanto Juvenil Programa de Adolescencia	Prof Dr Jose Maria Mendez Ribas	Cordova 2351. (1120), Capital, Argentina; Fax: 541 7841105/54.1.7867590; Email: mr@consultoriointegral.com.ar
Allegheny University Hopsitals I/II	Dr JS Sanfilippo	320 East North Avenue, Pittsburgh, PA, 15212-4772; Phone: 1.412-3596326; Fax: 1.412-3595133; email: jsanfili@alienf.edu
Ottawa Civic Hospital	Prof JEH Spence	1053 Carling Ottawa Ontario, Canada, K1 Y4E9; Phone: 1.613 761-4573: Fax: 1.613 724-4942
Gynakologische Gemeinschaftspraxis Institute of Endocrinology and Reproductive Center	Prof A Wolf	Frauenstrasse 51 89073 Ulmm Germany Tel: 49 731966510, Fax: 497319665730
AG kinder-und Jugendgynakologie e. V.	Dr mde Marlene Heiz	Postfach 101303, D-40004 Dusseldorf, Germany Secretary: Phone: +49(0)2114305233; Fax: +49(0)2114305352 Email: MBRANDENcscde.jnj.com; marheinz@debitel.net
Philippine Children's Medical Center	Dr Corazon Yabes-Almirante	Quezon Avenue, Quezon City, Philippines; Phone: 924-6601 local 236 or 322 Email: pagsphil@yahoo.com
Dept Pediatric Adolescent Gynecology, Royal Children's Hospital	Assoc Professor Sonia Grover	Flmington Rd, Parkville 3052, Victoria, Australia Phone: +61 3 93455890; Fax: +61 3 93456343; Email: sonia.grover@rch.org.au
Baylor College of Medicine	Dr Jennifer E Dietrich	6620 Main St, Ste 1450; Houston, TX 77030 713-798-5295 (office); 713-798-7957 (fax) Email: jedietri@bcm.edu

The pediatric and Adolescent Gynecology Unit of the Philippine Children's Medical Center was established in April 22, 2002. Figures 19.1 to 19.3 shows cutting of the ribbon to the outpatient clinic.

The head of the unit Dr Corazon Yabes Almirante and the training officer Dr Blanca de Guia took the IFEPAG Exam in Santiago, Chile in October 2003 and passed (Fig. 19.4). The first fellow graduate of the training program took the IFEPAG exam in Athen's Greece in 2004 and passed (Fig. 19.5).

In November 4, 2004, the President of FIGU visited the Philippines and accredited the PAG unit as a PAG training

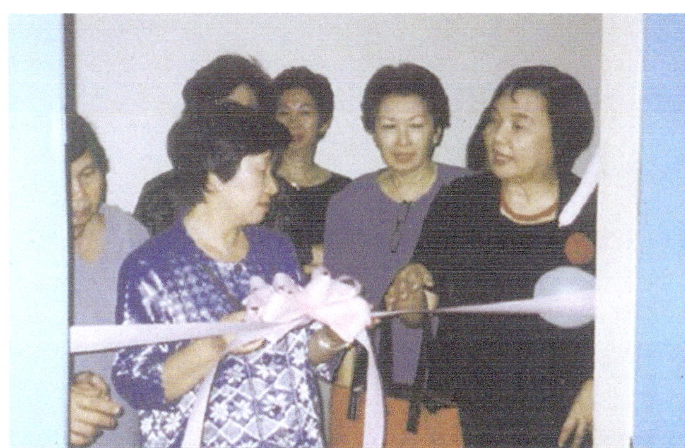

Fig. 19.1

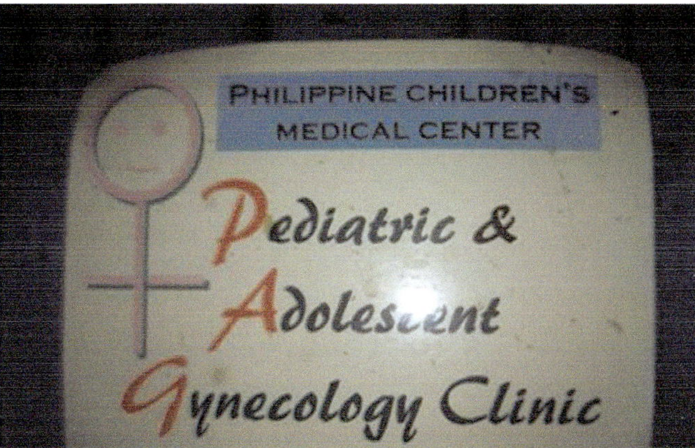

Fig. 19.2

Figs 19.1 and 19.2: Ribbon-cutting to the out-patient clinic by the executive director of the Philippine Children's Medical Center, Dr Lillian Lee, assisted by heads of the different subspecialties involved. Date: April 22, 2002

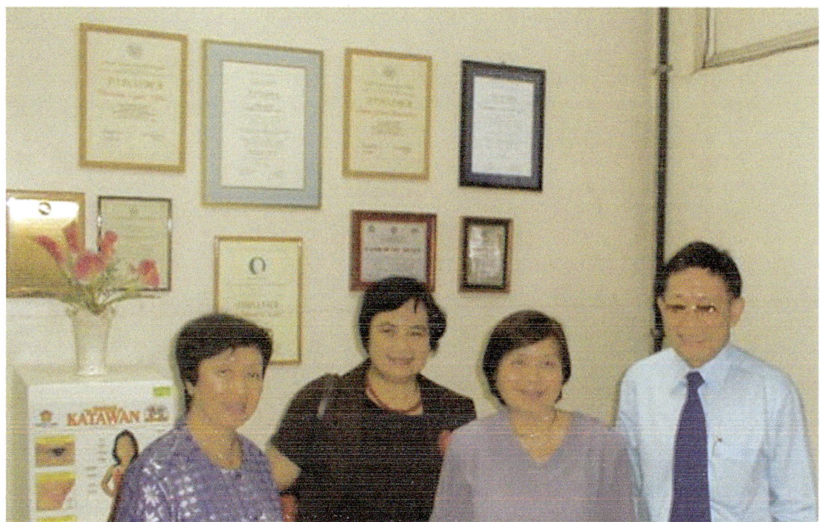

Fig. 19.3: Inside the out-patient clinic with Dr Lillian Lee (Executive Director), Dr Corazon Almirante, Dr Alicia Tamesis, Dr Franklin Atencio

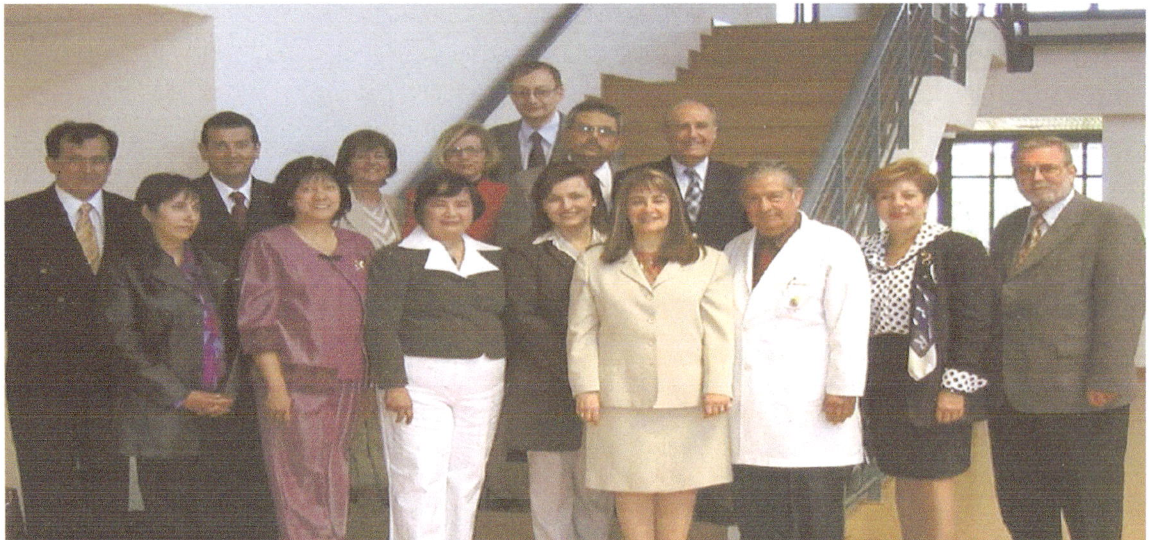

Fig. 19.4: IFEPAG exam passers in Santiago, Chile, October 2003, Drs Corazon Almirante and Blanca de Guia

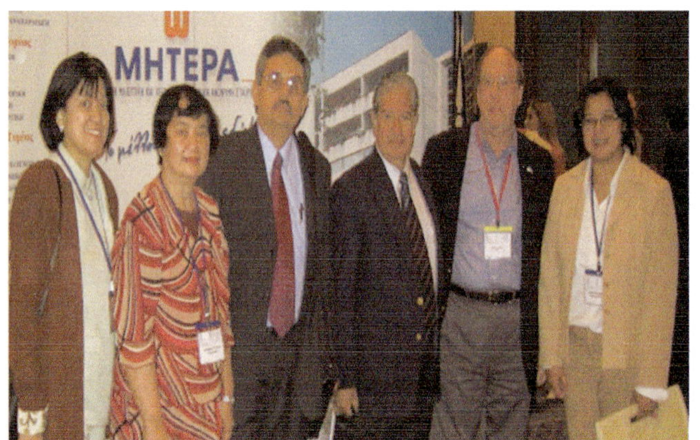

Fig. 19.5: IFEPAG exams in Athens, Greece. Dr Socorro Bernardino, 1st PAG fellow passes exams. May 2004

center (Figs 19.6A and B). The Pediatric and Adolescent Gynecology Society of the Philippines was established and the officers headed by the President Corazon Yabes Almirante were inducted into office by Dr Dan Apter, President of FIGU (Figs 19.7 and 19.8).

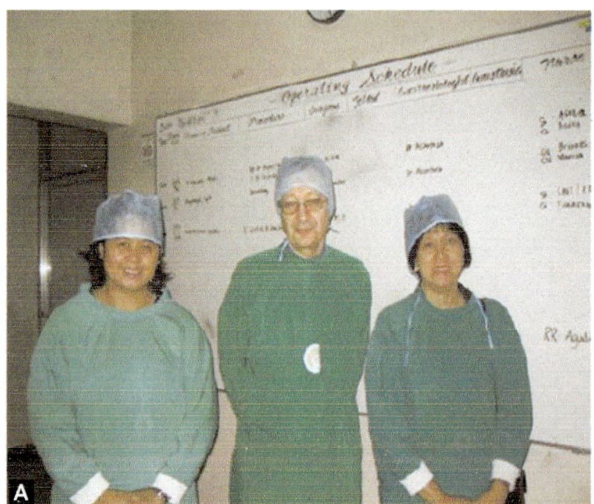

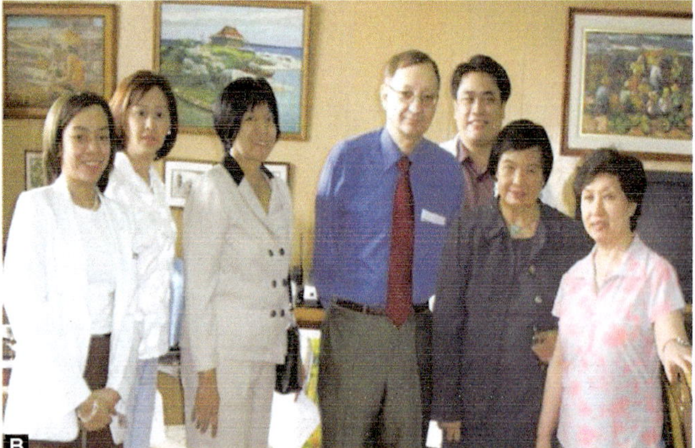

Figs 19.6A and B: Pediatric adolescent gynecology unit undergoes assessment as Training Center of PAG by Dr Dan Apter, President of Federation Internationale Gynecologie Infantile et Juvenile (FIGIJ). Date: November 4, 2004

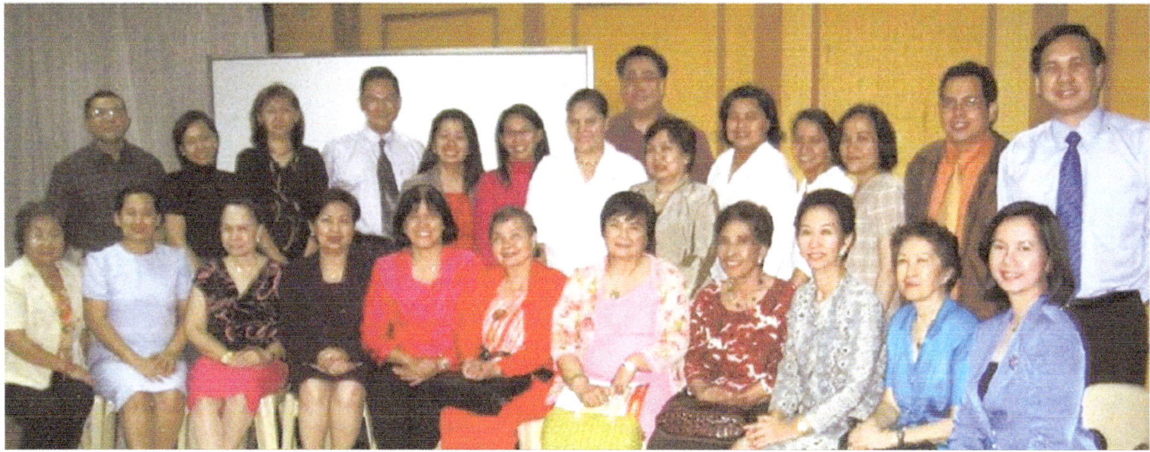

Fig. 19.7: Pediatric and adolescent gynecology society of the Philippines (PAGSPHIL) is established with 76 founding members. Date: April 2004. Subsequent acceptance of members of the society will be passers of IFEPAG

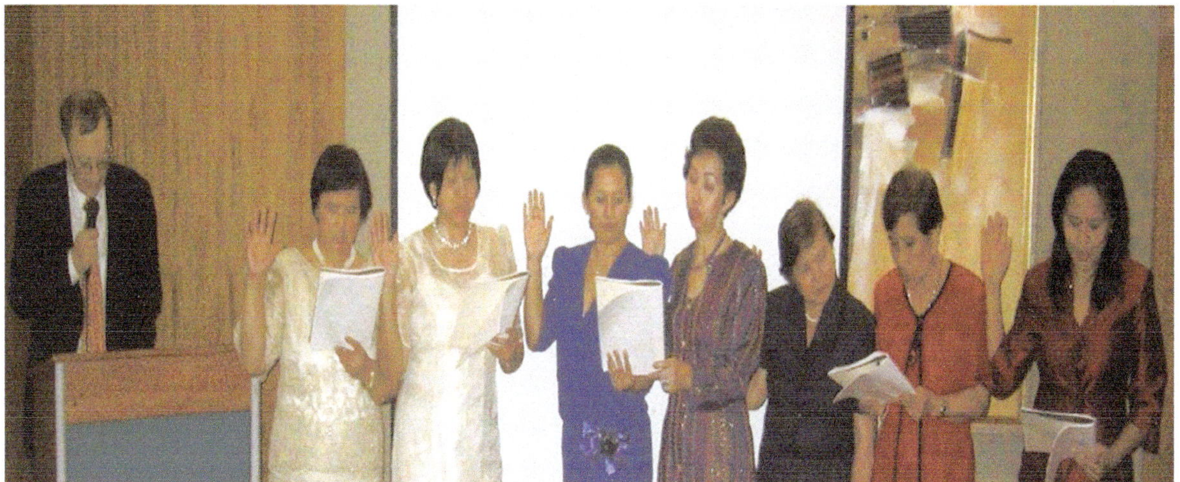

Fig. 19.8: Induction of officers of the pediatric and adolescent gynecology society of the Philippines (PAGSPHIL) headed by Dr Corazon Yabes-Almirante, President; Dr Blanca de Guia, Secretary; and Dr Dan Apter, President, FIGIJ

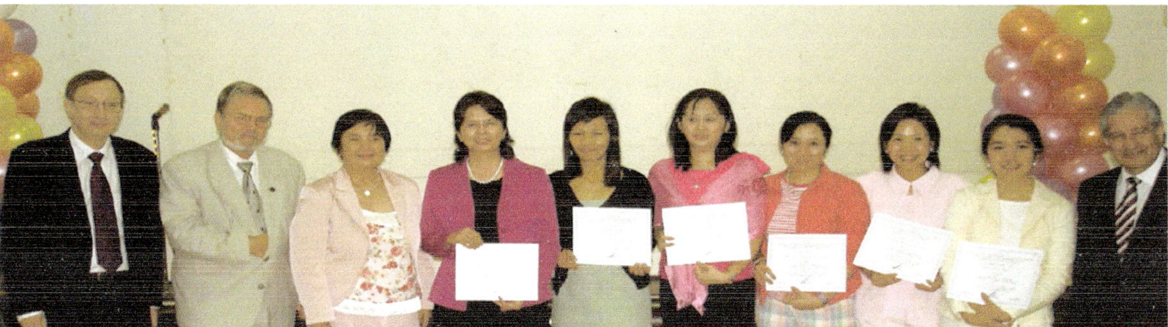

Fig. 19.9: IFEPAG passers in Manila 2006 with examiners Dr Dan Apter, Pres FIGIJ, Dr Jan Horejsi, Treas FIGIJ, Dr Corazon Yabes-Almirante, Pres PAGSPHIL and on the extreme right Prof Ramiro Molina Cartres, current Pres FIGIJ. Successful examinees: Drs Marietta Sapaula, Rosa Ma Nancho, Christine Dizon, Dianalyn Sazon-Carlos, Annebelle Aherrera, and Angela Aguilar

During the first convention of the Pediatric and Adolescent Gynecology Society of the Philippines, Officers of FIGU were invited as speakers. Dr Dan Apter, President, Dr Ramiro Molina, Pres of IFEPAG and Dan Horejsi Treasurer. They conducted the IFEPAG exam, where 7 members of PAGSPHIL took the exam, 6 passed the (Fig. 19.9) for the IFEPAG passers with their certificates and the 4 examiners.

There were 5 other graduates of the PAG fellowship training program of the Philippine Children's Medical Center. Figures 19.10 to 19.12 shows these graduates identified by numbers.

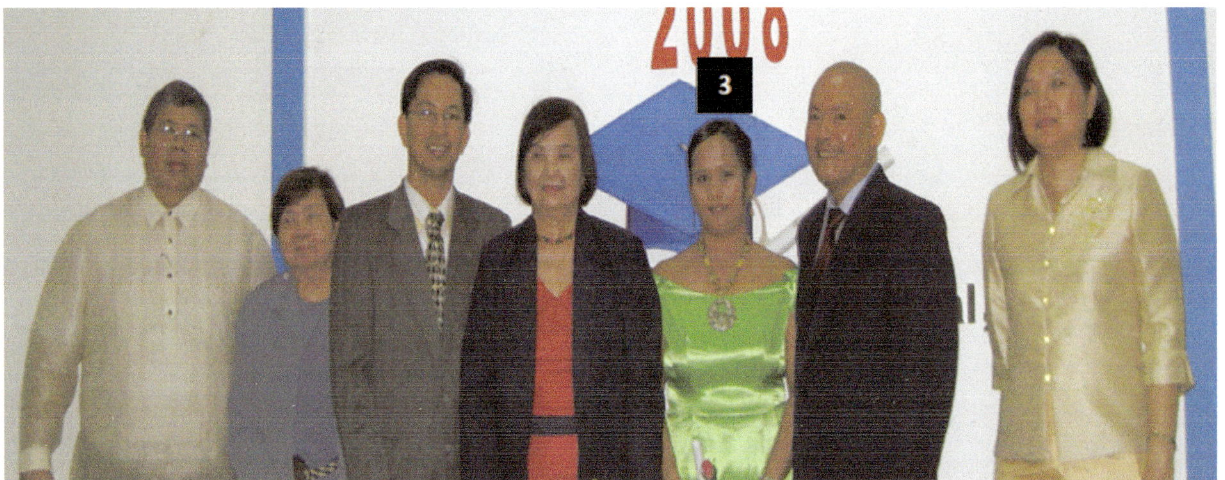

Fig. 19.10: Recognition rites at the Philippine Children's Medical Center. From left, Dr Joel Elises, (training officer) Dr Alicia Tamesis, Mr Butaran, Dr Corazon Almirante, Dr Marites Butaran, Dr Julius Lecciones (Executive Medical Director), and Dr Sonia Gozales (training officer)

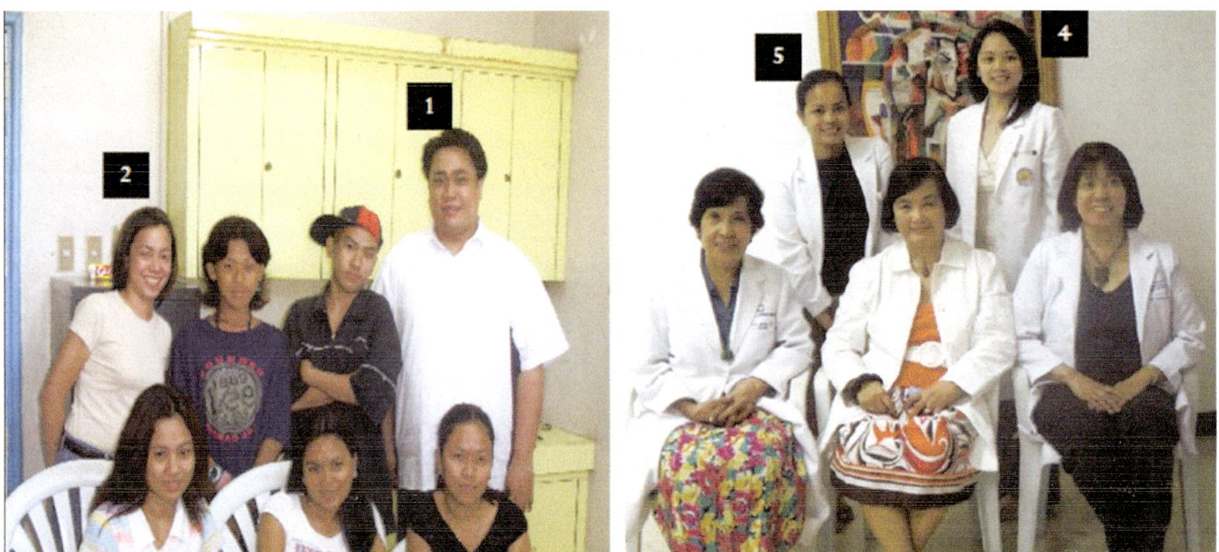

Fig. 19.11 **Fig. 19.12**

Figs 19.11 and 19.12: Previous and current fellows-in-training of the pediatric and adolescent gynecology unit: Drs Ryan Capitulo (1), Cathy Canonizado-Donato (2), Marites Butaran (3), Maria Therese Mallen (4), and Julie Christine de Torres (5)

BIBLIOGRAPHY

1. Goldfarb AF, Creatsas G, Mastorakos G, Chroousos GP (Eds). *The future of Pediatric and Adolescent Gynecology.* Annals of the New York Academy of Sciences 1997;816:1-3.

Index

Page numbers followed by *f* refer to figure and *t* refer to table

R

S

T

U